Basic Research in Endocrinology: A Modern Strategy for the Development and Technologies of Personalized Medicine

Basic Research in Endocrinology: A Modern Strategy for the Development and Technologies of Personalized Medicine

Editors

Yuliya I. Ragino
Mikhail I. Voevoda

MDPI • Basel • Beijing • Wuhan • Barcelona • Belgrade • Manchester • Tokyo • Cluj • Tianjin

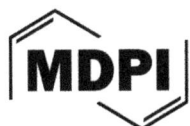

Editors

Yuliya I. Ragino
Laboratory of Biochemistry
Institute of Internal and
Preventive Medicine–Branch of
Institute of Cytology and
Genetics, Siberian Branch of
Russian Academy of Sciences
Novosibirsk
Russia

Mikhail I. Voevoda
Laboratory of Genetics
Institute of Internal and
Preventive Medicine–Branch
of Institute of Cytology and
Genetics, Siberian Branch of
Russian Academy of Sciences
Novosibirsk
Russia

Editorial Office
MDPI
St. Alban-Anlage 66
4052 Basel, Switzerland

This is a reprint of articles from the Special Issue published online in the open access journal *Journal of Personalized Medicine* (ISSN 2075-4426) (available at: www.mdpi.com/journal/jpm/special_issues/Endocrinology_Russia).

For citation purposes, cite each article independently as indicated on the article page online and as indicated below:

LastName, A.A.; LastName, B.B.; LastName, C.C. Article Title. *Journal Name* **Year**, *Volume Number*, Page Range.

ISBN 978-3-0365-2997-4 (Hbk)
ISBN 978-3-0365-2996-7 (PDF)

© 2022 by the authors. Articles in this book are Open Access and distributed under the Creative Commons Attribution (CC BY) license, which allows users to download, copy and build upon published articles, as long as the author and publisher are properly credited, which ensures maximum dissemination and a wider impact of our publications.

The book as a whole is distributed by MDPI under the terms and conditions of the Creative Commons license CC BY-NC-ND.

Contents

About the Editors . . . . **vii**

Preface to "Basic Research in Endocrinology: A Modern Strategy for the Development and Technologies of Personalized Medicine" . . . . **ix**

Elena Shakhtshneider, Alla Ovsyannikova, Oksana Rymar, Yuliya Ragino and Mikhail Voevoda
Basic Research in Endocrinology: A Modern Strategy for the Development and Technologies of Personalized Medicine
Reprinted from: *J. Pers. Med.* **2021**, *11*, 895, doi:10.3390/jpm11090895 . . . . **1**

Julia Samoilova, Mariia Matveeva, Olga Tonkih, Dmitry Kudlau, Oxana Oleynik and Aleksandr Kanev
A Prospective Study: Highlights of Hippocampal Spectroscopy in Cognitive Impairment in Patients with Type 1 and Type 2 Diabetes
Reprinted from: *J. Pers. Med.* **2021**, *11*, 148, doi:10.3390/jpm11020148 . . . . **5**

Svetlana V. Mustafina, Oksana D. Rymar, Liliya V. Shcherbakova, Evgeniy G. Verevkin, Hynek Pikhart and Olga V. Sazonova et al.
The Risk of Type 2 Diabetes Mellitus in a Russian Population Cohort According to Data from the HAPIEE Project
Reprinted from: *J. Pers. Med.* **2021**, *11*, 119, doi:10.3390/jpm11020119 . . . . **13**

Olga E. Redina, Svetlana E. Smolenskaya, Yulia K. Polityko, Nikita I. Ershov, Michael A. Gilinsky and Arcady L. Markel
Hypothalamic Norepinephrine Concentration and Heart Mass in Hypertensive ISIAH Rats Are Associated with a Genetic Locus on Chromosome 18
Reprinted from: *J. Pers. Med.* **2021**, *11*, 67, doi:10.3390/jpm11020067 . . . . **29**

Olga I. Kiseleva, Viktoriia A. Arzumanian, Ekaterina V. Poverennaya, Mikhail A. Pyatnitskiy, Ekaterina V. Ilgisonis and Victor G. Zgoda et al.
Does Proteomic Mirror Reflect Clinical Characteristics of Obesity?
Reprinted from: *J. Pers. Med.* **2021**, *11*, 64, doi:10.3390/jpm11020064 . . . . **45**

Dinara E. Ivanoshchuk, Elena V. Shakhtshneider, Oksana D. Rymar, Alla K. Ovsyannikova, Svetlana V. Mikhailova and Veniamin S. Fishman et al.
The Mutation Spectrum of Maturity Onset Diabetes of the Young (MODY)-Associated Genes among Western Siberia Patients
Reprinted from: *J. Pers. Med.* **2021**, *11*, 57, doi:10.3390/jpm11010057 . . . . **59**

Irina N. Grigor'eva
Gallstone Disease, Obesity and the Firmicutes/Bacteroidetes Ratio as a Possible Biomarker of Gut Dysbiosis
Reprinted from: *J. Pers. Med.* **2020**, *11*, 13, doi:10.3390/jpm11010013 . . . . **73**

Dinara E. Ivanoshchuk, Elena V. Shakhtshneider, Oksana D. Rymar, Alla K. Ovsyannikova, Svetlana V. Mikhailova and Pavel S. Orlov et al.
Analysis of APPL1 Gene Polymorphisms in Patients with a Phenotype of Maturity Onset Diabetes of the Young
Reprinted from: *J. Pers. Med.* **2020**, *10*, 100, doi:10.3390/jpm10030100 . . . . **91**

Yulia I. Ragino, Veronika I. Oblaukhova, Yana V. Polonskaya, Natalya A. Kuzminykh, Liliya V. Shcherbakova and Elena V. Kashtanova
The Blood Cytokine Profile of Young People with Early Ischemic Heart Disease Comorbid with Abdominal Obesity
Reprinted from: *J. Pers. Med.* **2020**, *10*, 87, doi:10.3390/jpm10030087 . . . . **101**

Elena Mazurenko, Oksana Rymar, Liliya Shcherbakova, Ekaterina Mazdorova and Sofia Malyutina
The Risk of Osteoporotic Forearm Fractures in Postmenopausal Women in a Siberian Population Sample
Reprinted from: *J. Pers. Med.* **2020**, *10*, 77, doi:10.3390/jpm10030077 . . . . **113**

Nadezhda N. Musina, Tatiana V. Saprina, Tatiana S. Prokhorenko, Alexander Kanev and Anastasia P. Zima
Correlations between Iron Metabolism Parameters, Inflammatory Markers and Lipid Profile Indicators in Patients with Type 1 and Type 2 Diabetes Mellitus
Reprinted from: *J. Pers. Med.* **2020**, *10*, 70, doi:10.3390/jpm10030070 . . . . **125**

Margarita V. Kruchinina, Andrey A. Gromov, Vladimir M. Generalov and Vladimir N. Kruchinin
Possible Differential Diagnosis of the Degrees of Rheological Disturbances in Patients with Type 2 Diabetes Mellitus by Dielectrophoresis of Erythrocytes
Reprinted from: *J. Pers. Med.* **2020**, *10*, 60, doi:10.3390/jpm10030060 . . . . **139**

About the Editors

Yuliya I. Ragino

Ph.D. and Sc.D. in medicine, Main Accreditation Commission (VAK) professor, Russian Academy of Sciences (RAS) professor, corresponding member of the RAS, head of the Institute of Internal and Preventive Medicine –a branch of a federal publicly funded scientific institution, the federal research center Institute of Cytology and Genetics, the Siberian Branch of the RAS (IIPM –a branch of the ICG SB RAS). Ragino Yu.I. is an expert in the fields of medical biochemistry and pathophysiology and an author or coauthor of more than 350 scientific publications, including 8 books, 10 patents of the Russian Federation, and 4 patents of the Eurasian Patent Organization. In the Russian Scientific Citation Index (RSCI): h-index: 24. In Scopus: h-index: 10. In the Web of Science: h-index: 8. The main basic-research accomplishments of Ragino Yu.I.: A study on the key biochemical markers and mechanisms of formation of unstable atherosclerotic plaquesand of their various types in atherosclerosis. The development of methods for early biochemical diagnosis of atherosclerosis and risk assessment of acute coronary syndrome. Conceptualization of the one-directionality of highly atherogenic changes of oxidation-modified and structurally altered lipoproteins of the blood, including small high-density atherogenic subfractions of lipoproteins, in clinically significant atherosclerosis and in the presence of its major risk factors; in this regard, novel evaluation criteria of pharmacotherapy effectiveness have been proposed. Research into atherogenic properties of oxidized proteins and their role in atherogenesis. Creation and investigation of experimental animal models (in vitro, in vivo), new lipid-containing coordination compounds of HMG-CoA reductase inhibitors with glycyrrhizin. Significant antiatherogenic effects of the obtained compounds have been demonstrated.

Mikhail I. Voevoda

Ph.D. and Sc.D. in medicine, Main Accreditation Commission (VAK) professor, Russian Academy of Sciences (RAS) professor, academician of the RAS. Voevoda M.I. is an expert in the fields of the molecular and medical genetic and an author or coauthor of more than 800 scientific publications, including 13 books, 16 patents of the Russian Federation. In the Russian Scientific Citation Index (RSCI): 935 publications, 8414 citations, h-index: 35. In Scopus: 281 publications, 6578 citations, h-index: 23. In the Web of Science: 283 publications, 4429 citations, h-index: 21. The main basic-research accomplishments of Voevoda M.I.: A study on the key on molecular biological, organism level, and populational patterns of development of major internal diseases in the Siberian population and designing a scientific basis for their prevention, diagnosis, and treatment. Voevoda M.I. supervises graduate courses in the Medical Genetics specialty and the Endocrinology specialty. Under him tutelage, 20 Ph.D. dissertations and 10 Sc.D. dissertations have been defended.

Preface to "Basic Research in Endocrinology: A Modern Strategy for the Development and Technologies of Personalized Medicine"

The first all-Russia conference with international participation "Basic Research in Endocrinology: A Modern Strategy for the Development and Technologies of Personalized Medicine" was held in Novosibirsk on 26–27 November 2020. The purpose of this conference was to disseminate the latest basic and clinical findings in the fields of etiology, clinical characteristics, and modern diagnostics and treatments of endocrine disorders among various relevant specialists. The conference was intended for practicing endocrinologists, primary care physicians, medical geneticists, pediatric endocrinologists, pediatricians, and physician–scientists. The conference included plenary sessions, specialty sessions, satellite symposia, an open competition for young scientists, and the first-in-Russia educational course for physicians: "Maturity Onset Diabetes of the Young (MODY): Molecular Genetic Determinants and a Personalized Approach to Patient Management."

The main topics included epidemiology and pathogenesis of endocrine disorders; genomic research in endocrinology; biochemical characteristics of endocrine aberrations; immunology and immunogenetics in endocrinology; cellular technologies in endocrinology; metabolomic research in endocrinology; pharmacogenetics; basic pathomorphology; high-tech care of patients with endocrine disorders; iodine-deficiency–related, autoimmune, and oncological diseases of the thyroid; modern diagnostic and therapeutic strategies for diabetes mellitus; osteoporosis and osteopenias; polyendocrinopathies; an interdisciplinary approach to the diagnosis and treatment of obesity and metabolic syndrome; hypo- and hyperparathyroidism, vitamin D; neuroendocrine disorders; reproductive health; rehabilitation of patients with endocrine disorders; health resort and spa treatments of endocrine disorders and comorbid conditions.

Scientists from Siberian cities, from Moscow, St. Petersburg, and Kazan, as well as Kazakhstan and Great Britain, delivered presentations at the conference. The conference was organized by the Institute of Internal and Preventive Medicine –a branch of the Institute of Cytology and Genetics, the Siberian Branch of the Russian Academy of Sciences (IIPM –a branch of the ICG SB RAS). The objectives and subject areas of the IIPM are basic, exploratory, and applied scientific studies in priority areas of molecular medicine and human genetics as well as safeguarding and improvement of human health, the development of health care and medical science, and preparation of advanced specialists in science and medicine.

Yuliya I. Ragino, Mikhail I. Voevoda

Editors

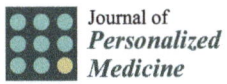

Editorial

Basic Research in Endocrinology: A Modern Strategy for the Development and Technologies of Personalized Medicine

Elena Shakhtshneider [1,2], Alla Ovsyannikova [1], Oksana Rymar [1], Yuliya Ragino [1,*] and Mikhail Voevoda [2,*]

[1] Institute of Internal and Preventive Medicine—Branch of Institute of Cytology and Genetics, Siberian Branch of Russian Academy of Sciences (SB RAS), 175/1 Borisa Bogatkova Str., Novosibirsk 630089, Russia; 2117409@mail.ru (E.S.); aknikolaeva@bk.ru (A.O.); orymar23@gmail.com (O.R.)
[2] Institute of Cytology and Genetics, Siberian Branch of Russian Academy of Sciences (SB RAS), 10 Prospect Ak. Lavrentyeva, Novosibirsk 630090, Russia
* Correspondence: ragino@mail.ru (Y.R.); mvoevoda@yandex.ru (M.V.)

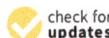

Citation: Shakhtshneider, E.; Ovsyannikova, A.; Rymar, O.; Ragino, Y.; Voevoda, M. Basic Research in Endocrinology: A Modern Strategy for the Development and Technologies of Personalized Medicine. *J. Pers. Med.* **2021**, *11*, 895. https://doi.org/10.3390/jpm11090895

Received: 3 September 2021
Accepted: 6 September 2021
Published: 8 September 2021

Publisher's Note: MDPI stays neutral with regard to jurisdictional claims in published maps and institutional affiliations.

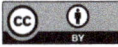

Copyright: © 2021 by the authors. Licensee MDPI, Basel, Switzerland. This article is an open access article distributed under the terms and conditions of the Creative Commons Attribution (CC BY) license (https://creativecommons.org/licenses/by/4.0/).

The first all-Russia conference with international participation, "Basic Research in Endocrinology: A Modern Strategy for the Development and Technologies of Personalized Medicine", was held in Novosibirsk on 26–27 November 2020. The purpose of this conference was to disseminate the latest basic and clinical findings in the fields of etiology, clinical characteristics, and modern diagnostics and treatments of endocrine disorders among various relevant specialists. The conference was intended for practicing endocrinologists, primary care physicians, medical geneticists, pediatric endocrinologists, pediatricians, and physician–scientists. The conference included plenary sessions, specialty sessions, satellite symposia, an open competition for young scientists, and the first-in-Russia educational course for physicians: "Maturity Onset Diabetes of the Young (MODY): Molecular Genetic Determinants and a Personalized Approach to Patient Management." This Special Issue on "Basic Research in Endocrinology: A Modern Strategy for the Development and Technologies of Personalized Medicine" includes a review and 10 original studies about diabetes mellitus, hypothalamic norepinephrine, obesity, and osteoporosis.

Six of the special-issue articles, Samoilova et al. [1], Mustafina et al. [2], Ivanoshchuk et al. [3,4], Musina et al. [5], and Kruchinina et al. [6], focus on the detection and characterization of various types of diabetes mellitus. Samoilova et al. [1] evaluated the specificity of hippocampal spectroscopy for parameters of type 1 and type 2 diabetes mellitus (T1DM and T2DM) and cognitive dysfunction. The authors analyzed 65 T1DM patients with cognitive deficits and 20 T1DM patients without, as well as 75 T2DM patients with cognitive deficits and 20 T2DM patients without. They determined that patients with diabetes possessed an altered hippocampal metabolism, which may serve as an early predictive marker of neurometabolic changes. The main modifiable risk factors whose correction may slow down the progression of cognitive dysfunction were identified. Mustafina et al. [2] investigated the 14-year risk of T2DM and developed a risk score for T2DM in a Siberian cohort. A random population sample (males/females, 45–69 years old) was examined at baseline in 2003–2005 (Health, Alcohol, and Psychosocial Factors in Eastern Europe [HAPIEE] project, n = 9360, Novosibirsk) and re-examined in 2006–2008 and 2015–2017. After the exclusion of subjects with baseline T2DM, the final analysis included 7739 participants. In addition, secondary education, low physical activity, and a history of cardiovascular disease were significantly associated with T2DM in females. Ivanoshchuk et al. [3] researched the genetic characteristics of MODY. The authors analyzed 14 MODY genes in 178 patients with a MODY phenotype in Western Siberia. A multiplex ligation-dependent probe amplification analysis of DNA samples from 50 randomly selected patients without detectable mutations did not reveal large rearrangements in the MODY genes. In 38 patients (among them, 37% males) out of the 178, mutations were identified in *HNF4A*, *GCK*, *HNF1A*, and *ABCC8*. The authors of ref. [4] investigated the *APPL1* gene, which is associated with MODY 14. Thirteen variants were found in *APPL1*, three of which (rs79282761, rs138485817, and rs11544593) were located in exons. There were no statistically significant differences in the frequencies of rs11544593 alleles and genotypes between T2DM patients and the general population. In the MODY group, AG rs11544593 genotype carriers were significantly more frequent (AG vs. AA + GG: odds ratio 1.83, confidence interval 1.15–2.90, $p = 0.011$) compared with the control group. Musina et al. [5] established relations among inflammatory status, ferrokinetics, and lipid metabolism in patients with diabetes mellitus. The discovered relations among lipid profile indices, inflammatory status, and microalbuminuria confirmed the mutual influences of hyperlipidemia, inflammation, and nephropathy in diabetes patients. Their results justify the strategy involving early hypolipidemic therapy for patients with diabetes mellitus to prevent the development and progression of microvascular complications. Kruchinina et al. [6] investigated the feasibility of a differential diagnosis of degrees of rheological disturbances in patients with T2DM by dielectrophoresis of erythrocytes. The proposed experimental approach features a low invasiveness, high productivity, shorter duration, and vividness of the results. The method allows one to evaluate not only the local (renal and ocular) but also systemic status of microcirculation using more than 20 parameters of erythrocytes.

Redina et al. [7] addressed the role of hypothalamic norepinephrine in the activation of the sympathetic nervous system. They carried out genetic mapping by quantitative trait loci analysis and identified loci associated both with an increased hypothalamic norepinephrine concentration and with an increase of the heart weight in Inherited Stress-Induced Arterial Hypertension (ISIAH) rats, a model of the stress-sensitive type of arterial hypertension. The contribution to the development of heart hypertrophy in ISIAH rats is controlled by different genetic loci, one of which is associated with hypothalamic norepinephrine concentration (on chromosome 18) and the other correlating with high blood pressure (on chromosome 1).

Kiseleva et al. [8] investigated correlations between the parameters of classic clinical blood tests and the proteomic profiles of 104 lean and obese subjects. As a result, the authors compiled patterns of the proteins whose presence or absence allowed one to predict the weight of a patient fairly well. Ragino et al. [9] studied the blood cytokine/chemokine profile of 25–44 year old patients with early ischemic heart disease comorbid with abdominal obesity. Their findings related to Flt3 ligand, granulocyte macrophage–colony stimulating factor (GM-CSF), and interleukin 4 (IL-4) are consistent with the international literature. The results of that study are partly confirmative and partly hypothesis-generating.

Mazurenko et al. [10] examined the frequency of osteoporotic forearm fractures in postmenopausal women to assess their association with risk factors of chronic noncommunicable diseases. In the studied population sample of postmenopausal women, a high total cholesterol level and a history of smoking were cross-sectional determinants of osteoporotic forearm fractures, whereas the body–mass index was a protective factor against the risk of osteoporotic fractures.

Grigor'eva [11] wrote a review about the relation of gallstone disease, obesity, and the Firmicutes/Bacteroidetes ratio as a possible biomarker of gut dysbiosis. This review presents and summarizes recent findings of studies on the gut microbiota in patients with gallstone disease.

The articles in this special issue cover interesting topics in endocrinology that are also related to gastroenterology, genetics, hematology, and cardiology. The presented data expand our knowledge about basic endocrinology.

Author Contributions: E.S. and A.O. were responsible for the preparation of the scientific program and overall organization of the conference; O.R. chaired the sessions and was in charge of the conference content; Y.R. and M.V. conceived the conference. All authors have read and agreed to the published version of the manuscript.

Funding: This work received no external funding.

Conflicts of Interest: The authors declare that they have no conflicts of interest.

References

1. Samoilova, J.; Matveeva, M.; Tonkih, O.; Kudlau, D.; Oleynik, O.; Kanev, A. A Prospective Study: Highlights of Hippocampal Spectroscopy in Cognitive Impairment in Patients with Type 1 and Type 2 Diabetes. *J. Pers. Med.* **2021**, *11*, 148. [CrossRef] [PubMed]
2. Mustafina, S.V.; Rymar, O.D.; Shcherbakova, L.V.; Verevkin, E.G.; Pikhart, H.; Sazonova, O.V.; Ragino, Y.I.; Simonova, G.I.; Bobak, M.; Malyutina, S.K.; et al. The Risk of Type 2 Diabetes Mellitus in a Russian Population Cohort According to Data from the HAPIEE Project. *J. Pers. Med.* **2021**, *11*, 119. [CrossRef] [PubMed]
3. Ivanoshchuk, D.E.; Shakhtshneider, E.V.; Rymar, O.D.; Ovsyannikova, A.K.; Mikhailova, S.V.; Fishman, V.S.; Valeev, E.S.; Orlov, P.S.; Voevoda, M.I. The Mutation Spectrum of Maturity Onset Diabetes of the Young (MODY)-Associated Genes among Western Siberia Patients. *J. Pers. Med.* **2021**, *11*, 57. [CrossRef] [PubMed]
4. Ivanoshchuk, D.E.; Shakhtshneider, E.V.; Rymar, O.D.; Ovsyannikova, A.K.; Mikhailova, S.V.; Orlov, P.S.; Ragino, Y.I.; Voevoda, M.I. Analysis of APPL1 Gene Polymorphisms in Patients with a Phenotype of Maturity Onset Diabetes of the Young. *J. Pers. Med.* **2020**, *10*, 100. [CrossRef] [PubMed]
5. Musina, N.V.; Saprina, T.S.; Prokhorenko, T.; Kanev, A.P.; Zima, A. Correlations between Iron Metabolism Parameters, Inflammatory Markers and Lipid Profile Indicators in Patients with Type 1 and Type 2 Diabetes Mellitus. *J. Pers. Med.* **2020**, *10*, 70. [CrossRef] [PubMed]
6. Kruchinina, M.V.; Gromov, A.A.; Generalov, V.M.; Kruchinin, V.N. Possible Differential Diagnosis of the Degrees of Rheological Disturbances in Patients with Type 2 Diabetes Mellitus by Dielectrophoresis of Erythrocytes. *J. Pers. Med.* **2020**, *10*, 60. [CrossRef] [PubMed]
7. Redina, O.E.; Smolenskaya, S.E.; Polityko, Y.K.; Ershov, N.I.; Gilinsky, M.A.; Markel, A.L. Hypothalamic Norepinephrine Concentration and Heart Mass in Hypertensive ISIAH Rats Are Associated with a Genetic Locus on Chromosome 18. *J. Pers. Med.* **2021**, *11*, 67. [CrossRef] [PubMed]
8. Kiseleva, O.I.; Arzumanian, V.A.; Poverennaya, E.V.; Pyatnitskiy, M.A.; Ilgisonis, E.V.; Zgoda, V.G.; Plotnikova, O.A.; Sharafetdinov, K.K.; Lisitsa, A.V.; Tutelyan, V.A.; et al. Does Proteomic Mirror Reflect Clinical Characteristics of Obesity? *J. Pers. Med.* **2021**, *11*, 64. [CrossRef] [PubMed]
9. Ragino, Y.I.; Oblaukhova, V.I.; Polonskaya, Y.V.; Kuzminykh, N.A.; Shcherbakova, L.V.; Kashtanova, E.V. The Blood Cytokine Profile of Young People with Early Ischemic Heart Disease Comorbid with Abdominal Obesity. *J. Pers. Med.* **2020**, *10*, 87. [CrossRef] [PubMed]
10. Mazurenko, E.; Rymar, O.; Shcherbakova, L.; Mazdorova, E.; Malyutina, S. The Risk of Osteoporotic Forearm Fractures in Postmenopausal Women in a Siberian Population Sample. *J. Pers. Med.* **2020**, *10*, 77. [CrossRef]
11. Grigor'eva, I.N. Gallstone Disease, Obesity and the Firmicutes/Bacteroidetes Ratio as a Possible Biomarker of Gut Dysbiosis. *J. Pers. Med.* **2021**, *11*, 13. [CrossRef]

Article

A Prospective Study: Highlights of Hippocampal Spectroscopy in Cognitive Impairment in Patients with Type 1 and Type 2 Diabetes

Julia Samoilova [1], Mariia Matveeva [1,*], Olga Tonkih [1], Dmitry Kudlau [2], Oxana Oleynik [1] and Aleksandr Kanev [1]

1. Medical Faculty, Siberian State Medical University, 634050 Tomsk, Russia; samoilova_y@inbox.ru (J.S.); ostonkih@mail.ru (O.T.); oleynikoa@mail.ru (O.O.); alexkanev92@gmail.com (A.K.)
2. Institute of Immunology, Federal Medical and Biological Agency of Russia, 115478 Moscow, Russia; dakudlay@generiumzao.ru
* Correspondence: matveeva.mariia@yandex.ru; Tel.: +7-913-8152-552

Abstract: Diabetes mellitus type 1 and 2 is associated with cognitive impairment. Previous studies have reported a relationship between changes in cerebral metabolite levels and the variability of glycemia. However, the specific risk factors that affect the metabolic changes associated with type 1 and type 2 diabetes in cognitive dysfunction remain uncertain. The aim of the study was to evaluate the specificity of hippocampal spectroscopy in type 1 and type 2 diabetes and cognitive dysfunction. Materials and methods: 65 patients with type 1 diabetes with cognitive deficits and 20 patients without, 75 patients with type 2 diabetes with cognitive deficits and 20 patients without have participated in the study. The general clinical analysis and evaluation of risk factors of cognitive impairment were carried out. Neuropsychological testing included the Montreal Scale of Cognitive Dysfunction Assessment (MoCA test). Magnetic resonance spectroscopy (MRS) was performed in the hippocampal area, with the assessment of N-acetylaspartate (NAA), choline (Cho), creatine (Cr), and phosphocreatine (PCr) levels. Statistical processing was performed using the commercially available IBM SPSS software. Results: Changes in the content of NAA, choline Cho, phosphocreatine Cr2 and their ratios were observed in type 1 diabetes. More pronounced changes in hippocampal metabolism were observed in type 2 diabetes for all of the studied metabolites. Primary risk factors of neurometabolic changes in patients with type 1 diabetes were episodes of severe hypoglycemia in the history of the disease, diabetic ketoacidosis (DKA), chronic hyperglycemia, and increased body mass index (BMI). In type 2 diabetes, arterial hypertension (AH), BMI, and patient's age are of greater importance, while the level of glycated hemoglobin (HbA1c), duration of the disease, level of education and insulin therapy are of lesser importance. Conclusion: Patients with diabetes have altered hippocampal metabolism, which may serve as an early predictive marker. The main modifiable factors have been identified, correction of which may slow down the progression of cognitive dysfunction.

Keywords: type 1 diabetes mellitus; type 2 diabetes mellitus; proton spectroscopy; hippocampus; cognitive dysfunction

1. Introduction

Clinical studies indicate that type 1 and type 2 diabetes are risk factors for cognitive decline, while structural and functional deficits are associated with synaptic plasticity processes. Experimental data derived from rodent model of diabetes demonstrate the decline in learning and memory of varying extent, owing to the hippocampus dysfunction. These changes are associated with an increase in oxidative stress, levels of pro-inflammatory cytokines, β-amyloid, as well as dysfunction of the hypothalamic-pituitary-adrenal axis [1]. The hippocampus is a vital structure for learning and memory. High density of insulin receptors has been found in this area of the brain [2]. Magnetic resonance spectroscopy (MRS), the latest biochemical analysis method, detects changes in metabolic neurochemical levels and energy metabolism in different areas of the brain in vivo [3–5]. Considering that MRS is both safe and non-invasive, researchers have used MRS to investigate the underlying causes of many neurological conditions, such as Alzheimer's disease and diabetes mellitus [6]. Monitoring changes in the level of each metabolite and metabolite ratios can provide information on neuronal damage, membrane metabolic dysfunctions, and transmission defects that occur in neurological diseases [7,8]. The purpose of the present study was to evaluate the features of spectroscopy of the hippocampus in patients with type 1 and 2 diabetes. Hypothesis: patients with type 1 and type 2 diabetes have risk factors for impaired neurometabolism in the hippocampus, which is clinically manifested by cognitive impairment.

2. Materials and Methods

All patients included in the study signed an informed consent, which was approved by an ethics committee (No. 265 from 2 May 2017). Sixty-five patients with type 1 diabetes with cognitive deficits and 20 patients without, 75 patients with type 2 diabetes with cognitive deficits and 20 patients without have participated in the study. According to the design, the study is characterized as an observational, cross-sectional, single-center, continuous, comparative study. Inclusion criteria for the study: diabetes type 1 and 2, age 18–65 years with varying degrees of disease compensation, carbohydrate metabolism, severity of vascular changes, the duration of the disease, and the type of therapy; obligatory presence of voluntary informed consent. Exclusion criteria: non-compliance with the inclusion criteria; presence of organic brain damage (tumors, stroke); of drugs or substances that alter cognitive functions (psychotropic, narcotic drugs); chronic alcoholism (anamnestic, ambulatory history); vitamin B12 deficiency (determined at study inclusion); condition after severe trauma and surgery; presence of hematologic, oncologic, and severe infectious diseases; decompensation of chronic heart failure with pronounced clinical symptoms, functional class of chronic heart failure functional class higher than II; acute coronary syndrome and transient ischemic attack in previous 6 months.

2.1. Sample Characteristics

The cohort of patients examined is presented below (Table 1).

Table 1. Characteristics of patients with type 1 and type 2 diabetes; M (interquartile range—Q1–Q3).

Parameters	Type 1 Diabetes and Cognitive Dysfunction	Type 1 Diabetes and Normal Cognitive Functions	Type 2 Diabetes and Cognitive Dysfunction	Type 2 Diabetes and Normal Cognitive Function
Age, years	44 (42–48)	45 (43–48)	53 (37–69)	53 (31–71)
Disease duration, years	13 (10–21)	13 (6–23)	10 (4–14)	9 (2–13)
HbA1, %	8.4 (6.6–9.3)	7.4 (5.4–10.1)	8.2 (6.3–9.9)	7.9 (6.2–9.1)
Glycemia, mmol/l	8 (5.6–18.3)	8 (7–9)	7.5 (5.6–9.0)	7.2 (7.0–7.5)

Patients with type 1 diabetes were younger and had longer duration of the disease. However, inside of type 1 and type 2 diabetes groups, no statistically significant differences in patients' characteristics were noted between subgroups with and without cognitive dysfunction.

2.2. Risk Factors

Each patient underwent the assessment of risk factors for cognitive impairment, including metabolic parameters, acute complications of diabetes, hypertension, Body Mass Index (BMI), duration of the disease, age, level of education, smoking status, alcohol abuse, insulin therapy.

2.3. Cognitive Function

For the diagnosis of cognitive impairment, the generally accepted test is the Montreal cognitive assessment (MoCA) (Copyright 2019, Ziad Nasreddine, MD) [9]. The test assesses eight cognitive domains: executive and visual-constructive skills, naming, memory, attention, speech, abstraction, delayed memory, and orientation. The maximum score is 30 points; borderline—26 points. The specificity of MoCA in detecting mild cognitive impairment is 90%, the sensitivity is 87%. A MoCA survey takes up to 10 min. This scale is now recommended by most modern experts in the field of cognitive impairment for widespread use in everyday clinical practice.

2.4. Proton Spectroscopy of the Brain

MRS of the brain with an echo time (TE) of 135 ms, and the volume of one voxel of 1.5 cm^3 was performed immediately after MRI of the brain. This technique was carried out in a multi-voxel mode, which allows placing 64 voxels on one slice simultaneously. In the areas of interest, the main spectra of N-acetylaspartate (NAA), choline (Cho), creatine (Cr), and phosphocreatine (PCr), as well as their ratios, were recorded. The protocol of proton magnetic resonance spectroscopy of the brain included the following steps (the total time of the study is approximately 35–40 min): (1) positioning of the examined patient (supine); (2) conducting a standard MRI of the brain; (3) performing sighting slices on the hippocampus area, T2 3 mm hippocampus; (4) MRS on the area of interest—frontal and temporal lobes area of the hippocampus (the camera serial interface protocol was used); (5) obtaining MR spectra of NAA, Cho, Cr, PCr in multivoxel mode; (6) postprocessing of the results of proton magnetic resonance spectroscopy including the analysis of spectrograms and the construction of color maps of the distribution of the main metabolites, as well as their ratios. The Turbo Spin Echo (Turbo SE) method with the parameters: recovery time—1500 ms, TE—135 ms, field of view—160 mm, matrix—192 × 256, slice thickness—5 mm, scanning time—12 min, was used. The quantitative characteristics of the studied metabolites and their ratios in the gray matter of the cerebral cortex, white matter of the brain, subcortical structures, and in the hippocampus on both sides were assessed. Using a regional approach, data were selected for NAA, Cho, Cr, PCr, localized in the left and right hippocampus, as shown in Figure 1. There were no missing data in our selection of patients.

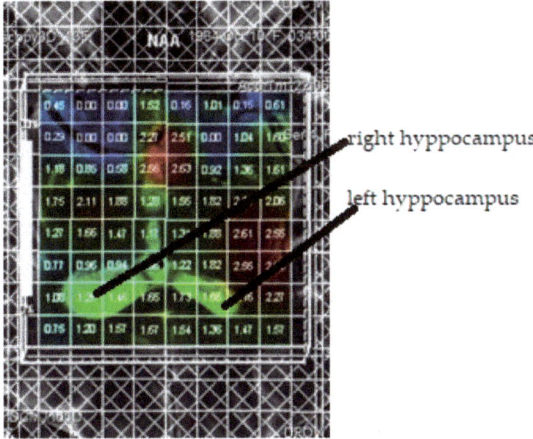

Figure 1. A Regional approach to assessing metabolite content in the hippocampus.

To calculate sample size, we used the formula calculating the minimum sample size. As previous studies investigating hippocampal metabolism parameters in diabetes patients are lacking, the required sample size was estimated based on the results of two studies that were assessing the NAA/Cr ratio in patients with type 2 diabetes mellitus [10] (NAA/Cr ratio 1.36 ± 0.15) and mild cognitive impairment, which also included diabetes patients (NAA/Cr ratio 1.58 ± 0.14) [6]. According to the aforementioned data, should we pursue the power of 0.9, the sample size of 11 in each group would be sufficient to prove the initial hypothesis.

The statistical processing was performed using the IBM SPSS Statistics software (USA), 19.0.0 Russian version. The following coefficients were evaluated: Shapiro–Wilk W-test, distribution estimate. Differences were determined by Student's t-test for normal, Mann–Whitney Z-test for non-normal distribution, Wilcoxon's test for dependent data. Descriptive analysis included the determination of the arithmetic mean X, error of the mean m, and calculation of median and quartiles (Me, Q1–Q3) depending on the type of distribution. The critical level of significance p when testing statistical hypotheses in the study was taken equal to 0.05. Qualitative data were analyzed using frequency analysis. For definition of accuracy, we used Pearson χ^2 test. Spearman test was used for the correlation analysis [11].

3. Results

As a result of randomization, 15 people each from the group with type 1 and type 2 diabetes dropped out of the study (Figure 2).

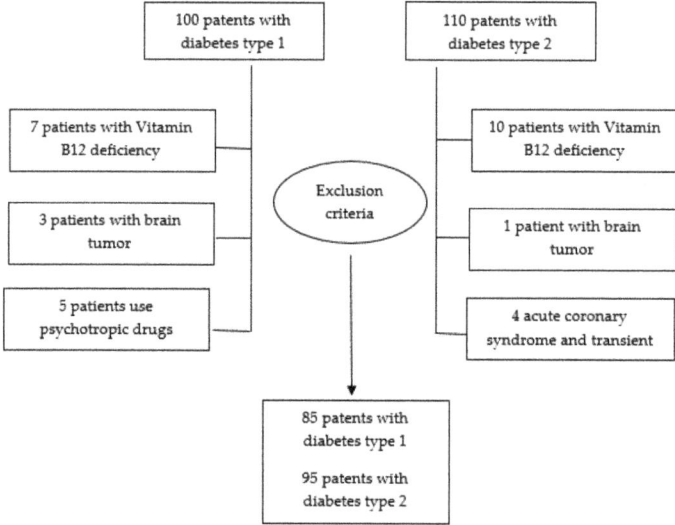

Figure 2. A Flowchart of randomized process.

In patients with type 1 diabetes presenting with cognitive impairment, an increase in NAA and PCr, and a decrease in the Cho content was noted. NAA/Cho, Cho/Cr ratios were also decreased, while the Cho/Cr ratio was increased. In patients with type 2 diabetes, more pronounced metabolic impairments were evidenced (Table 2).

Table 2. The content of metabolites of the hippocampus in patients with type 1 and type 2 diabetes with different cognitive functions.

Hippocampal Metabolites	Type 1 Diabetes and Cognitive Dysfunction	Type 1 Diabetes and Normal Cognitive Functions	Type 2 Diabetes and Cognitive Dysfunction	Type 2 Diabetes and Normal Cognitive Function
NAA left	1.796 ± 0.418 *	1.5705 ± 0.317	1.723 ± 0.427 *	0.768 ± 0.472
NAA right	1.851 ± 0.320	1.848 ± 0.204	1.966 ± 0.580 *	0.574 ± 0.158
Cho left	0.854 ± 0.255	0.946 ± 0.088	2.028 ± 1.333 *	0.949 ± 0.223
Cho right	0.919 ± 0.239 *	1.312 ± 0.496	1.119 ± 0.699	1.101 ± 0.257
Cr left	0.901 ± 0.212	0.905 ± 0.190	0.924 ± 0.137 *	0.741 ± 0.233
Cr right	0.900 ± 0.116	0.939 ± 0.136	1.567 ± 0.429 *	0.582 ± 0.246
PCr left	1.419 ± 0.297 *	1.219 ± 0.271	1.162 ± 0.483 *	0.667 ± 0.175
PCr right	2.025 ± 0.723	1.466 ± 0.450	2.147 ± 0.740 *	0.523 ± 0.167
NAA/Cr left	0.544 ± 0.293	0.596 ± 0.161	1.787 ± 0.406 *	0.616 ± 0.226
NAA/Cr right	0.498 ± 0.102	0.513 ± 0.087	1.980 ± 0.913 *	0.536 ± 0.140
NAA/Cho left	0.568 ± 0.217	0.624 ± 0.117	0.970 ± 0.138	0.913 ± 0.388
NAA/Cho right	0.592 ± 0.123 *	0.723 ± 0.304	1.332 ± 0.684 *	1.106 ± 0.342
Cho/Cr left	1.118 ± 0.358 *	1.087 ± 0.249	1.820 ± 1.246	1.700 ± 0.456
Cho/Cr right	1.204 ± 0.216 *	1.437 ± 0.615	1.017 ± 0.184 *	1.998 ± 0.785

Note: * $p \leq 0.05$.

The correlation analysis was carried out between the content of basic metabolites in brain cells and the basic indicators of glycemic variability (Figure 3).

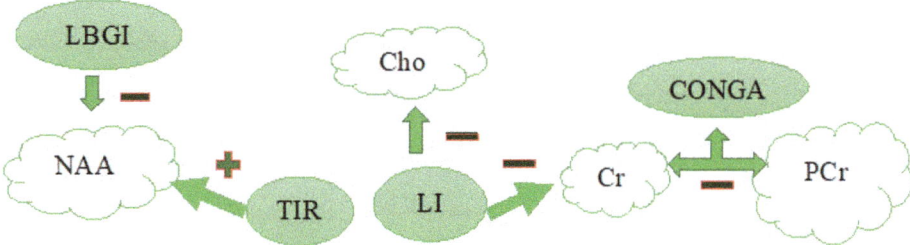

Figure 3. Correlation analysis of the relationship between brain metabolites and glycemic variability indicators. Note. NAA—N-acetylaspartate, Cho—choline, Cr—creatine, PCr—creatine phosphate, LBGI—low blood glucose index, LI—lability index, TIR—time in range, CONGA—glycemia long-term increase index, <<+>>—positive correlation, <<−>>—negative correlation.

As a result of the study on the relationship between metabolite content and glycemic variability indices, a number of significant positive correlations were registered: the level of NAA with the index of hypoglycemic risk/low blood glucose index (LBGI), Cho with the index of glycemic lability/liability index (LI), the duration and the time in range level (TIR), Cr with the index of prolonged glycemic increase (CONGA), and PCr with LI, CONGA and TIR.

In addition, the elevated HbA1c level, the glycemic lability index, and the mean glucose value were correlated in patients with Type 2 diabetes with reduced creatine levels in the hippocampus region. A decrease in the Cho creatine to NAA/Cr ratio was recorded in patients with increased LI and average glycemia level, when the Cho/Cr increase was more frequently noted when the long-term glycemic increase index (CONGA) was increased (Table 3).

Table 3. Correlation of brain metabolites, carbohydrate metabolism parameters, and serum protein taupe in patients with Table 2. diabetes mellitus.

Parameters	Spearman's Criterion	p
Cr and HbA1	−0.8	0.007
Cr and LI	−0.7	0.03
Cr and mean	−0.8	0.007
NAA-Cr & mean	−0.6	0.048
Cho-Cr and CONGA	−0.6	0.04
Cho-Cr & LI	−0.6	0.03

Note: NAA—N-acetylaspartate, Cho—choline, Cr—creatine, PCr—creatine phosphate, mean—average value of glycemia, LI—glycemia lability index, CONGA—glycemia long-term increase index.

When assessing the influence of risk factors for cognitive impairment on brain metabolism in type 1 diabetes, there was a relationship between NAA left and HbA1c level (−0.247, $p \leq 0.05$), Cho on the right and age, history of diabetic ketoacidosis and degree of cognitive impairment (−0.237, −0.230, 0.216, $p \leq 0.05$), Cr on the right and a history of severe hypoglycemia (0.220, $p \leq 0.05$), Cr2 on the left and body mass index (−0.218, $p \leq 0.05$), NAA/Cr on the right and a history of severe hypoglycemia episodes (0.210, $p \leq 0.05$).

When assessing the influence of risk factors for cognitive impairment on brain metabolism in type 2 diabetes, associations between NAA on the left and HbA1c level (−0.733, $p \leq 0.05$), NAA on the left and the level of arterial hypertension (0.511, $p \leq 0.05$), Cho on the left and the level of arterial hypertension (0.682, $p \leq 0.05$), Cho on the right and age and the degree of cognitive impairment (0.785, 0.576, −0.561, $p \leq 0.05$), Cr on the right and the duration of the disease and the degree of cognitive impairment (0.445, −0.508, 0.619, $p \leq 0.05$), Cr2 on the left and the degree of arterial hypertension (0.577694, $p \leq 0.05$), NAA/Cr on the left and a history of episodes of diabetic ketoacidosis in the anamnesis, and the level of HbA1c (0.451, 0.733, $p \leq 0.05$), NAA/Cr on the left and the presence of higher education and insulin therapy (0.424, −0.596, $p \leq 0.05$), NAA/Chon the left and body mass index, and degree of arterial hypertension (−0.562, −0.481, $p \leq 0.05$), NAA/Chon the left and body mass index (−0.529, $p \leq 0.05$), Ch/Cr on the left and age, and glycemic level (−0.457, −0.733, $p \leq 0.05$), Ch/Cr on the right and the degree of arterial hypertension (−0.512, $p \leq 0.05$) were noted.

For the purpose of timely detection of cognitive dysfunction at the earliest stage of the pathological process development, a method of early prediction of cognitive dysfunction in patients with type 1 and 2 diabetes using neuroimaging methods was developed.

For this aim, the data obtained by MRS were processed by the program on the platform of IBM Watson Studio 1.2.2.0, 2018, Armonk, NY, USA, 2018, to build a neural network model, which is a decision support system. This program is used to generalize a large number of complexly structured data using non-linear mathematical operations and allows you to build a model for predicting cognitive disorders in diabetes patients.

The predicted value of the cognitive test was used as the output parameter. The accuracy of this model for type 1 diabetes was 73%, error 1.7%, and for type 2 diabetes—79%, error 1.3%.

4. Discussion and Conclusions

With a change in the modern lifestyle, the incidence of diabetes increases from year to year [12]. The prevalence of cognitive dysfunction caused by diabetes is 10.8–65.0%, and its occurrence is associated with hippocampal atrophy [13–15]. In patients with diabetes, the literature suggests lower values of NAA of the hippocampus on both sides in patients with diabetic retinopathy, which is in accordance with our results, as in our study, patients with cognitive impairment also had a decrease in this metabolite [16]. These data indicate a common effect of complications of diabetes on metabolism in hippocampal cells, which is associated with the loss of neurons or axons and is independently associated with the development of diabetes.

Obesity combined with type 2 diabetes is an important factor of brain damage. The available knowledge demonstrates that in patients with obesity, there are a number of cerebral disorders, either associated with or preceding diabetes, including impaired substrate processing, insulin resistance, and impaired organ interconnections [17]. In keeping with that, in our study, it is BMI that is a risk factor for neurometabolic disorders.

In experimental models of diabetes, the role of dysglycemia on the change in the level of metabolites of the hippocampus was shown, along with the violation of glucose oxidation and an increase in creatinine levels [18]. Another study demonstrated the acute effect of hyperglycemia, i.e., in fact, DKA, on a decrease in NAA, which was combined with hyperphosphorylation of the tau protein, which supports the results of our study and the role of acute complications in the dysfunction of the hippocampus at the stage of manifestation [19]. Currently, data are scant on the effects of hypoglycemia on hippocampal metabolism. In a recent study, Wiegers et al. performed a two-stage hyperinsulinemic euglycemic (5 mmol/L)—hypoglycemic (2.8 mmol/L) test in 7 patients with poor hypoglycemic awareness and in seven patients with normal awareness of hypoglycemia, Hypoglycemia, and in healthy controls. The results showed that all metabolites were reduced by 20% in patients with poor awareness ($p < 0.001$) [20]. In the same study, patients with DM type 1 and frequent hypoglycemia had altered metabolism of the hippocampus.

Cao et al. investigated brain metabolites in the frontal and parietal cortex in 33 patients with diabetes and hypertension and noted the significant decrease in NAA/Cr and Cho/Cr ratios [21]. In our study, hypertension was an important determinant of changes in the hippocampal region.

Other risk factors, such as duration of the disease and age, naturally impair cognitive function and cannot be corrected [22].

A limitation of the study was the non-randomized nature of their comparisons. However, in the future, these points will be taken into account.

In this study, when performing proton spectroscopy, patients with type 1 diabetes showed an increase of NAA, Cho, and Cr2 levels in the hippocampus area, which are responsible for normal neuronal functioning. In type 2 diabetes, NAA levels were increased, as well, Cho, Cr, and Cr2 content decreased. According to several authors, such changes occur in gliosis and membrane necrosis and when oxidative stress is activated [23,24]. MRS of the brain in patients with diabetes shows changes associated with neurodegenerative processes [25]. In this connection, we determined non-invasive markers of metabolic and structural brain changes in patients with diabetes by means of various MRI techniques.

Author Contributions: Conceptualization, J.S. and M.M.; methodology, M.M.; software, O.T. and M.M.; validation, J.S., O.O. and M.M.; formal analysis, J.S. and M.M.; investigation, D.K., J.S. and M.M.; resources, D.K. and O.T.; supervision, D.K. and J.S.; data curation, J.S., O.O., O.T., A.K. and M.M.; writing—original draft preparation, J.S., O.O., O.T., A.K. and M.M.; writing—review and editing, M.M. and A.K.; visualization, O.T.; supervision, D.K. and J.S.; project administration, M.M.; funding acquisition, M.M. All authors have read and agreed to the published version of the manuscript.

Funding: This research was funded with the support of a grant from the President, agreement 075-15-2020-192 dated 03.2019.

Institutional Review Board Statement: The study was conducted according to the guidelines of the Declaration of Helsinki, and approved by the Ethics Committee of Siberian State Medical University (265 from 2 May 2017).

Informed Consent Statement: Informed consent was obtained from all subjects involved in the study.

Data Availability Statement: The data presented in this study are available on request from the corresponding author. The data are not publicly available due to ethical restrictions.

Conflicts of Interest: The authors declare no conflict of interest.

References

1. Biessels, G.J.; Reagan, L.P. Hippocampal insulin resistance and cognitive dysfunction. *Nat. Rev. Neurosci.* **2015**, *16*, 660–671. [CrossRef] [PubMed]
2. Santhakumari, R.; Reddy, I.Y.; Archana, R. Effect of Type 2 Diabetes Mellitus on Brain Metabolites by Using Proton Magnetic Resonance Spectroscopy—A Systematic Review. *Int. J. Pharma Bio Sci.* **2014**, *5*, 1118–1123. [PubMed]
3. Duarte, J.M.; De Lausanne, E.P.F. Metabolism in the Diabetic Brain: Neurochemical Profiling by 1H Magnetic Resonance Spectroscopy. *DMD* **2016**, *3*, 1–6. [CrossRef]
4. Sherry, E.B.; Lee, P.; Choi, I.-Y. In Vivo NMR Studies of the Brain with Hereditary or Acquired Metabolic Disorders. *Neurochem. Res.* **2015**, *40*, 2647–2685. [CrossRef] [PubMed]
5. Duarte, J.M.; Do, K.Q.; Gruetter, R. Longitudinal neurochemical modifications in the aging mouse brain measured in vivo by 1H magnetic resonance spectroscopy. *Neurobiol. Aging* **2014**, *35*, 1660–1668. [CrossRef]
6. Kantarci, K.; Jack, C.R.; Xu, Y.C. Regional metabolic patterns in mild cognitive impairment and Alzheimer's disease. A 1H MRS study. *Neurology* **2000**, *55*, 210–217. [CrossRef]
7. Lin, A.-L.; Rothman, D.L. What have novel imaging techniques revealed about metabolism in the aging brain? *Future Neurol.* **2014**, *9*, 341–354. [CrossRef]
8. Samoilova, I.G.; Rotkank, M.A.; Kudlay, D.A.; Zhukova, N.G.; Matveeva, M.V.; Tolmachev, I.V. A prognostic model of cognitive impairment in patients with type 1 diabetes mellitus. *Zhurnal Nevrol. Psikhiatr.* **2020**, *120*, 19–22. [CrossRef]
9. Nasreddine, Z.S. MoCA Test Mandatory Training and Certification: What Is the Purpose? *J. Am. Geriatr. Soc.* **2020**, *68*, 444–445. [CrossRef]
10. Kreis, R.; Ross, B.D. Cerebral metabolic disturbances in patients with subacute and chronic diabetes mellitus: Detection with proton MR spectroscopy. *Radiology* **1992**, *184*, 123–130. [CrossRef] [PubMed]
11. Gerget, O.M. Bionic models for identification of biological systems. *J. Phys. Conf. Ser.* **2017**, *803*, 12046. [CrossRef]
12. Nathan, D.M.; DCCT/Edic Research Group. The diabetes control and complications trial/epidemiology of diabetes interventions and complications study at 30 years: Overview. *Diabetes Care* **2014**, *37*, 9–16. [CrossRef]
13. Tong, J.; Geng, H.; Zhang, Z.; Zhu, X.; Meng, Q.; Sun, X.; Zhang, M.; Qian, R.; Sun, L.; Liang, Q. Brain metabolite alterations demonstrated by proton magnetic resonance spectroscopy in diabetic patients with retinopathy. *Magn. Reson. Imaging* **2014**, *32*, 1037–1042. [CrossRef]
14. Zhang, J.; Liu, Z.; Li, Z.; Wang, Y.; Chen, Y.; Li, X.; Chen, K.; Shu, N.; Zhang, Z. Disrupted White Matter Network and Cognitive Decline in Type 2 Diabetes Patients. *J. Alzheimer's Dis.* **2016**, *53*, 185–195. [CrossRef]
15. Matveeva, M.V.; Samoilova, Y.G.; Zhukova, N.G.; Tolmachov, I.V.; Brazovskiy, K.S.; Leiman, O.P.; Fimushkina, N.Y.; Rotkank, M.A. Neuroimaging methods for assessing the brain in diabetes mellitus (literature review). *Bull. Sib. Med.* **2020**, *19*, 189–194. [CrossRef]
16. Lu, X.; Gong, W.; Wen, Z.; Hu, L.; Peng, Z.; Zha, Y. Correlation Between Diabetic Cognitive Impairment and Diabetic Retinopathy in Patients with T2DM by 1H-MRS. *Front. Neurol.* **2019**, *10*, 1068. [CrossRef] [PubMed]
17. Ma, X.C.; Wang, G.Z.; Wang, Y.C.; Fang, Q.; Wang, K.L. Clinical analysis of hydrogen proton spectroscopy in hippocampus of type 2 diabetic patients. *Modern J. Integr. Tradit. Chin. Western Med.* **2010**, *32*, 45–48.
18. van der Graaf, M.; Janssen, S.W.; van Asten, J.J. Metabolic profile of the hippocampus of Zucker Diabetic Fatty rats assessed by in vivo 1H magnetic resonancespectroscopy. *NMR Biomed.* **2004**, *17*, 405–410. [CrossRef]
19. Zhang, H.; Huang, M.; Gao, L.; Lei, H. Region-Specific Cerebral Metabolic Alterations in Streptozotocin-Induced Type 1 Diabetic Rats: An in vivo Proton Magnetic Resonance Spectroscopy Study. *Br. J. Pharmacol.* **2015**, *35*, 1738–1745. [CrossRef]
20. Wiegers, E.C.; Rooijackers, H.M.; Tack, C.J.; Heerschap, A.; De Galan, B.E.; Van Der Graaf, M. Brain Lactate Concentration Falls in Response to Hypoglycemia in Patients with Type 1 Diabetes and Impaired Awareness of Hypoglycemia. *Diabetes* **2016**, *65*, 1601–1605. [CrossRef]
21. Bejide, M.; Contreras, P.; Homm, P.; Duran, B.; García-Merino, J.A.; Rosenkranz, A.; DeNardin, J.C.; Del Río, R.; Hevia, S.A. Nickel Nanopillar Arrays Electrodeposited on Silicon Substrates Using Porous Alumina Templates. *Molecules* **2020**, *25*, 5377. [CrossRef] [PubMed]
22. Biessels, G.J.; Deary, I.J.; Ryan, C.M. Cognition and diabetes: A lifespan perspective. *Lancet Neurol.* **2008**, *7*, 184–190. [CrossRef]
23. Hansen, T.M.; Brock, B.; Juhl, A.; Drewes, A.M.; Vorum, H.; Andersen, C.U.; Jakobsen, P.E.; Karmisholt, J.; Frøkjær, J.B.; Brock, C. Brain spectroscopy reveals that N-acetylaspartate is associated to peripheral sensorimotor neuropathy in type 1 diabetes. *J. Diabetes Its Complicat.* **2019**, *33*, 323–328. [CrossRef]
24. Zhao, X.; Han, Q.; Gang, X.; Wang, G. Altered brain metabolites in patients with diabetes mellitus and related complications—Evidence from 1H MRS study. *Biosci. Rep.* **2018**, *38*. [CrossRef] [PubMed]
25. Seaquist, E.R. The Impact of Diabetes on Cerebral Structure and Function. *Psychosom. Med.* **2015**, *77*, 616–621. [CrossRef] [PubMed]

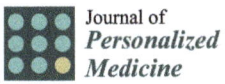

Article

The Risk of Type 2 Diabetes Mellitus in a Russian Population Cohort According to Data from the HAPIEE Project

Svetlana V. Mustafina [1,*], Oksana D. Rymar [1], Liliya V. Shcherbakova [1], Evgeniy G. Verevkin [1], Hynek Pikhart [2], Olga V. Sazonova [3], Yuliya I. Ragino [1], Galina I. Simonova [1], Martin Bobak [2], Sofia K. Malyutina [1,3] and Mikhail I. Voevoda [1]

[1] Institute of Internal and Preventive Medicine–Branch of Institute of Cytology and Genetics, Siberian Branch of Russian Academy of Sciences, 630089 Novosibirsk, Russia; orymar23@gmail.com (O.D.R.); 9584792@mail.ru (L.V.S.); ewer@mail.ru (E.G.V.); ragino@mail.ru (Y.I.R.); yu.p.nikitin@gmail.com (G.I.S.); smalyutina@hotmail.com (S.K.M.); mvoevoda@ya.ru (M.I.V.)
[2] Institute of Epidemiology and Health Care, University College London, Gower Street, London WC1E6BT, UK; h.pikhart@ucl.ac.uk (H.P.); m.bobak@ucl.ac.uk (M.B.)
[3] Novosibirsk State Medical University, 630091 Novosibirsk, Russia; ov_sazonova@mail.ru
* Correspondence: svetlana3548@gmail.com; Tel.: +7-923-228-97-57

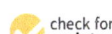

Citation: Mustafina, S.V.; Rymar, O.D.; Shcherbakova, L.V.; Verevkin, E.G.; Pikhart, H.; Sazonova, O.V.; Ragino, Y.I.; Simonova, G.I.; Bobak, M.; Malyutina, S.K.; et al. The Risk of Type 2 Diabetes Mellitus in a Russian Population Cohort According to Data from the HAPIEE Project. *J. Pers. Med.* **2021**, *11*, 119. https://doi.org/10.3390/jpm11020119

Academic Editor: Mikhail Ivanovich Voevoda

Received: 10 December 2020
Accepted: 8 February 2021
Published: 11 February 2021

Publisher's Note: MDPI stays neutral with regard to jurisdictional claims in published maps and institutional affiliations.

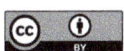

Copyright: © 2021 by the authors. Licensee MDPI, Basel, Switzerland. This article is an open access article distributed under the terms and conditions of the Creative Commons Attribution (CC BY) license (https://creativecommons.org/licenses/by/4.0/).

Abstract: The aim of this study is to investigate the 14-year risk of type 2 diabetes mellitus (T2DM) and develop a risk score for T2DM in the Siberian cohort. A random population sample (males/females, 45–69 years old) was examined at baseline in 2003–2005 (Health, Alcohol, and Psychosocial Factors in Eastern Europe (HAPIEE) project, *n* = 9360, Novosibirsk) and re-examined in 2006–2008 and 2015–2017. After excluding those with baseline T2DM, the final analysis included 7739 participants. The risk of incident T2DM during a 14-year follow-up was analysed using Cox regression. In age-adjusted models, male and female hazard ratios (HR) of incident T2DM were 5.02 (95% CI 3.62; 6.96) and 5.13 (95% CI 3.56; 7.37) for BMI ≥ 25 kg/m^2; 4.38 (3.37; 5.69) and 4.70 (0.27; 6.75) for abdominal obesity (AO); 3.31 (2.65; 4.14) and 3.61 (3.06; 4.27) for fasting hyperglycaemia (FHG); 2.34 (1.58; 3.49) and 3.27 (2.50; 4.26) for high triglyceride (TG); 2.25 (1.74; 2.91) and 2.82 (2.27; 3.49) for hypertension (HT); and 1.57 (1.14; 2.16) and 1.69 (1.38; 2.07) for family history of diabetes mellitus (DM). In addition, secondary education, low physical activity (PA), and history of cardiovascular disease (CVD) were also significantly associated with T2DM in females. A simple T2DM risk calculator was generated based on non-laboratory parameters. A scale with the best quality included waist circumference >95 cm, HT history, and family history of T2DM (area under the curve (AUC) = 0.71). The proposed 10-year risk score of T2DM represents a simple, non-invasive, and reliable tool for identifying individuals at a high risk of future T2DM.

Keywords: diabetes mellitus; risk factor; diabetes risk scale; diabetes risk model

1. Introduction

In the last decades, the prevalence of diabetes mellitus (DM) has consistently risen in the general world population, thus making DM a medical and social problem worldwide [1]. According to the International Diabetes Federation forecast in 2019, the number of subjects with diabetes is expected to reach 578 million by 2030 and 700 million by 2045 [2]. In the Russian Federation, the prevalence of DM is also rising. According to the Federal Register of Diabetes Mellitus, in Russia by the end of 2016, 4.35 million subjects (3.0% of the population) had been registered in a dispensary as DM patients, of which 92% (4 million) had type 2 diabetes mellitus (T2DM), 6% (255,000) had type 1 diabetes mellitus, and 2% (75,000) other types of diabetes [3]. According to the NATION study, among the adult Russian population of 20–79 years old, 5.4% have T2DM. Moreover, approximately one-half of patients with diagnosed DM (54%) were unaware of this disease [4]. In our baseline survey within the Health, Alcohol, and Psychosocial Factors in Eastern Europe (HAPIEE) project, 2003–2005, we found a high prevalence of T2DM (11.3%) in the population sample aged 45–69 years old in Novosibirsk [5]. The rate is close to the data on compatible age groups in the NATION study conducted in Russia in 2013–2015 [4].

T2DM is known to be a multifactorial disease, and environmental factors are important for T2DM pathogenesis. The risk factors of T2DM are well established and include abdominal obesity (waist circumference (WC) ≥ 94 cm in males and ≥ 80 cm in females), a family history of DM, age >45 years old, hypertension and major cardiovascular diseases (CVDs), gestational diabetes, the use of drugs that contribute to hyperglycaemia, and weight gain. Early identification of T2DM risk factors and their clusters with the aim of modification can help to prevent T2DM [6,7]. At present, preventive strategies rely on the identification of risk factors and their combinations and subsequent lifestyle intervention. Appropriate lifestyle changes, including the normalisation of diet, increased physical activity, and weight loss can reduce the risk of T2DM by as much as 56% [8].

One of the first tools to identify individuals at high risk for T2DM is the Finnish diabetes risk score (FINDRISC) [9,10]. This tool was later successfully validated in other countries, including Germany, Holland, Denmark, Sweden, England, and Australia, [10,11]. The results show good sensitivity (Se) and specificity (Sp) in Germany, the USA, Switzerland, and Canada [12–15], although it did not perform well among the Omani Arabs [16].

To prevent further increase in the prevalence of diabetes, the identification of individuals at high risk for hyperglycaemia using inexpensive and available methods is crucial. Using risk score methods of prediction allows us to set the level of total risk, identify high-risk patients, and prescribe the necessary preventive measures.

Risk factors of T2DM have been studied in healthcare institutions and cross-sectional studies in Russia. Nonetheless, we are not aware of a Russian prospective cohort analysis of the long-term risk of T2DM in the general population. In this study, we aimed to investigate the 14-year risk of T2DM in a Russian population cohort in order to develop a risk scale to predict the development of T2DM over 10 years in people aged 45–69 years old.

2. Materials and Methods

2.1. Study Population and Methods

The data came from the Russian arm of the HAPIEE project [17]. The cohorts in this multicentre project were randomly selected from population registers or electoral lists and stratified by sex and five year age groups. The planned sample size was 10,000 persons in each country. At baseline, a cross-sectional analysis of the random age- and sex-stratified population sample of males and females aged 45–69 years old was performed in 2003–2005 in Novosibirsk (Russia) (n = 9360, response rate 61%). In the Russian arm of the study, both the questionnaire and the examination have been completed in an outpatient clinic. The details of sampling have been described elsewhere [17]. The cohort was re-examined in 2006–2008 and in 2015–2017. Follow-up data were collected between 2003 and 2017; the average follow-up period comprised 13.7 (0.7) years (mean (SD)). The last survey and follow-up were supported by Russian Science Foundation. We excluded from the analysis those who have no baseline glucose assessment and those with T2DM at baseline defined as fasting plasma glucose (FPG) ≥ 7.0 mmol/L or current treatment with insulin or oral hypoglycaemic agents (1621 subjects excluded). In total, the final analysis included 7739 participants (3376 males; 4363 females). Incident DM in any wave of follow-up was registered as the endpoint.

2.2. Baseline Examination

The baseline and repeated examinations involved standardised questionnaires, objective measurements, and blood sampling for biomarker assays. Details of the baseline protocol of the HAPIEE project have been published previously [17,18]. The participants did an interview with trained technicians regarding sociodemographic characteristics, behavioural risk factors (including smoking and alcohol intake), a history of DM and hypertension and their treatment, a history of major CVDs and other chronic diseases, physical activity (PA), a family history of T2DM and CVDs, meal frequency and other health, lifestyle, and social characteristics.

Objective measurements included anthropometry (body weight, height, WC, and hip circumference) and blood pressure (BP) determination. The body weight was measured on a weighing scale with a participant wearing one layer of clothes (accuracy to 0.1 kg). The height was measured using a vertical stadiometer (accuracy 0.1 cm). WC and hip circumference were measured by means of a tape with 0.1 cm accuracy. The body–mass index (BMI) was calculated as weight in kilograms divided by the square of height in meters and categorised as BMI < 25.0 kg/m^2 and BMI $\geq$ 25 kg/m^2 [18]. Abdominal obesity was defined as a WC of $\geq$94 cm for males and $\geq$80 cm for females [3].

BP was measured after 5-min rest on the right hand in a sitting position using Omron M5-I (Omron Co. Ltd., Terado-cho, Muko, Kyoto, Japan). The measurement of BP was carried out three times with an interval of 2 min. For the present analysis, the average of the three values of BP was used. Hypertension was defined as systolic BP (SBP) $\geq$140 mmHg or diastolic BP (DBP) $\geq$90 mmHg and/or antihypertensive medication use during the last two weeks.

Blood samples were drawn after overnight fasting (at least 8 h). Serum levels of glucose, total cholesterol (TC), triglycerides (TGs), and high-density lipoprotein cholesterol (HDL-C) were determined by enzymatic methods on a KoneLab 30i automated analyser (Thermo Fisher Scientific Inc., Waltham, MA, USA). The fasting serum glucose value was converted to fasting plasma glucose (FPG) via the formula of the European Association for the Study of Diabetes in 2007 [19]:

FPG (mmol/L) = $-0.137 + 1.047 \times$ serum glucose concentration (mmol/L). Impaired fasting glucose was defined as FPG of 6.1–6.9 mmol/L.

Hypertriglyceridemia was defined as a serum TG level of $\geq$2.8 mmol/L, and abnormal HDL-C was defined as HDL cholesterol of $\leq$0.9 mmol/L for males and females [3].

We followed the cohort from the baseline survey up to 31 December 2017; the average period of follow-up comprised 13.7 (0.7) years (mean (SD)). The incident cases of T2DM were ascertained using overlapping sources—the cases registered by the municipal diabetes register and new cases identified by the repeated surveys in 2006–2008 and 2015–2017. Baseline T2DM was defined as FPG of $\geq$7.0 mmol/L or current treatment with insulin or oral hypoglycaemic agents [20]; these persons were excluded from the study. An incident case of DM was defined as a new case registered by the T2DM register during the 2003–2017 period or a new case identified in the second or third survey as FPG $\geq$7.0 mmol/L or current treatment with insulin or oral hypoglycaemic agents.

2.3. Statistical Analyses

These analyses were carried out using the statistical package SPSS for Windows Version 13.0, (SPSS Inc., Chicago, IL, USA). Baseline characteristics of the study participants are given as means (SD) and were compared by the χ^2 test, unpaired Student's *t* test (2-tailed), or Mann–Whitney test, depending on the type of distribution of the variables.

First, the association between potential risk factors and incident T2DM was assessed by Cox regression analysis in age- and sex-adjusted Model 1 and in age-adjusted Model 2 split by sex. Incident T2DM served as a dependent variable. Independent variables tested sequentially included the education level (categorised into three groups—higher education, secondary, or primary education); marital status (categorised into two groups—married or cohabitating/single); SBP and DBP (as continuous variables); hypertension (dichotomised as yes/no); TC, TG, HDL-C, and FPG (as continuous variables); high TG concentration (dichotomised as $\geq$2.8 mmol/L and <2.8 mmol/L); low HDL-C concentration (dichotomised as cholesterol $\leq$0.9 mmol/L for males and females and cholesterol >0.9 mmol/L for males and females); fasting hyperglycaemia (dichotomised as $\geq$6.1 and <6.1 mmol/L); obesity (categorised into two groups—BMI < 25 kg/m^2 and $\geq$25 kg/m^2); abdominal obesity (categorised into two groups—WC $\geq$ 94 cm for males and $\geq$80 cm for females and <94 cm for males and <80 cm for females); smoking (categorised into three groups—current smokers, past smokers, or never smoked); alcohol consumption was rated in two versions—as a continuous variable (the mean dose of ethanol per occasion, in grams) and as a dichotomised variable (higher than a calculated sex-specific mean amount of alcohol intake per session in the population sample, yes/no; the lack of leisure time PA weekly or daily (PA in a previous week was categorised into three groups—none, insufficient (1–179 min), and sufficient ($\geq$180 min); everyday PA was categorised into three groups—none, insufficient (1–29 min), and sufficient ($\geq$30 min)), and a dichotomised variable 'low PA' was generated based on weekly or daily insufficient PA at leisure time (yes/no); fruit and vegetable consumption (dichotomised as every day/not every day); a family history of DM (dichotomised as a T2DM history in first-degree relatives and no family history of T2DM); and a history of major CVDs (dichotomised as yes/no). Covariates were age (as a continuous variable, per year) and sex (male or female).

Among the tested factors, for subsequent Cox regression analysis, we selected those significantly associated with T2DM, and in a set of similar variables, we selected the ones with greater hazard ratios (HRs). The selected variables included age, BMI, abdominal obesity, hypertension, dyslipidaemia (high TG and low HDL-C levels), FPG, the history of CVDs, smoking status, alcohol intake, the education level, marital status, PA, fruit and vegetable consumption, and the family history of DM.

At the second stage, we applied Cox proportional hazards regression analysis to assess the association between risk factors and incident T2DM in age-adjusted and multivariable-adjusted models separately in males and females.

HRs with a 95% confidence interval (CI) were calculated for the above factors selected as independent variables. In males, the multivariable model included age, BMI $\geq$ 25 kg/m^2, hypertension, high TG concentration, FPG, a family history of DM, and a history of CVD. In females, the model included age, BMI $\geq$ 25 kg/m^2, hypertension, high TG concentration, FPG, education level, PA, marital status, a family history of DM, and a history of CVD.

At the third stage, we used dichotomised variables based on cut-off points for risk factors of T2DM obtained using receiver-operating characteristic (ROC) analysis. These cut-offs were applied further to build a 10-year risk score for T2DM using Cox regression and ROC analysis and select a model which includes a minimum number of prognostic parameters and has the maximum positive predictive power for T2DM risk.

Logistic regression was used to compute β-coefficients for significant risk factors for T2DM. Coefficients (β) of the model were used to assign a score value for each variable, and the composite diabetes risk score was calculated as the sum of those scores. The sensitivity (the probability that the test is positive for subjects who will receive drug-treated diabetes in the future) and the specificity (the probability that the test is negative for subjects without drug-treated diabetes) with 95% CIs were calculated for each diabetes risk score level in differentiating subjects developed incident T2DM from those who did not. Then, ROC curves were plotted for the diabetes risk score; the sensitivity was plotted on the y-axis, and the false-positive rate (1-specificity) was plotted on the x-axis. The more accurately discriminatory the test, the steeper the upward portion of the ROC curve and the higher the area under the curve (AUC), the optimal cut point being the peak of the curve.

3. Results

The population sample of males and females aged 45–69 years old was examined at baseline in 2003–2005 in Novosibirsk (n = 9360 subjects). The present analysis was limited to those without T2DM at baseline (n = 7739). The baseline characteristics of this sample are presented in Table 1.

3.1. The 14-Year Risk of T2DM

During the follow-up of 13.7 (0.7) years (mean (SD)), 915 participants developed T2DM for the first time (11.8%). Among males, the frequency of incident cases of T2DM was 1.8-fold lower than that among females, 9.7% and 15.5%, respectively (p < 0.0001).

Table 1. Characteristics of the studied population sample (aged 45–69 years old at baseline, n = 7739).

	Males and Females	Males	Females	p
Examined	7739	3376	4363	
Age (years)	57.7 (7.1)	57.8 (7.0)	57.6 (7.1)	0.211
Height (cm)	164.0 (8.9)	171.3 (6.3)	158.4 (6.0)	<0.001
Weight (kg)	75.8 (14.2)	77.3 (13.8)	74.7 (14.4)	<0.001
BMI (kg/m^2)	28.3 (5.3)	26.3 (4.2)	29.8 (5.6)	<0.001
Waist circumference (cm)	91.7 (12.4)	93.0 (11.6)	90.7 (12.9)	<0.001
Abdominal obesity •, n(%)	5014 (64.8)	1563 (46.3)	3451 (79.1)	<0.001
SBP (mmHg)	142.8 (24.5)	142.4 (22.6)	143.1 (25.8)	0.202
DBP (mmHg)	90.0 (13.3)	90.0 (13.0)	89.9 (13.5)	0.899
FPG (mmol/L)	5.61 (0.6)	5.63 (0.6)	5.59 (0.6)	0.003
TC (mmol/L)	6.2 (1.2)	5.9 (1.1)	6.4 (1.2)	<0.001
TG (mmol/L)	1.4 (0.7)	1.4 (0.7)	1.5 (0.6)	<0.001
HDL-C (mmol/L)	1.5 (0.4)	1.5 (0.4)	1.6 (0.3)	<0.001
Hypertension * n(%)	4910 (63.5)	2082 (61.7)	2828 (64.8)	0.005
Low HDL-C ■, n(%)	43 (0.6)	26 (0.8)	17 (0.4)	0.026
High TG ♦, n(%)	296 (3.8)	125 (3.7)	171 (3.9)	0.609
Fasting hyperglycaemia •, n(%)	1541 (20.2)	708 (21.2)	833 (19.4)	0.045
BMI ≥ 25 kg/m^2, n(%)	5510 (71.2)	1993 (59.0)	3517 (80.6)	<0.001
Alcohol, mean dose per occasion (g)	35.8 (36.5)	54.2 (45.6)	21.7 (17.3)	<0.001
Smoking, n(%)				<0.001
Never smoked	4624 (59.8)	917 (27.2)	3707 (85.0)	
Former smoker	973 (12.6)	786 (23.3)	187 (4.3)	
Current smoker	2141 (27.7)	1672 (49.5)	469 (10.7)	
Marital status, n(%)				<0.001
Single	2145 (27.7)	387 (11.5)	1758 (40.3)	
Married or cohabitating	5594 (72.3)	2989 (88.5)	2605 (59.7)	
Education level, n(%)				<0.001
Only primary	719 (9.3)	335 (9.9)	384 (8.8)	
Any secondary	4722 (61.0)	1927 (57.1)	2795 (64.1)	
University	2298 (29.7)	1114 (33.0)	1184 (27.1)	
Family history of T2DM (%)	863 (11.2)	300 (9.0)	563 (12.9)	<0.001
History of CVD, n(%)	832 (10.8)	475 (14.1)	357 (8.2)	<0.001
Fruit and vegetable consumption less than every day ˆ, n(%)	833 (10.8)	361 (10.7)	472 (10.8)	0.856
Leisure-time PA in previous week #, min	6260 (80.9)	2803 (83.0)	3457 (79.2)	<0.001

• Abdominal obesity: waist circumference (WC) ≥94 cm for males and ≥80 cm for females. * Hypertension is defined as systolic blood pressure (SBP) ≥140 mmHg or diastolic blood pressure (DBP) ≥90 mmHg or antihypertensive drug treatment during the last two weeks; ■ Low high-density lipoprotein cholesterol (HDL-C) ≤0.9 mmol/L for males and females. ♦ High triglyceride (TG): serum TG concentration ≥2.8 mmol/L. • Fasting hyperglycaemia: glucose ≥6.1 mmol/L. ˆ Fruit and vegetable consumption (every day/not every day); # Leisure time physical activity (PA) in a previous week (insufficient: 1–179 min or sufficient: ≥180 min).

We compared 26 factors potentially related to T2DM between the participants who developed T2DM and those who remained free of T2DM; the results are summarised in Table 2. Individuals of both sexes who developed T2DM were younger, had a greater BMI, greater WC, more frequent abdominal obesity, higher SBP and DBP, more frequent hypertension, a more frequent family history of DM, and higher FPG, TG, and HDL-C levels as compared to those without T2DM.

Males with incident T2DM had higher TC levels were less frequently current smokers and more frequently smokers in the past than their counterparts without T2DM. Females with incident T2DM had a more frequent history of CVD, engaged in less PA, and more frequently had a secondary-education level than their counterparts without T2DM.

The results of the Cox regression analysis are presented in Table 3. In the age-adjusted model for males, the 14-year risk of incident T2DM was associated with BMI ≥ 25 kg/m^2, abdominal obesity, fasting hyperglycaemia, a high TG level, hypertension, and a family history of DM (Table 3). In the age-adjusted model for females, the 14-year risk of incident T2DM was associated with abdominal obesity, BMI ≥ 25 kg/m^2, fasting hyperglycaemia, a high TG level, hypertension, a family history of DM, any secondary-education level, low PA (1–179 min/week or 1–29 min/day), and a history of CVD (Table 3).

Table 2. Baseline characteristics of groups with incident T2DM and without T2DM stratified by sex (mean (SD), and n(%)).

	Males			Females		
	T2DM (+)	T2DM (−)	p	T2DM (+)	T2DM (−)	p
Examined	328	3048		587	3776	
Age (years)	57.2 (6.7)	57.8 (7.1)	0.154	57.3 (6.7)	57.6 (7.2)	0.347
Height (cm)	171.5 (6.4)	171.3 (6.3)	0.572	158.2 (5.7)	158.4 (6.1)	0.595
Weight (kg)	87.1 (14.5)	76.2 (13.3)	<0.001	83.0 (14.7)	73.4 (14.0)	<0.001
BMI (kg/m^2)	29.6 (4.2)	25.9 (4.0)	<0.001	33.1 (5.5)	29.3 (5.4)	<0.001
Waist circumference (cm)	101.9 (11.1)	92.1 (11.2)	<0.001	98.9 (11.8)	89.4 (12.6)	<0.001
Abdominal obesity •, n(%)	255 (78.0)	1308 (42.9)	<0.001	556 (94.7)	2895 (76.7)	<0.001
SBP (mmHg)	146.9 (22.8)	142.0 (22.5)	<0.001	149.7 (25.6)	142.1 (25.7)	<0.001
DBP (mmHg)	93.9 (13.1)	89.6 (13.0)	<0.001	94.1 (13.0)	89.3 (13.5)	<0.001
FPG (mmol/L)	6.0 (0.6)	5.6 (0.6)	<0.001	5.9 (0.6)	5.5 (0.6)	<0.001
TC (mmol/L)	6.1 (1.1)	5.9 (1.1)	0.003	6.5 (1.2)	6.4 (1.2)	0.181
TG (mmol/L)	1.7 (0.9)	1.3 (0.6)	<0.001	1.8 (0.9)	1.4 (0.6)	<0.001
HDL-C (mmol/L)	1.4 (0.3)	1.5 (0.4)	<0.001	1.5 (0.3)	1.6 (0.3)	<0.001
Hypertension *, n(%)	248 (75.6)	1834 (60.2)	<0.001	479 (81.6)	2349 (62.2)	<0.001
Low HDL-C ■, n(%)	3 (0.9)	23 (0.8)	0.754	4 (0.7)	13 (0.3)	0.216
High TG ♦, n(%)	29 (8.8)	96 (3.2)	<0.001	62 (10.7)	109 (2.9)	<0.001
Fasting hyperglycaemia •, n(%)	149 (47.2)	559 (18.5)	<0.001	247 (43.5)	586 (15.7)	<0.001
BMI ≥ 25 kg/m^2, n(%)	287 (87.5)	1706 (56.0)	<0.001	556 (94.7)	2961 (78.4)	<0.001
Alcohol, mean dose per occasion (g)	54.3 (46.1)	54.2 (45.5)	0.953	22.3 (19.2)	21.6 (17.0)	0.322
Smoking, n(%)			0.001			0.423
Never smoked	101 (30.9)	816 (26.8)		509 (86.7)	3198 (84.7)	
Former smoker	96 (29.4)	690 (22.6)		21 (3.6)	166 (4.4)	
Current smoker	130 (39.8)	1542 (50.6)		57 (9.7)	412 (10.9)	
Marital status, n(%)			0.229			0.294
Single	31 (9.5)	356 (11.7)		230 (39.2)	1528 (40.5)	
Married or cohabitating	297 (90.5)	2692 (88.3)		357 (60.8)	2248 (59.5)	
Education level, n(%)			0.287			0.001
Primary	26 (7.9)	309 (10.1)		43 (7.3)	341 (9.0)	
Any secondary	184 (56.1)	1743 (57.2)		417 (71.0)	2378 (63.0)	
University	118 (36.0)	996 (32.7)		127 (21.6)	1057 (28.0)	
Family history of T2DM (%)	44 (13.5)	256 (8.5)	0.002	117 (20.0)	446 (11.9)	<0.001
History of CVD, n(%)	52 (15.9)	423 (13.9)	0.328	61 (10.4)	296 (7.8)	0.036
Fruit and vegetable consumption less than every day ˆ, n(%)	35 (10.7)	326 (10.7)	0.993	66 (11.2)	406 (10.8)	0.740
Leisure-time PA in previous week #, min	276 (84.1)	2527 (82.9)	0.570	490 (83.5)	2967 (78.6)	0.006

• Abdominal obesity: WC ≥ 94 cm for males and ≥80 cm for females. * Hypertension is defined as SBP ≥ 140 mmHg or DBP ≥ 90 mmHg or antihypertensive drug treatment during the last 2 weeks; ■ Low HDL-C: ≤0.9 mmol/L for males and females. ♦ High TG: serum TG level ≥2.8 mmol/L. • Fasting hyperglycaemia: glucose concentration ≥6.1 mmol/L. ˆ Fruit and vegetable consumption (every day/not every day); # Leisure time PA in a previous week (insufficient: 1–179 min or sufficient: ≥180 min).

The results of multivariable-Cox regression analysis are given in Table 3. In the multivariable-adjusted model, BMI ≥ 25 kg/m^2 made the greatest contribution to the development of T2DM, with HR = 3.34 (2.60; 4.30); besides, the risk of incident T2DM was independently associated with fasting hyperglycaemia (HR = 2.70 (2.35; 3,10)), hypertension (HR = 1.86 (1.57; 2.21)), a high TG level (HR = 1.59 (1.26; 2.01)), a family history of DM (HR = 1.53 (1.28; 1.83)), a low leisure-time PA (HR = 1.22 (1.02; 1.46)) (Table 3).

Table 3. The preliminary assessment of the relationship between the 14-year risk of T2DM and risk factors by age-adjusted and age- and sex-adjusted Cox regression.

Risk Factors	Model 1 HR (95% CI) *	Model 2 HR (95% CI) **		Model 3 HR (95% CI) ***
	Males and Females	Males	Females	Males and Females
Smoking				
Never	1.0	1.0	1.0	1.0
Former	1.02 (0.81; 1.27)	1.10 (0.83; 1.45)	0.74 (0.48; 1.15)	0.84 (0.67; 1.06)
Current	0.72 (0.60; 0.88)	0.66 (0.50; 0.85)	0.87 (0.66; 1.15)	0.83 (0.68; 1.02)
Alcohol intake above sex-specific mean amount per session in study population				
Alcohol, <mean dose per occasion (g)	1.0	1.0	1.0	
Alcohol, ≥mean dose per occasion (g)	0.99 (0.87; 1.13)	0.93 (0.74; 1.16)	1.02 (0.87; 1.21)	
Education level				
University	1.0	1.0	1.0	1.0
Any secondary	1.21 (1.04; 1.40)	0.91 (0.72; 1.15)	1.44 (1.18; 1.76)	1.05 (0.79; 1.38)
Primary	0.95 (0.73; 1.25)	0.80 (0.52; 1.22)	1.10 (0.77; 1.57)	1.25 (0.96; 1.62)
Marital status				
Single	1.0	1.0	1.0	
Married or cohabitating	1.07 (0.92; 1.25)	1.21 (0.83; 1.75)	1.05 (0.89; 1.24)	
Family history of DM				
No	1.0	1.0	1.0	1.0
Yes	1.65 (1.34; 1.96)	1.57 (1.14; 2.16)	1.69 (1.38; 2.07)	1.53 (1.28; 1.83)
History of CVD				
No	1.0	1.0	1.0	1.0
Yes	1.31 (1.07; 1.61)	1.22 (0.90; 1.66)	1.40 (1.07; 1.84)	1.04 (0.85; 1.28)
Hypertension *				
No	1.0	1.0	1.0	1.0
Yes	2.56 (2.17; 3.01)	2.25 (1.74; 2.91)	2.82 (2.27; 3.49)	1.86 (1.57; 2.21)
Abdominal obesity				
No	1.0	1.0	1.0	
Yes	4.62 (3.74; 5.71)	4.38 (3.37; 5.69)	5.13 (3.56; 7.37)	
BMI ≥ 25 kg/m^2				
No	1.0	1.0	1.0	1.0
Yes	4.87 (3.82; 6.21)	5.02 (3.62; 6.96)	4.70 (3.27; 6.75)	3.34 (2.60; 4.30)
High TG level				
No	1.0	1.0	1.0	1.0
Yes	2.93 (2.35; 3.65)	2.34 (1.58; 3.49)	3.27 (2.50; 4.26)	1.59 (1.26; 2.01)
Low HDL-C concentration				
No	1.0	1.0	1.0	1.0
Yes	1.49 (0.70; 3.15)	1.29 (0.41; 4.02)	1.68 (0.61; 4.64)	1.48 (0.70; 3.12)
Fasting hyperglycaemia				
No	1.0	1.0	1.0	1.0
Yes	3.51 (3.07; 4.02)	3.31 (2.65; 4.14)	3.61 (3.06; 4.27)	2.70 (2.35; 3.10)

Table 3. Cont.

Risk Factors	Model 1 HR (95% CI) *	Model 2		Model 3 HR (95% CI) ***
		HR (95% CI) **	HR (95% CI)	
	Males and Females	Males	Females	Males and Females
Smoking				
Low PA at leisure time				
≥180 min per week	1.0	1.0	1.0	1.0
1–179 min per week	1.29 (1.08; 1.53)	1.11 (0.83; 1.50)	1.39 (1.12; 1.73)	1.22 (1.02; 1.46)
Fruit and vegetable consumption				
every day	1.0	1.0	1.0	1.0
not every day	0.97 (0.79; 1.19)	0.92 (0.65; 1.31)	0.99 (0.77; 1.28)	1.05 (0.85; 1.29)

* Model 1: age- and sex-adjusted model. ** Model 2: age-adjusted model split by sex. *** Model 3: The model is multivariable and adjusted for age, sex, a family history of diabetes mellitus (DM), fasting hyperglycaemia, a history of cardiovascular disease (CVD), hypertension, abdominal obesity, high TG level, low HDL-C concentration, education level, smoking, low PA, and fruit and vegetable consumption.

3.2. Development of the Type 2 Diabetes Risk Scale

In many countries, 10-year risk scales for T2DM have been created on the basis of epidemiological studies [11]. These scales are based on the most specific risk factors of T2DM in a population under study. To build models for assessing the risk of T2DM, we used cut-off points (cut-off) which were calculated for the Siberian population in the age group under study. This allowed us to take into account the regional characteristics of the studied cohort. Different values were obtained for males and females: for males, the BMI (cut-off) was 27 kg/m^2, WC (cut-off) 95.0 cm, SBP (cut-off) 150 mmHg, DBP (cut-off) 90 mmHg, TG (cut-off) 1.4 mmol/L, HDL-C (cut-off) 0.9 mmol/L, and FPG (cut-off) 6.0 mmol/L; for females, the BMI (cut-off) 32 kg/m^2, WC (cut-off) 95 cm, SBP (cut-off) 135 mmHg, DBP (cut-off) 90 mmHg, TG (cut-off) 1.5 mmol/L, HDL-C (cut-off) 0.9 mmol/L, and FPG (cut-off) 5.7 mmol/L.

We designed a model for assessing the 10-year risk of T2DM on the basis of the cut-offs and multivariate Cox regression analysis. To create a risk scale, a new variable was created—arterial hypertension (HT)$_1$ BP ≥ 150/90 mmHg for males and BP ≥ 135/90 mmHg for females. During the 10 years of follow-up, 463 (5%) new cases of T2DM were registered. The average age at first diagnosis of T2DM in the study population was 61.3 (6.7) years old.

Having studied the association between dichotomised risk factors and the 10-year risk of T2DM by multivariable-adjusted Cox regression analysis.

In males, the final version of the T2DM risk model includes significant risk factors dichotomised by the cut-off as T2DM predictors: FPG (cut-off) ≥6.0 mmol/L (HR = 3.79 (2.6; 5.6)), the BMI (cut-off) ≥27 kg/m^2 (HR = 3.03 (2.0; 4.7)), HDL-C (cut-off) ≤0.9 mmol/L (HR = 2.20 (1.2; 3.9)), TG (cut-off) ≥1.4 mmol/L (HR = 1.55 (1.0; 2.3)), and HT$_1$ ≥150/90 mmHg (HR = 1.57 (1.0; 2.4). The model for males is adjusted for FPG (cut-off), BMI (cut-off), HDL-C (cut-off), TG (cut-off), HT$_1$. For females, predictors were included that were different from those in the model for males: WC (cut-off) ≥95 cm (HR = 2.25 (1.6; 3.1)), FPG (cut-off) ≥5.7 mmol/L (HR = 2.58 (2.0; 3.3)), TG (cut-off) ≥1.5 mmol/L (HR = 1.81 (1.4; 2.3)), HT$_1$ ≥135/90 mmHg (HR = 1.64 (1.2; 2.2)), a family history of T2DM (HR = 1.50 (1.1; 2.0)), and the BMI (cut-off) ≥32 kg/m^2 (HR = 1.47 (1.1; 1.9)). The model for females is adjusted for WC (cut-off), FPG (cut-off), TG (cut-off), HT$_1$, age, family history of T2DM, BMI (cut-off).

Exp(B) measures served as weights to create the risk scale. Each predictor included in the regression model was scored by rounding out Exp(B) to a whole number (Table 4). The maximum total number of points on the created T2DM risk scale of the model is 13 for males and 12 for females.

Table 4. The 10-year risk scale for incident T2DM.

	T2DM Predictor	Interval Scale (Category)	Points
	Males		
1	Fasting plasma glucose level >6.0 mmol/L	No	0
		Yes	4
2	BMI ≥ 27 kg/m^2	No	0
		Yes	3
3	HDL-C level ≤ 0.9 mmol/L	No	0
		Yes	2
4	TG level ≥ 1.4 mmol/L	No	0
		Yes	2
5	BP level $\geq 150/90$ mmHg	No	0
		Yes	2
	Females		
1	WC ≥ 95 cm	No	0
		Yes	2
2	Fasting plasma glucose level ≥ 5.7 mmol/L	No	0
		Yes	3
3	TG level ≥ 1.5 mmol/L	No	0
		Yes	2
4	BP level $\geq 135/90$ mmHg	No	0
		Yes	2
5	family history of T2DM	No	0
		Yes	2
6	BMI ≥ 32 kg/m^2	No	0
		Yes	1

To determine the threshold of the total score associated with a high risk of T2DM, a receiver-operating characteristic (ROC) curve was constructed. The optimal cut-off for the sum of points that allowed to divide the analysed groups into two subgroups was 7 points (sensitivity (Se) 76.0%, specificity (Sp) 71.5%) for males and 6 points (Se 71.7%, Sp 69.2%) for females. When cross-checking the adequacy of the model in the population of Novosibirsk, we calculated the actual incidence of T2DM. Among the males who scored 7 or more points, T2DM developed in 10.2% of cases, and in the group of people who scored less than 7 points, only in 1.4% of cases; females who scored 6 or more points developed T2DM in 15.8% of cases, and among those who scored less than 6 points, incident cases of DM were detected only in 3.2% of cases.

Clinical testing of the newly developed model and of the Finnish model predicting the 10-year risk of T2DM on persons of retirement age in Novosibirsk revealed difficulties with independent filling out of the questionnaire [21]. Determination of the BMI, blood lipid levels, and in some cases, of own BP was difficult for the elderly. Accordingly, the next aim was to develop a simple T2DM risk calculator that would be convenient to use in primary health care and for self-completion for both sexes. Our model had to include only the parameters that can be easily assessed without laboratory tests or other measurements that require specialised medical skills. Predictors of the 10-year risk of T2DM selected for the best scale included history of hypertension 1.6 (HR = 1.6 (1.3; 1.8)), family history of T2DM (HR = 1.8 (1.1; 1.9)), WC (cut-off) (HR = 3.6 (1.9; 3.8)).

As a result of the analysis of various multivariate models, a scale with the best quality was selected (Table 5), where the area under the curve (AUC) was 0.71; this scale included such risk factors as WC, a history of arterial hypertension, and a family history of T2DM.

The relative risk scores obtained in the Cox regression analysis were chosen as variables to create a risk scale. Each of the three predictors included in the regression model was scored by rounding out to a whole number (Table 5). The highest total score on the created T2DM risk scale is 8 points. The cut-off of the scale was found to be 4 points—Se 74.7% and Sp 60.0%.

Table 5. The risk scale predicting the development of T2DM within 10 years (both females and males).

	T2DM Predictor	Interval Scale (Category)	Points
1	WC ≥ 95 cm	No	0
		Yes	4
2	Have you been told that you have high BP?	No	0
		Yes	2
3	Family history of T2DM	No	0
		Yes	2

Note: WC of 95 cm was obtained by receiver-operating characteristic (ROC) analysis for those surveyed who experienced the first onset of type 2 diabetes mellitus (T2DM) within 10 years of observation in Novosibirsk.

In the group that scored ≥4 points during 10 years, T2DM developed in 10.7% of cases, and in the group with <4 points, T2DM developed in 2.6% of cases.

4. Discussion

According to our analysis of the study population aged 45–69 years old, the prevalence of T2DM was 11.0% in both the male and female samples [22]. During 14 years of observation, new cases of T2DM occurred in 9% of the population more often among females than among males, 328 (9.7%) and 587 (15.5%), respectively ($p < 0.001$).

The results were subjected to Cox univariate proportional hazards regression analysis with adjustment for age. This analysis revealed significant risk factors for T2DM among males and females: BMI ≥ 25 kg/m^2, abdominal obesity, fasting hyperglycaemia, a high TG level, hypertension, a family history of DM, and a history of CVD. Among females, additional predictors were vocational- or primary-education level and leisure-time PA reported for the previous week (insufficient: 1–179 min per week or 1–29 min every day).

An increased BMI and WC indicate the presence of increased intra-abdominal visceral fat, which disrupts insulin metabolism through a release of serum-free fatty acids [23]. Nonetheless, according to a meta-analysis in 2018, not all obese individuals are at the same risk of T2DM; it seems that the risk is affected by their metabolic profile—the metabolically unhealthy obese have a ~10-fold higher risk of T2DM, whereas the metabolically healthy obese have a ~4.5-fold higher risk of T2DM, as compared to nonobese individuals. Moreover, in that study, weight gain during early adulthood was found to be more harmful than weight gain after the age of 25. On the contrary, peripheral fat accumulation has been linked to a better metabolic profile, which manifests itself in the observed protective effect of the greater hip circumference on T2DM [24].

Hypertension is known to be associated with the development of T2DM [25,26]. Persons with hypertension have an increased activity of the renin–angiotensin system, which causes systemic inflammatory processes leading to T2DM [27].

The presence of a family history of DM indicates a genetic contributor to DM but can also reflect the lifestyle or environmental conditions people were exposed to during their upbringing [28].

Impaired lipid metabolism with insulin resistance is characterised by an increase in TG levels, lower concentration of HDL-C, and an increase in free fatty acid levels. Diabetic dyslipidaemia also includes qualitative and kinetic lipid disorders, which are more atherogenic in nature, because cholesterol ester transfer protein (CETP) increases the production of small particles of low-density lipoproteins (LDL) [29]. Earlier studies in mice have shown dyslipidaemia to be a factor contributing to the apoptosis of pancreatic β-cells, to insulin biosynthesis, defective insulin secretion, and altered glucose metabolism. Fatty acid metabolism is known to be affected by ceramide formation, endoplasmic reticulum stress, oxidative stress, inflammation, the insulin signalling pathway, and protein kinase B, associated with damage to pancreatic β-cells. According to observational studies, there is a correlation between the level of TGs and the risk of T2DM [30,31].

High PA at leisure time reduces the relative risk of T2DM. Regular PA improves blood glucose control and can prevent or delay the onset of T2DM. [32,33]. Observational studies suggest that greater physical performance is associated with a reduced risk of T2DM [23], even if only as moderate-intensity exercises.

A 2018 meta-analysis revealed an association of lower educational attainment with a higher risk of T2DM [34]. The education level constitutes a component of socioeconomic status. Lower socioeconomic status correlates with higher stress levels, leading to a disruption of endocrine function through perturbations in the neuroendocrine system. Additionally, people with low socioeconomic status are more prone to an unhealthy lifestyle and have limited access to healthcare facilities [35].

In a multivariate regression analysis, we identified gender differences in the risk factors of T2DM. Among males, the best predictors were BMI, fasting hyperglycaemia, hypertension, and a family history of DM. Among females, the best predictors were BMI, fasting hyperglycaemia, hypertension, and fasting hyperglycaemia.

In 2016, Kautzky-Willer et al. analysed sex dimorphism in diabetes risk factors and found that T2DM is more often diagnosed at an earlier age in males, whereas the best predictors of T2DM are the BMI and WC in males and the BMI and WC in females. Limited mobility increases the risk of T2DM in females, and fasting hyperglycaemia in males [36]. The obtained data are explained by those authors as the influence of sex hormones on energy metabolism, body composition, vascular function, and inflammatory reactions. An endocrine imbalance denotes adverse cardiometabolic symptoms in females or males. Furthermore, genetic effects, epigenetic mechanisms, nutritional factors, and a sedentary lifestyle have different effects on the risk of T2DM and complications in both sexes [36].

According to the literature, the risk of DM increases with age [37], although in our models no such increase in risk was found. A possible explanation is that other factors such as WC or physical inactivity also increase with age [38], thus cancelling out the age-specific increase in DM risk.

According to a prospective study in Turkey with an average follow-up of 5.9 years, significant independent predictors of DM are abdominal obesity (risk ratio = 2.61 (95% CI 1.87–3.63)) and age in both sexes, hypertension (risk ratio = 1.81 (95% CI 1.10–2.98)), and low HDL-C in males only [39].

In the FINDRISK study, 38,689 participants aged 30–59 years old were analysed to estimate the prevalence of T2DM at the start and within 10 years. Among males, the frequency of diagnosed pharmacologically controlled T2DM increased over time. Compared to males surveyed in the 1970s, the incidence of diabetes was higher among males in the 1980s (adjusted HR = 1.44, 95% CI: 1.13–1.84) and in the 1990s (adjusted HR = 1.72, 95% CI: 1.32–2.24). The BMI explained some but not all of this variance. The increase occurred predominantly among males with a low education level (adjusted HR in the 1980s = 2.07, 95% CI: 1.28–3.35; adjusted HR in the 1990s = 2.12, 95% CI: 1.28–3.53) and an average education level (adjusted HR in the 1980s = 1.30, 95% CI: 0.85–1.99; adjusted HR in the 1990s = 1.65, 95% CI: 1.05–2.60). The female subgroup showed no dependence of DM incidence on education [40].

In a study conducted in Iran, after observation for an average of six years, 237 new cases of diabetes were identified, which corresponded to an age- and sex-adjusted cumulative incidence of 6.4% (95% CI: 5.6–7.2). In that study, in addition to the classic risk factors of DM, female sex and low levels of education significantly increased the risk of DM in the age-adjusted models. In the full model, independent predictors were age (odds ratio = 1.2 (95% CI: 1.1–1.3), family history of DM (1.8 (1.3–2.5)), BMI $\geq$ 30 kg/m^2 (2.3 (1.5–3.6)), abdominal obesity (1.9 (1.4–2.6)), high TG concentration (1.4 (1.1–1.9)), impaired fasting glucose (7.4 (3.6–15.0)), impaired glucose tolerance (5.9 (4.2–8.4)), and combined impaired fasting glucose and impaired glucose tolerance (42.2 (23.8–74.9)) [41].

In Australia, among 554 adults who completed the study with a six-year follow-up, 100 developed DM. Abdominal obesity increased the risk of DM for aboriginal people (risk ratio = 2.0 (95% CI: 1.1–3.6)) and for residents of the Torres Strait Islands (odds ratio = 6.3 (95% CI: 2.5–16.1)) as compared to subjects with normal weight. Metabolic syndrome was a strong predictor of DM (corrected risk ratio = 2.4 (CI 95% 1.6–3.7)). For both groups, the ratio of WC to hip circumference and the presence of metabolic syndrome predicted DM better than did WC or the BMI [42].

Risk models and calculators were first developed for cardiovascular diseases and are widely used in clinical practice and public health.

Diabetes risk scales in various countries have been actively designed since the 2000s. Most risk scales are based on the most sensitive and easily identifiable risk factors of T2DM such as age, sex, BMI, WC, T2DM in relatives, PA level, hypertension or regular use of antihypertensive drugs, and occasionally detectable hyperglycaemia. According to a 2011 review, 145 T2DM risk scales had been published, of which 94 risk models were consistent with qualitative studies—overall, 55 were inferences from risk models based on population studies and 39 were based on validation in new populations [10]. Millions of participants worldwide have already taken part in epidemiological studies assessing the risk of DM. A greater number of possible risk scales are now available to those wishing to use them clinically, but none of them is perfect, all have strengths and weaknesses.

The study has several limitations. One potential limitation is related to non-responders at baseline who might differ from responders by the distribution of DM2 risk factors or poor health; but, the response rate (61%) was a commonly accepted level for population studies and it is unlikely to influence the estimates of outcome risk. Against potential 'recall' bias in the survey, we applied standardised questionnaires/personnel/interview procedures, duplicated questions, and definitions of diseases by few sources (e.g., T2DM by interview of DM history and treatment, and fasting plasma glucose). We could not exclude the attrition bias at the follow-up stage due to those who dropped-out from the follow-up as non-responders for waves 2 or 3 or missed from the DM register, and those who died from competing causes. However, we used overlapping sources for diabetic endpoints in the cohort (DM register, CVD and mortality register, two repeated surveys, phone calls for non-responders) which minimised the chance for missing new cases of T2DM. The study was conducted in an urban Siberian population and has limited generalisability. However, it fits well for the risk of T2DM in the region and provides an excellent approach from the point of personalised medicine for region-specific preventive measures.

The validation of the FINDRISC questionnaire in Novosibirsk demonstrated the good quality of the model, which provides support for its use in Siberian populations. The cut-off risk score of 11 using the FINDRISC questionnaire to identify diabetes had a sensitivity and specificity (76.0% and 60.2%, respectively). The area under the receiver-operating curve for T2DM was 0.73 (0.73 in men and 0.70 in women) [43]. The T2DM risk model that includes three risk factors has several advantages over existing models. The cut-off of the scale was found to be 4 points—Se 74.7% and Sp 60.0%. Thus, the indicators of sensitivity and specificity of the cut-off values of the FINDRISK risk scale and the short Siberian risk scale are comparable and can be used in the medical practice.

5. Conclusions

Millions of people around the world have already participated in epidemiological studies aimed at assessing the risk of DM. A large number of risk scales are now available to those who seek to apply them clinically, but none of these instruments is ideal; each has strengths and shortcomings. In 2015, validation of the FINDRISC risk scale was conducted on a population sample in Novosibirsk [43]. During the validation, we obtained data suggestive of good quality of the model, which allows us to recommend its use in the Siberian population. Nevertheless, according to our data, not all risk factors included in the FINDRISC scale are widespread among patients with newly diagnosed T2DM, and the incidence of newly diagnosed DM in the very-high-risk group is lower than that predicted in Finland (22.6% versus 50%) [43]. Thus, the task of creating a risk scale for DM remains urgent, as does the issue of finding risk factors with a pronounced contribution to the development of T2DM in the Siberian population representing the appropriate approach from the point of personalised medicine. In addition, the revealed risk determinants might be validated on a wider sample for generalisability. In this study, for the first time in Russia, as part of a cohort study, an assessment of the risk factors of T2DM in males and females was carried out via multivariate risk models for the development of T2DM. This approach allowed us to identify significant risk factors and direct preventive measures for correcting these factors.

The T2DM risk model that includes three risk factors has several advantages over existing models. It is based on a questionnaire, which takes little time to complete and enables a person to independently determine their risk of T2DM and then visit a healthcare institution for examination, determination of carbohydrate metabolism disorders or T2DM, and preventive measures.

6. Patents

Patent No. 030585 (EAPO), issued on 31.08.2018. "A method for predicting the risk of developing type 2 diabetes".

Author Contributions: Conceptualization M.I.V., G.I.S., M.B. and S.K.M.; methodology H.P., M.B., S.V.M. and S.K.M.; validation L.V.S., E.G.V. and S.V.M.; formal analysis S.V.M., S.K.M., L.V.S. and O.D.R.; investigation S.K.M., Y.I.R., S.V.M. and O.V.S.; data curation S.K.M.; writing—original draft preparation S.V.M., O.D.R., S.K.M.; writing—review and editing H.P., M.B.,Y.I.R., M.I.V.; supervision S.K.M., M.B.; project administration M.B. and S.K.M.; funding acquisition S.K.M., M.B. All authors have read and agreed to the published version of the manuscript.

Funding: This research was funded by the Russian Science Foundation (grant No. 20-15-00371) and the Russian Academy of Science (state assignment No. AAAA-A17-117112850280-2); the HAPIEE study was funded by the Welcome Trust (WT064947, WT081081) and the US National Institute of Aging (1RO1AG23522).

Institutional Review Board Statement: The study was conducted according to the guidelines of the Declaration of Helsinki and approved by the Ethics Committee of Research Institute of Internal and Preventive Medicine–Branch of the Institute of Cytology and Genetics, Siberian Branch of Russian Academy of Sciences (protocol № 1 from 14.mar.2002).

Informed Consent Statement: Informed consent was obtained from all subjects involved in the study.

Data Availability Statement: The data presented in this study are available in tabulated form on request. The data are not publicly available due to ethical restrictions and project regulations.

Acknowledgments: The authors acknowledge A. Peasey, M. Holmes, D. Stefler, and J. Hubacek for valuable advice on manuscript planning and discussion.

Conflicts of Interest: The authors declare no conflict of interest. The funders had no role in the design of the study; in the collection, analyses, or interpretation of the data; in the writing of the manuscript; or in the decision to publish the results.

References

1. Kaiser, A.B.; Zhang, N.; Pluijm, V.W. Global Prevalence of Type 2 Diabetes over the Next Ten Years (2018–2028). *Diabetes* **2018**, *67* (Suppl. S1). [CrossRef]
2. IDF Diabetes Atlas, 9th ed. 2019, p. 176. Available online: https://www.diabetesatlas.org/upload/resources/material/20200302_133351_IDFATLAS9e-final-web.pdf (accessed on 9 December 2020).
3. Dedov, I.I.; Shestakova, M.V.; Mayorova, A.Y. Algorithms for specialized medical care for patients with diabetes mellitus, 8th edition. *Diabetes Mellit.* **2019**, *20*, 1–112. [CrossRef]
4. Dedov, I.I.; Shestakova, M.V.; Galstyan, G.R. The prevalence of type 2 diabetes mellitus in the adult population of Russia (NATION study). *Diabetes Mellit.* **2016**, *19*, 113–118. [CrossRef]
5. Mustafina, S.V.; Rymar, O.D.; Malyutina, S.K.; Denisova, D.V.; Shcherbakova, L.V.; Voevoda, M.I. Prevalence of diabetes in the adult population of Novosibirsk. *Diabetes Mellit.* **2017**, *20*, 329–334. [CrossRef]
6. Herder, C.; Peltonen, M.; Koenig, W.; Kräft, I.; Müller-Scholze, S.; Martin, S.; Lakka, T.; Ilanne-Parikka, P.; Eriksson, J.G.; Hämäläinen, H.; et al. Systemic immune mediators and lifestyle changes in the prevention of type 2 diabetes: Results from the Finnish Diabetes Prevention Study. *Diabetes* **2006**, *55*, 2340–2346. [CrossRef]

7. Kuntsevich, A.K.; Mustafina, S.V.; Malyutina, S.K.; Verevkin, E.G.; Rymar, O.D. Population-based nutrition study on an urban population with type 2 diabetes mellitus. *Diabetes Mellit.* **2015**, *4*, 33–39. Available online: https://www.dia-endojournals.ru/jour/article/view/7174/5557# (accessed on 10 February 2021). [CrossRef]
8. Lindstrom, J.; Tuomilehto, J. The Diabetes Risk Score: A practical tool to predict type 2 diabetes risk. *Diabetes Care* **2003**, *26*, 725–731. [CrossRef]
9. Saaristo, T.; Peltonen, M.; Lindstrom, J.; Saarikoski, L.; Sundvall, J.; Eriksson, J.G.; Tuomilehto, J. Cross-sectional evaluation of the Finnish Diabetes Risk Score: A tool to identify undetected type 2 diabetes, abnormal glucose tolerance and metabolic syndrome. *Diabetes Vasc. Dis. Res.* **2005**, *2*, 67. [CrossRef]
10. Noble, D.; Mathur, R.; Dent, T.; Meads, C.; Greenhalgh, T. Risk models and scores for type 2 diabetes: Systematic review. *BMJ* **2011**, *343*. [CrossRef]
11. Mustafina, S.V.; Simonova, G.I.; Rymar, O.D. Comparative characteristics of diabetes risk scores. *Diabetes Mellit.* **2014**, *17*, 17–22. [CrossRef]
12. Bergmann, A.; Li, J.; Wang, L.; Schulze, J.; Bornstein, S.R.; Schwarz, P.E.H. A simplified Finnish diabetes risk score to predict type 2 diabetes risk and disease evolution in a German population. *Horm. Metab. Res.* **2007**, *39*, 677–682. [CrossRef] [PubMed]
13. Zhang, L.; Zhang, Z.; Zhang, Y.; Hu, G.; Chen, L. Evaluation of Finnish Diabetes Risk Score in screening undiagnosed diabetes and prediabetes among U.S. adults by gender and race: NHANES 1999–2010. *PLoS ONE* **2014**, *9*, e97865. [CrossRef] [PubMed]
14. Schmid, R.; Vollenweider, P.; Bastardot, F.; Waeber, G.; Marques-Vidal, P. Validation of 7 type 2 diabetes mellitus risk scores in a population-based cohort: CoLaus study. *Arch. Intern. Med.* **2012**, *172*, 188–189. [CrossRef]
15. Robinson, C.A.; Agarwal, G.; Nerenberg, K. Validating the CANRISK prognostic model for assessing diabetes risk in Canada's multi-ethnic population. *Chronic Dis. Inj. Can.* **2011**, *32*, 19–31. Available online: https://pubmed.ncbi.nlm.nih.gov/22153173/ (accessed on 9 December 2020).
16. Al-Lawati, J.A.; Tuomilehto, J. Diabetes risk score in Oman: A tool to identify prevalent type 2 diabetes among Arabs of the Middle East. *Diabetes Res. Clin. Pract.* **2007**, *77*, 438–444. [CrossRef]
17. Peasey, A.; Bobak, M.; Kubinova, R.; Malyutina, S.; Pajak, A.; Tamosiunas, A.; Pikhart, H.; Nicholson, A.; Marmot, M. Determinants of cardiovascular disease and other non-communicable diseases in Central and Eastern Europe: Rationale and design of the HAPIEE study. *BMC Public Health* **2006**, *6*, 255. [CrossRef]
18. *Obesity: Preventing and Managing the Global Epidemic—Report of a WHO Consultation*; WHO Technical Report series 894; World Health Organization: Geneva, Switzerland, 2000; p. 252. Available online: https://www.who.int/nutrition/publications/obesity/WHO_TRS_894/en/ (accessed on 5 December 2020).
19. Members, F.; Ryden LCo-Chairperson Standl, E. Guidelines on diabetes, pre-diabetes, and cardiovascular diseases: Executive summary. *Eur. Heart J.* **2007**, *28*, 88–136. [CrossRef]
20. *World Health Organization: Definition and Diagnosis of Diabetes Mellitus and Intermediate Hyperglycemia: Report of a WHO/IDF Consultation*; World Health Organization: Geneva, Switzerland, 2006; p. 50. Available online: https://www.who.int/diabetes/publications/diagnosis_diabetes2006/en/ (accessed on 8 December 2020).
21. Mustafina, S.V.; Rymar, O.D.; Dolinskaya, Y.A.; Astrakova, K.S.; Voevoda, S.M.; Esipenko, O.V. Evaluation of the 10-year risk of developing type 2 diabetes in elderly people using the Finnish risk scale (FINDRISK), VII All-Russian Diabetes Congress. In Proceedings of the Diabetes Mellitus in the 21st Century-Time for Uniting Efforts, Moscow, Russia, 25–27 May 2015; p. 244.
22. Kahn, B.B.; Flier, J.S. Obesity and insulin resistance. *J. Clin. Investig.* **2000**, *106*, 473–481. [CrossRef]
23. Bellou, V.; Belbasis, L.; Tzoulaki, I.; Evangelou, E. Risk factors for type 2 diabetes mellitus: An exposure-wide umbrella review of meta-analyses. *PLoS ONE* **2018**, *13*, e0194127. [CrossRef] [PubMed]
24. Izzo, R.; Simone, G.; Chinali, M.; Iaccarino, G.; Trimarco, V.; Rozza, F.; Giudice, R.; Trimarco, B.; Luca, N. Insufficient control of blood pressure and incident diabetes. *Diabetes Care* **2009**, *32*, 845–850. [CrossRef] [PubMed]
25. Kim, M.J.; Lim, N.K.; Choi, S.J.; Park, H.Y. Hypertension is an independent risk factor for type 2 diabetes: The Korean genome and epidemiology study. *Hypertens. Res.* **2015**, *38*, 783–789. [CrossRef]
26. Emdin, C.A.; Anderson, S.G.; Woodward, M.; Rahimi, K. Usual Blood Pressure and Risk of New-Onset Diabetes: Evidence From 4.1 Million Adults and a Meta-Analysis of Prospective Studies. *J. Am. Coll. Cardiol.* **2015**, *66*, 1552–1562. [CrossRef]
27. Kolb, H.; Martin, S. Environmental/lifestyle factors in the pathogenesis and prevention of type 2 diabetes. *BMC Med.* **2017**, *15*, 131. [CrossRef] [PubMed]
28. Verges, B. Pathophysiology of diabetic dyslipidemia: Where are we? *Diabetologia* **2015**, *58*, 886–899. [CrossRef]
29. Beshara, A.; Cohen, E.; Goldberg, E.; TShochat MGarty Krause, I. Hypertriglyceridemia a risk factor for diabetes: A large cohort study. *Eur. J. Intern. Med.* **2013**, *24*, e94. [CrossRef]
30. Kwon, Y.H.; Kim, S.K.; Cho, J.H.; Kwon, H.; Park, S.E.; Oh, H.G.; Park, C.Y.; Lee, W.Y.; Oh, K.W.; Park, S.W.; et al. The Association Between Persistent Hypertriglyceridemia and the Risk of Diabetes Development: The Kangbuk Samsung Health Study. *Endocrinol. Metab.* **2018**, *33*, 55–61. [CrossRef] [PubMed]
31. Li, G.; Zhang, P.; Wang, J.; Gregg, E.W.; Yang, W.; Gong, Q.; Li, H.; Jiang, Y.; An, Y.; Shuai, Y.; et al. The long-term effect of lifestyle interventions to prevent diabetes in the China Da Qing Diabetes Prevention Study: A 20-year follow-up study. *Lancet* **2008**, *371*, 1783–1789. [CrossRef]
32. Wang, Y.; Simar, D.; Fiatarone, M.A. Singh Adaptations to exercise training within skeletal muscle in adults with type 2 diabetes or impaired glucose tolerance: A systematic review. *Diabetes Metab. Res. Rev.* **2009**, *25*, 13–40. [CrossRef]

33. Sui, X.; Hooker, S.P.; Lee, I.M.; Church, T.S.; Colabianchi, N.; Lee, C.D.; Blair, S.N. A prospective study of cardiorespiratory fitness and risk of type 2 diabetes in women. *Diabetes Care* **2008**, *31*, 550–555. [CrossRef]
34. Agardh, E.; Allebeck, P.; Hallqvist, J.; Moradi, T.; Sidorchuk, A. Type 2 diabetes incidence and socio-economic position: A systematic review and meta-analysis. *Int. J. Epidemiol.* **2011**, *40*, 804–818. [CrossRef]
35. Kautzky-Willer, A.; Harreiter, J.; Pacini, G. Sex and Gender Differences in Risk, Pathophysiology and Complications of Type 2 Diabetes Mellitus. *Endocr. Rev.* **2016**, *37*, 278–316. [CrossRef]
36. Wild, S.; Roglic, G.; Green, A.; Sicree, R.; King, H. Global prevalence of diabetes: Estimates for the year 2000 and projections for 2030. *Diabetes Care* **2004**, *27*, 1047–1053. [CrossRef]
37. Stevens, J.; Katz, E.G.; Huxley, R.R. Associations between gender, age and waist circumference. *Eur. J. Clin. Nutr.* **2010**, *64*, 6–15. [CrossRef]
38. Ford, E.S.; Mokdad, A.H.; Giles, W.H. Trends in waist circumference among U.S. adults. *Obes. Res.* **2003**, *11*, 1223–1231. [CrossRef]
39. Onat, A.; Hergenç, G.; Uyarel, H.; Can, G.; Özhan, H. Prevalence, incidence, predictors and outcome of type 2 diabetes in Turkey. *Anadolu Kardiyol. Derg.* **2006**, *6*, 314–321. Available online: https://www.anatoljcardiol.com/jvi.aspx?un=AJC-13549, (accessed on 9 December 2020). [PubMed]
40. Abouzeid, M.; Wikström, K.; Peltonen, M.; Lindström, J.; Borodulin, K.; Rahkonen, O.; Laatikainen, T. Secular trends and educational differences in the incidence of type 2 diabetes in Finland, 1972–2007. *Eur. J. Epidemiol.* **2015**, *30*, 649–659. [CrossRef] [PubMed]
41. Harati, H.; Hadaegh, F.; Saadat, N.; Azizi, F. Population-based incidence of Type 2 diabetes and its associated risk factors: Results from a six-year cohort study in Iran. *BMC Public Health* **2009**, *9*, 186. [CrossRef] [PubMed]
42. McDermott, R.A.; Li, M.; Campbell, S.K. Incidence of type 2 diabetes in two Indigenous Australian populations: A 6-year follow-up study. *Med. J. Aust.* **2010**, *192*, 562–565. [CrossRef] [PubMed]
43. Mustafina, S.V.; Rymar, O.D.; Sazonova, O.V.; Shcherbakova, L.V.; Voevoda, M.I. Validation of the Finnish diabetes risk score (FINDRISC) for the Caucasian population of Siberia. *Diabetes Mellit.* **2016**, *19*, 113–118. [CrossRef]

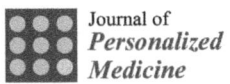

Article

Hypothalamic Norepinephrine Concentration and Heart Mass in Hypertensive ISIAH Rats Are Associated with a Genetic Locus on Chromosome 18

Olga E. Redina [1,*], Svetlana E. Smolenskaya [1], Yulia K. Polityko [1,2], Nikita I. Ershov [1], Michael A. Gilinsky [2] and Arcady L. Markel [1,3]

[1] Federal Research Center Institute of Cytology and Genetics, Siberian Branch of the Russian Academy of Sciences, 10 Lavrentieva ave., 630090 Novosibirsk, Russia; svsmol@ngs.ru (S.E.S.); polityko.yulia@gmail.com (Y.K.P.); nikotinmail@mail.ru (N.I.E.); markel@bionet.nsc.ru (A.L.M.)

[2] Scientific Research Institute of Physiology and Basic Medicine, 4 Timakova Street, 630117 Novosibirsk, Russia; m.a.gilinsky@physiol.ru

[3] Department of Natural Sciences, Novosibirsk State University, 2 Pirogova Street, 630090 Novosibirsk, Russia

* Correspondence: oredina@bionet.nsc.ru or oredina@ngs.ru

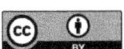

Citation: Redina, O.E.; Smolenskaya, S.E.; Polityko, Y.K.; Ershov, N.I.; Gilinsky, M.A.; Markel, A.L. Hypothalamic Norepinephrine Concentration and Heart Mass in Hypertensive ISIAH Rats Are Associated with a Genetic Locus on Chromosome 18. *J. Pers. Med.* **2021**, *11*, 67. https://doi.org/10.3390/jpm11020067

Academic Editor: Mikhail Ivanovich Voevoda

Received: 1 December 2020
Accepted: 21 January 2021
Published: 23 January 2021

Publisher's Note: MDPI stays neutral with regard to jurisdictional claims in published maps and institutional affiliations.

Copyright: © 2021 by the authors. Licensee MDPI, Basel, Switzerland. This article is an open access article distributed under the terms and conditions of the Creative Commons Attribution (CC BY) license (https://creativecommons.org/licenses/by/4.0/).

Abstract: The relationship between activation of the sympathetic nervous system and cardiac hypertrophy has long been known. However, the molecular genetic basis of this association is poorly understood. Given the known role of hypothalamic norepinephrine in the activation of the sympathetic nervous system, the aim of the work was to carry out genetic mapping using Quantitative Trait Loci (QTL) analysis and determine the loci associated both with an increase in the concentration of norepinephrine in the hypothalamus and with an increase in heart mass in Inherited Stress-Induced Arterial Hypertension (ISIAH) rats simulating the stress-sensitive form of arterial hypertension. The work describes a genetic locus on chromosome 18, in which there are genes that control the development of cardiac hypertrophy associated with an increase in the concentration of norepinephrine in the hypothalamus, i.e., genes involved in enhanced sympathetic myocardial stimulation. No association of this locus with the blood pressure was found. Taking into consideration previously obtained results, it was concluded that the contribution to the development of heart hypertrophy in the ISIAH rats is controlled by different genetic loci, one of which is associated with the concentration of norepinephrine in the hypothalamus (on chromosome 18) and the other is associated with high blood pressure (on chromosome 1). Nucleotide substitutions that may be involved in the formation or absence of association with blood pressure in different rat strains are discussed.

Keywords: norepinephrine concentration in the hypothalamus; heart mass; QTL analysis; SNPs; ISIAH hypertensive rat strain

1. Introduction

Hypertension is known to contribute to the development of such often fatal complications as cerebral stroke and myocardial infarction. Myocardial hypertrophy associated with hypertension, although not so pronounced in its initial clinical manifestations, ultimately leads to the development of cardiosclerosis, dangerous arrhythmias and heart failure. The development of myocardial hypertrophy in arterial hypertension is produced mainly by an increased afterload on the left ventricle. However, a lot of information has accumulated suggesting that the cause of myocardial hypertrophy in hypertension is far from unambiguous.

The dissociation between the blood pressure (BP) level and myocardial mass increase has been described both in patients with hypertension and in experimental hypertensive animals [1]. Thus, it was shown that the mass of the left ventricle in spontaneously hypertensive rats (SHR) is increased, not only in adult rats in which the blood pressure level is high, but also in young rat pups without obvious signs of arterial hypertension, which indicated the genetic origin of cardiac hypertrophy. Antihypertensive therapy in adult SHR rats led to a decrease in blood pressure. At the same time, there was some involution of myocardial mass, but only if the antagonist of the sympathetic system, alpha-methyldopamine, was used as a hypotensive drug. The use of another antihypertensive drug (hydralazine) led to an even greater decrease in blood pressure, but there was no involution of myocardial hypertrophy. The authors concluded that SHR rat myocardial hypertrophy is caused not only by an increase in blood pressure, but also by hormonal stimulation by the sympathetic adrenal and renin–angiotensin systems [2]. Another type of hypertension with myocardial hypertrophy was developed in rats receiving a high fructose diet (a condition similar to the metabolic syndrome of humans). It turned out that in this case the mechanism of cardiac hypertrophy is caused not so much by the degree of increase in blood pressure, but by an increase in the function of the sympathetic adrenal system [3]. When studying the role of adrenergic stimulation on the growth of cardiomyocytes in cell culture, it was shown that stimulation of α1-adrenergic receptors induces the growth and hypertrophy of neonatal cardiomyocytes and enhances the expression of contractile protein genes. Moreover, this effect did not depend on the mechanical activity of cells [4]. All this indicates the presence of additional factors, along with enhanced blood pressure, responsible for the development of myocardial hypertrophy in arterial hypertension, and these additional factors are directed to stimulation of the sympathetic adrenal and other neuroendocrine systems.

Recently, more and more attention has been paid to the role of the central nervous system and its sympathetic part as a kind of trigger in the pathogenesis of hypertension [5]. Using modern methods of visualizing the functioning of the brain (Fmri—functional magnetic resonance imaging) and constructing a neuroconnectome it has been shown that nerve connections between a number of brain structures, including the hypothalamus and the brainstem regions, are involved in maintaining the sympathetic tone and the regulation of blood pressure [6]. Hypothalamus, receiving extensive efferent information and having wide effector connections, is considered as the central integrating link of the nervous system. It functions as a regulatory center in maintaining the body's homeostasis, controlling endocrine, autonomic and somatic reactions. It is the hypothalamus that plays the role of coordinator of the neuroendocrine and sympathoadrenal systems' functions [7].

One of the most important hypothalamic neurotransmitters is norepinephrine. The paraventricular nucleus of the hypothalamus is thought to be the primary recipient of stress-related information, in particular, from the norepinephrine-releasing Locus Ceruleus (LC). The hypothalamus–LC axis controls input and output information from and to the peripheral autonomic nervous system, from and to the hypothalamic–adrenocortical and adrenomedullary systems with numerous brain-to-gland positive and negative (feedback) loops [8]. The neurons of the paraventricular nuclei, in which the central stimulator of the pituitary–adrenal system (stress system)—corticotropin releasing hormone (CRH) is synthesized, also receives noradrenergic stimulation [9,10]. Postganglionic sympathetic neurons innervate the myocardium, and myocardial hypertrophy associated with increased sympathetic tone is realized through stimulation of both myocardial alpha and beta adrenoreceptors [11].

The concentration of norepinephrine in the hypothalamus is an important factor in the regulation of the activity of the sympathetic nervous system and blood pressure [12,13]. The relationship between activation of the sympathetic nervous system and cardiac hypertrophy is shown in experimental rat models. Adult rats with spontaneously developing hypertension (SHR) are characterized by heart hypertrophy [14] and an increased content of norepinephrine in the hypothalamus [15,16]. Sympathetic hyperactivity in rats with heart failure is associated with an increase in norepinephrine in the paraventricular nucleus of the hypothalamus at rest, and in acute sympathetic activation under conditions of restraint stress in rats with heart failure, an impairment of the central noradrenergic system's response was observed [17].

Based on the available information, in Inherited Stress-Induced Arterial Hypertension (ISIAH) rats simulating the stress-sensitive form of arterial hypertension, one can also suggest a connection between sympathetic activation and pathological changes in the myocardium. In the medulla of the adrenal glands of the ISIAH rats, an increased amount of chromogranin A was shown [18], which is an indicator of the catecholamines synthesis activation [19]. In addition, an increased concentration of epinephrine in the adrenal glands has been shown [20], which indicates an enhanced function of the sympathoadrenal system in ISIAH rats. ISIAH rats are also characterized by increased reactivity of the sympathoadrenal and hypothalamic–pituitary–adrenal systems [20], as well as morphological changes in the peripheral target organs, including the heart. In early postnatal ontogenesis in ISIAH rats, specific morphometric changes were described, such as an increase in the thickness of the walls of the ventricles and interventricular septum, indicating the formation of structural remodeling of the ventricular myocardium [21], and in adult rats there is an increase in the absolute and relative mass of the heart and signs of left ventricular hypertrophy compared with normotensive control rats [22].

It is known that an increase in the activity of the sympathetic nervous system is associated with the development of pathophysiological processes in the cardiovascular system and the development of hypertension [23]. Taking into account that ISIAH rats have characteristic signs of increased sympathetic tone at rest and its increased reactivity under stress, including a sharp increase in norepinephrine and adrenaline in blood plasma, we can assume that cardiac hypertrophy in ISIAH rats is, at least in part, the result of sympathetic tension. This is also indicated by the high expression of mRNA of the *Adrb1* (beta 1-adrenergic receptor) gene in the myocardium of intact ISIAH rats [24]. The involvement of sympathetic activation both in the functioning of the heart and in the development of hypertension in ISIAH rats is also supported by the fact that intravenous administration of antisense oligonucleotides directed to mRNA of beta 1-adrenergic receptors resulted in a long-term decrease in the blood pressure in ISIAH rats [24].

One of the approaches to studying the genetic control of physiological and pathophysiological traits is Quantitative Trait Loci (QTL) analysis, which allows the determination of the genetic loci associated with phenotypic traits. QTL analysis is also an effective approach for determining common loci for several traits, where genes with pleiotropic effects on the traits under study can be located. Previously, using QTL analysis, we described the genetic loci associated with the level of blood pressure and the mass of the adrenal glands, kidneys, and heart [25,26], as well as the loci associated with the plasma corticosterone concentration in hypertensive ISIAH rats [27]. All the studied traits were associated with several loci suggesting polygenic control of the manifestation of the listed characters of ISIAH rats. In addition, it was previously shown using the linear regression method (ANOVA) that the trait "concentration of norepinephrine in the hypothalamus" can be associated with several genetic loci in ISIAH rats [28]. In addition, previously, using data from transcriptome (RNA-Seq) analysis of several organs/tissues of ISIAH and control (Wistar Albino Glaxo (WAG) rats, as well as the available sequencing data for the genomes of 42 other rat strains and substrains, ISIAH rat-specific single nucleotide polymorphisms (SNPs) have been described, and significant genetic distances between the genotype of ISIAH rats and the genotypes of all other rat strains and substrains were shown [29].

The aim of this work was to conduct a genome-wide analysis of the trait designated as "concentration of norepinephrine in the hypothalamus" using QTL analysis and to describe the complete list of genetic loci associated with this trait. In addition, the goal of this work was to identify the loci associated with both the concentration of norepinephrine in the hypothalamus and the increased myocardial mass in ISIAH rats, which may contain genes that lead to cardiac hypertrophy associated with increased sympathetic stimulation. In the QTL of interest, nucleotide substitutions specific to the ISIAH rat strain, which may possibly contribute to the phenotypes under consideration, were identified and discussed.

2. Results

2.1. Determination of Loci Associated with the Concentration of Norepinephrine in the Hypothalamus

Determination of loci associated with the concentration of norepinephrine in the hypothalamus was carried out using hypertensive ISIAH and normotensive control WAG rats. The concentration of norepinephrine in the hypothalamus of ISIAH rats is significantly higher than that of WAG rats (Table 1).

Table 1. Comparative characteristics of Inherited Stress-Induced Arterial Hypertension (ISIAH) and Wistar Albino Glaxo (WAG) rats aged 6 months.

Trait	ISIAH M ± SEM ($n = 10$)	WAG M ± SEM ($n = 14$)
Concentration of norepinephrine in the hypothalamus, ng/mg of tissue	1.698 ± 0.068 **	1.045 ± 0.068

** $p < 0.01$ in ISIAH as compared with WAG (Student's t-test). M—mean, SEM—standard error of mean.

A QTL analysis of this trait was performed using F_2(ISIAH × WAG) male rats at the age of 6 months. The trait "concentration of norepinephrine in the hypothalamus" was analyzed for the first time. Figure 1 shows the LOD (**logarithm of odds**) plots for chromosomes.

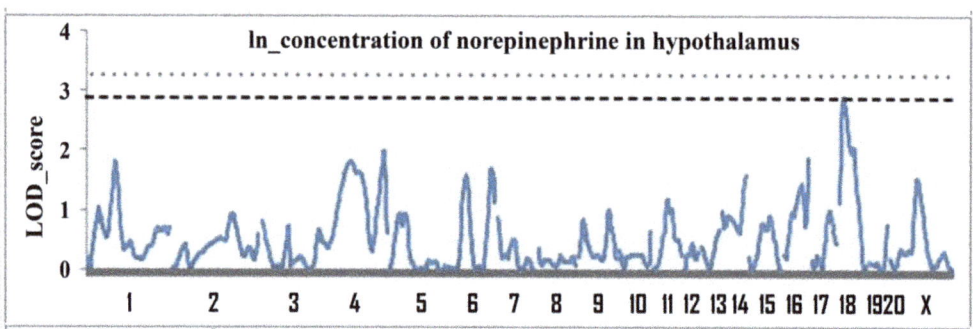

Figure 1. Genome-wide LOD (**logarithm of odds**) plots for concentration of norepinephrine in the hypothalamus in male rats F_2(ISIAH × WAG) aged 6 months. The X axis shows the chromosome numbers. Lines show the level of experimentwise threshold: the dashed line corresponds to $p = 0.05$, the dotted line corresponds to $p = 0.025$.

The genome scan revealed one significant and several suggestive loci associated with concentration of norepinephrine in the hypothalamus, indicating the polygenic control of the trait. The description of these QTL is given in Table 2.

The effects of alleles on the trait are shown in Table 3. In rats with two ISIAH alleles at the loci on chromosomes 18, 6 (in the region of the D6Rat143 marker) and X, the value of the trait "concentration of norepinephrine in the hypothalamus" was significantly increased in comparison with animals with both alleles of normotensive WAG rats in these QTL. At the loci, on chromosomes 4 and 16, the opposite effect was observed—a decrease in the value of the trait in the presence of two alleles of ISIAH rats. At two loci, a significant change in the concentration of norepinephrine in the hypothalamus was associated with a heterozygous genotype. At the locus on chromosome 6 (in the region of the marker D6Rat75), the value of the trait in animals with a heterozygous genotype decreased, and at the locus on chromosome 14 the value of the trait increased in heterozygotes. Accordingly, the obtained results show that the effects of alleles of hypertensive ISIAH rats at different loci have a specific modulating effect on the trait.

Table 2. Quantitative Trait Loci (QTL) associated with concentration of norepinephrine in the hypothalamus in male rats F₂(ISIAHxWAG) aged 6 months.

Chr.	Peak Marker (Mb)	Confidence Interval *, Mb	LOD Score	p	Variability, %
		Significant QTL			
18	D18Rat106 (13.2)	0–50	2.91	0.05	10.8
		Suggestive QTL			
1	D1Rat30 (107.1)	90–128	1.82	0.05	6.6
4	D4Rat27 (137.8)	84–186	1.80	0.05	8.0
4	D4Rat68 (233.3)	214–242	1.99	0.025	7.2
6	D6Rat143 (48.1)	40–72	1.60	0.05	10.7
6	D6Rat75 (136.6)	120–156.9	1.71	0.05	7.8
14	D14Rat18 (86.0)	68–115.1	1.58	0.025	6.3
16	D16Rat48 (79.7)	72–90	1.87	0.025	7.3
X	DXRat26 (45.1)	28–70	1.54	0.05	6.1

* Boundaries of a locus are defined in the respective one LOD interval; Mb—megabases.

Table 3. Allele effects in QTL associated with concentration of norepinephrine in the hypothalamus in male rats F₂(ISIAHxWAG) aged 6 months.

Trait Measurement in F₂ Hybrids (ISIAH × WAG) n	Chr.	Peak Marker (Mb)	Genotype			D [#]
			I/I M ± SEM n	I/W M ± SEM n	W/W M ± SEM n	
			Significant QTL			
	18	D18Rat106 (13.2)	2.21 ± 0.15 ** 29	1.97 ± 0.10 56	1.65 ± 0.11 38	0.1
			Suggestive QTL			
	1	D1Rat30 (107.1)	1.63 ± 0.12 [††] 27	2.05 ± 0.08 71	1.94 ± 0.18 24	−1.7
1.93 ± 0.07 123	4	D4Rat27 (137.8)	1.80 ± 0.11 * 31	1.79 ± 0.08 56	2.27 ± 0.16 [††] 36	1.0
	4	D4Rat68 (233.3)	1.87 ± 0.13 * 25	1.80 ± 0.07 74	2.39 ± 0.21 [††] 24	1.3
	6	D6Rat143 (48.1)	1.96 ± 0.11 * 50	2.01 ± 0.10 58	1.54 ± 0.13 [††] 15	1.2
	6	D6Rat75 (136.6)	2.11 ± 0.14 [†] 31	1.75 ± 0.08 59	2.09 ± 0.14 [†] 33	−35.0
	14	D14Rat18 (86.0)	1.72 ± 0.08 [††] 30	2.14 ± 0.12 58	1.76 ± 0.09 [†] 35	−20.0

Table 3. Cont.

Trait Measurement in F$_2$ Hybrids (ISIAH × WAG) n	Chr.	Peak Marker (Mb)	Genotype			D #
			I/I M ± SEM n	I/W M ± SEM n	W/W M ± SEM n	
	16	D16Rat48 (79.7)	1.61 ± 0.09 **†† 31	2.03 ± 0.10 60	2.06 ± 0.13 32	−0.9
	X	DXRat26 (45.1)	2.17 ± 0.13 ** 52		1.75 ± 0.06 71	

I/I—a homozygote for the ISIAH allele; W/W—a homozygote for the WAG allele; I/W—a heterozygote; Mb—megabases; * $p < 0.05$, ** $p < 0.01$—compared with W/W; † $p < 0.05$, †† $p < 0.01$—compared with H/W; #—degree of dominance.

2.2. Determination of Loci Associated with both the Concentration of Norepinephrine in the Hypothalamus and Heart Mass

Using the QTL Cartographer program, which allows one to determine the covariance of two or more characters, the character covariance of the norepinephrine concentration in the hypothalamus with heart mass was found at the locus on chromosome 18 in the region of marker D18Mgh1 (Figure 2). The description of the locus associated with the mass of the heart on chromosome 18 is given in Table 4.

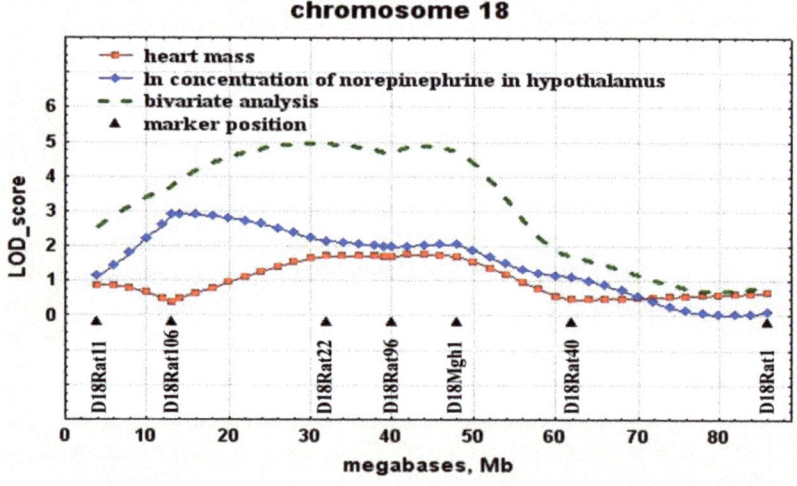

Figure 2. The covariance of two traits (in the hypothalamus and heart mass) at the locus on chromosome 18.

Table 4. QTL on chromosome 18 associated with heart mass in male rats F$_2$(ISIAHxWAG) aged 6 months.

Chr.	Peak Marker (Mb)	Confidence Interval *, Mb	LOD Score	p Chromosome-Wise	Variability, %
			Heart Mass		
18	D18Mgh1 (47.7)	18–60	1.76	0.025	6.5

* Boundaries of a locus are defined in the respective one LOD interval; Mb—megabases.

The presence of ISIAH alleles in QTL on chromosome 18 (in the region of marker D18Mgh1) is associated with an increase in both the concentration of norepinephrine in the hypothalamus and heart mass (Figure 3).

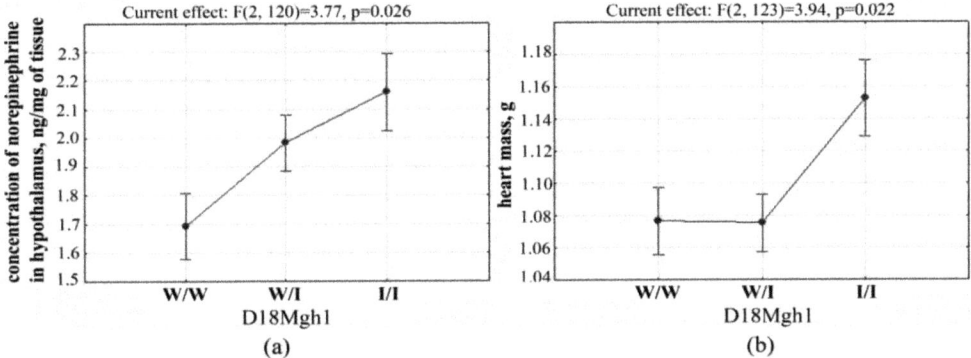

Figure 3. Allele effects on trait values in the QTL on chromosome 18 in the region of marker D18Mgh1: (**a**) concentration of norepinephrine in the hypothalamus; (**b**) heart mass; I/I—a homozygote for the ISIAH allele; W/W—a homozygote for the WAG allele; I/W—a heterozygote.

2.3. Nucleotide Substitutions (SNPs) Detected in ISIAH but not in WAG Rats

In the QTL associated with the concentration of norepinephrine in the hypothalamus and heart mass, 240 SNPs (Supplementary Table) were identified in the transcribed regions belonging to the sequences of 82 genes. None of the substitutions found at the locus were characterized as having a high impact effect, but most of them can have a modifying effect (Table 5).

Table 5. Classification of nucleotide substitutions (SNPs) effects.

SnpEff Classification	Number of SNPs	Effect
3_prime_UTR_variant	55	modifier
5_prime_UTR_premature_start_codon_gain_variant	3	low
5_prime_UTR_variant	3	modifier
downstream_gene_variant	67	modifier
intergenic_region	10	modifier
intron_variant	25	modifier
missense_variant	13	moderate
synonymous_variant	58	low
upstream_gene_variant	6	modifier

Nonsynonymous substitutions were analyzed using the Sorting Intolerant From Tolerant (SIFT) algorithm (Table 6). In two genes, *Slc4a9* (solute carrier family 4, member 9) and *Tcof1* (treacle ribosome biogenesis factor 1), nonsynonymous substitutions were characterized in the SIFT program as Deleterious, i.e., these substitutions are likely to have an effect on the structure and/or function of the proteins encoded by these genes. Comparison with the sequencing data of the genomes of 42 rat strains and substrains showed that a nonsynonymous substitution in the mRNA sequence of the *Slc4a9* gene (c.269C>T; p.Ala90Val) occurs only in ISIAH rats (Table 6). Several substitutions were found in the *Tcof1* gene (Table 6 and Supplementary Table) and the substitution c.1556C>A, leading to the replacement of the amino acid p.Ala519Glu, which is characterized as a Deleterious one, occurs in 20 out of 42 rat strains (Supplementary Table).

Table 6. Predicting the effects of missense variants on protein function using the Sorting Intolerant From Tolerant (SIFT) algorithm.

Gene Symbol	Position	ID	DP	SNP	Amino Acid Substitution	SIFT Score *	SIFT Classification
Slc4a9	29059899	novel	118	c.269C>T	p.Ala90Val	0.021	deleterious
Dcp2	35336920	novel	76	c.1109C>T	p.Ala370Val	0.718	tolerated
Megf10	51550880	rs199133377	131	c.3404C>G	p.Thr1135Ser	0.823	tolerated
RGD1312005	53356293	rs8169475	634	c.361A>G	p.Asn121Asp	1.000	tolerated
Synpo	55104621	rs63909326	331	c.1727T>C	p.Ile576Thr	0.378	tolerated
Synpo	55104676	rs198024246	253	c.1672C>T	p.His558Tyr	1.000	tolerated
Tcof1	55324879	rs198780519	351	c.2828A>G	p.Asn943Ser	1.000	tolerated
Tcof1	55334042	rs197009609	274	c.1556C>A	p.Ala519Glu	0.014	deleterious
Tcof1	55347410	rs199120971	231	c.126T>G	p.His42Gln	1.000	tolerated
Csf1r	55682600	rs198399348	798	c.1825C>A	p.Leu609Met	0.486	tolerated
Hmgxb3	55690668	rs198759766	350	c.3513T>G	p.His1171Gln	0.265	tolerated
Hmgxb3	55715142	rs197391293	293	c.1337G>A	p.Gly446Asp	0.087	tolerated
Napg	57562399	rs198931177	570	c.448T>A	p.Cys150Ser	0.157	tolerated

*—statistically significant values are given in bold; ID—identification number; DP—sequencing depth.

3. Discussion

The genome scan was carried out and QTL associated with the concentration of norepinephrine in the hypothalamus of ISIAH rats were identified. QTL analysis of this trait on other rat strains has not yet been performed. The obtained results unambiguously show that the manifestation of the trait "concentration of norepinephrine in the hypothalamus" in ISIAH rats is under polygenic control, like other earlier studied physiological traits (blood pressure, body weight and mass of the adrenal glands, kidneys, and heart, as well as plasma corticosterone concentration) [26,27]. We showed that the presence of ISIAH hypertensive rat alleles in some loci can lead to a decrease in the concentration of norepinephrine in the hypothalamus, and in other loci—to its increase. These data may be useful in selecting candidate genes for a specific modulating effect on the trait.

The most highly significant association of norepinephrine concentration in the hypothalamus was found with a genetic locus on chromosome 18. The significant extent of this QTL suggests that, in this region of chromosome 18, there are most likely several genes that may be involved in the genetic control of the norepinephrine concentration in the hypothalamus in ISIAH rats. In the central part of chromosome 18 in the region of marker D18Mgh1, this QTL overlaps with the locus previously described as associated with heart mass [26]. Despite the fact that the genetic control of heart mass in ISIAH rats was earlier associated with several genetic loci, only one of these was found to be associated with both heart mass and norepinephrine concentration in the hypothalamus (Figure 2). Accordingly, it is precisely in the central part of chromosome 18 in the region of the D18Mgh1 marker the closely linked genes controlling the manifestation of the studied traits, or genes with a pleiotropic effect on the traits "concentration of norepinephrine in the hypothalamus" and "heart mass" can be localized. Earlier, for this locus on chromosome 18, an association with the heart mass (Cardiac mass QTL 125, Cm125) was also found in the congenic rats SS.LEW-(D18Chm41-D18Rat92)/Ayd, in which the fragment of chromosome 18 (30.8—52.3 Mb) of Dahl salt-sensitive (DSS) rats, which are a model of the salt-sensitive hypertension, has been replaced by a fragment of the genome of normotensive Lewis (LEW) rats [30].

Increased sympathetic activity is considered a risk factor for cardiovascular problems and as a cause of the onset and maintenance of high blood pressure [23]. The central nervous system, in particular the nuclei of the hypothalamus, plays a vital role in the regulation of these processes [31]. The current work made it possible for the first time to determine the genetic loci associated with the concentration of norepinephrine in the hypothalamus and compare them with the loci previously associated with heart mass and blood pressure both in ISIAH rats and in other hypertensive rat strains. When studying SS hypertensive rat strains simulating salt-sensitive hypertension [30,32–34], and in SHR rats with spontaneously developing hypertension [35], this locus on chromosome 18 was also associated with the Blood pressure trait. We mapped the Blood pressure trait earlier in ISIAH rats [26]; however, no associations of the Blood pressure trait with the genetic locus on chromosome 18 discussed in this work was identified. This is not the first time that certain loci have been associated only with the weight parameters of target organs, but not with the level of blood pressure. It is believed that such results make it possible to identify the mechanisms that underlie the development of hypertrophy of target organs but independent of hypertension [30]. Accordingly, we assume that the genetic control of sympathetic activation, which affects the development of hypertension in ISIAH rats, differs from that in SHR rats and rats with salt-sensitive hypertension. The differences found in the genetic control of the traits in SS, SHR, and ISIAH rats are in good agreement with the fact that the genotype of ISIAH rats is significantly different from the genotypes of other hypertensive strains [29]. The fact that no association with blood pressure was found in ISIAH rats at this locus is in good agreement with the concept of the nature of hypertension in humans, when chronic activation of the sympathetic nervous system in hypertension has a diverse range of pathophysiological consequences independent of any increase in blood pressure [36].

It is known that various (hemodynamic and hormonal) factors can influence the functioning of the heart, which can cause left ventricular hypertrophy [37]. Our results are in good agreement with these ideas. Despite the fact that in ISIAH rats at the locus on chromosome 18, the value of heart mass is not associated with the level of blood pressure; such an association was found on other chromosomes. We previously showed that in the distal part of chromosome 1 there is a locus associated with both blood pressure and heart mass in ISIAH rats [26]. Moreover, at the locus common to these two traits on chromosome 1, the presence of ISIAH rat alleles was associated with an increase in the values of both characters. Our results allow us to conclude that in ISIAH rats the development of heart hypertrophy has a complex nature and is associated both with sympathetic activation, which is controlled by the locus on chromosome 18, and with increased blood pressure, which is controlled by the locus on chromosome 1. These data are in good agreement with the idea that the activation of the sympathetic nervous system plays an important role in the development and maintenance of arterial hypertension and development of cardiac hypertrophy and heart failure. In addition, our data emphasize that these processes can be controlled by different genetic loci. This is consistent with the opinion that pharmacological treatment of hypertension should be aimed not only at lowering blood pressure, but also at correcting the sympathetic nervous activity [38].

In ISIAH rats, numerous nucleotide substitutions were found at the discussed locus, which can have a modifying effect on the level of gene expression. As shown in a number of studies, nucleotide substitutions in the regulatory regions of mRNA [39–42] and in introns [43,44] can have a significant modifying effect on transcription and translation and lead to various pathologies. Accordingly, it can be assumed that some of the substitutions listed in Table 5 may be essential in the formation of phenotypes associated with the discussed locus.

However, it is believed that it is the single nucleotide polymorphisms that lead to nonsynonymous amino acid substitutions in protein molecules that can most significantly affect its function and have a significant impact on human health compared to SNPs in other regions of the genome [45]. Our analysis allowed us to identify two SNPs that lead to nonsynonymous amino acid substitutions and, according to the SIFT algorithm, can presumably lead to changes in the structure and/or function of proteins encoded by the *Slc4a9* and *Tcof1* genes.

Slc4a9 (solute carrier family 4, member 9) is encoding transmembrane anion exchange protein involved in chloride/bicarbonate exchange. However, according to the National Center for Biotechnology Information (NCBI) Database, this gene is expressed mainly in the kidneys, and its expression in brain and in heart is very low [46]. Accordingly, on the one hand, it can be assumed that the substitution found in the *Slc4a9* gene sequence may not play a key role in the formation of the discussed phenotypes. However, on the other hand, it can be assumed that the expression level of this gene may increase with sympathetic activation or other conditions and affect the function of the heart, which, however, has not been studied so far.

Tcof1 (treacle ribosome biogenesis factor 1) gene product is involved in ribosomal DNA gene transcription by interacting with upstream binding factor [47]. Mutations in the *TCOF1* gene cause Treacher Collins syndrome (TCS), which is an autosomal dominant disorder characterized by abnormalities of craniofacial development that arises during early embryogenesis. However, the nucleotide substitution c.1556C>A, detected in the genome of ISIAH rats, also occurs in 20 out of 42 analyzed rat strains and substrains (see Supplementary Table), the development of which corresponds to normal, which indicates that the discussed substitution in the mRNA sequence of the gene *Tcof1* is not associated with TCS. Interestingly, the *Tcof1* gene is considered the only function candidate for Blood pressure in QTL 319 also known as C18QTL3 (53.3–78.6 Mb), described in the study of genetic control of hypertension in salt-sensitive rats [48].

Could a missense mutation in the *Tcof1* gene sequence be the reason that no association with blood pressure was found at this locus in ISIAH rats? As we wrote above, this mutation was found in 20 out of 42 analyzed rat strains/substrains. These included both several rat strains used as a normotensive control (FHL/EurMcwi, WKY/N, WKY/Gla, WKY/NHsd), and several hypertensive strains (FHH/EurMcwi, SBH/Ygl, SHRSP/Gla, SHR/OlaIpcv, SHR/NCrlPrin, SHR/NHsd, SHR/OlaIpcvPrin). However, it should be noted that among the hypertensive strains with this substitution, there were no strains with salt-sensitive hypertension, in which arterial blood pressure-associated loci were described in the discussed genome locus, and rats with spontaneous hypertension (SHR/Mol), for which an association with blood pressure was found at the locus of chromosome 18 [35] were not included in SNPs analysis. For SHRSP rats on chromosome 18, the Blood pressure QTL2 locus was described in region 1–34.9 Mb [49], which does not include the *Tcof1* gene, and for FHH [50] and SBH rats [51], Blood pressure trait mapping showed associations with other chromosomes. Based on the foregoing, it can be concluded that the found substitution in the *Tcof1* gene deserves additional attention and subsequent study of its possible association with the manifestation of hypertensive status in rats of different strains. As shown earlier, the epistatic hierarchy may play an important role in the genetic regulation of blood pressure [52]. Perhaps for the manifestation of this polymorphism on the regulation of blood pressure, its effect must be combined with other genetic factors.

The results presented in this work add new information to the existing knowledge about the functional annotation of the genome, which is an important step in understanding the formation of external phenotype [53]. Undoubtedly, the QTL method has its limitations and is only the first stage in a long process of further experimental evidence of the relationship between the function of candidate genes found in loci and the manifestation of the phenotype. Nevertheless, this work was the first to analyze the QTL for an important trait—the concentration of norepinephrine in the hypothalamus, and for the first time, a genetic locus associated with both the concentration of norepinephrine in the hypothalamus and an increased heart mass was described. In addition, it was shown that the locus found on chromosome 18 may or may not be associated with the level of blood pressure in different strains of hypertensive rats. Accordingly, the results obtained in this study can be useful for identifying specific targets for the treatment of heart pathology associated with increased sympathetic activity at the identified genetic locus on chromosome 18. Nucleotide substitutions specific to ISIAH rats that were identified and discussed in this study can potentially be used in further studies of genetic control of the manifestation of the corresponding phenotypes in human populations.

4. Materials and Methods

4.1. Animals

We used hypertensive ISIAH/Icgn rats (abbreviation from the words Inherited Stress-Induced Arterial Hypertension) and the normotensive WAG/GSto-Icgn (Wistar Albino Glaxo) strain. This work was carried out on the basis of the *Center for Genetic Resources* of *Laboratory Animals*, Institute of Cytology and Genetics, Siberian Branch of the Russian Academy of Sciences, Novosibirsk, Russia. Rats were kept under standard conditions, water and balanced food were given without restriction. All manipulations with animals were carried out in accordance with the European Convention for the protection of Vertebrate Animals Used for experimental and Other Scientific Purposes (ETS 123), Strasbourg, 18 March 1986 and in compliance with the rules of the Animal Care and Use Committee of Institute of Cytology and Genetics SB RAS, and approved by the Bioethical Committee of the Scientific Research Institute of Physiology and Basic Medicine (protocol No. 7 of 9 October 2015), Novosibirsk, Russia.

4.2. Determination of Norepinephrine Concentration in the Hypothalamus

Rats were quickly decapitated, the hypothalamus was isolated and frozen in liquid nitrogen, and then stored at $-70\ °C$ until the norepinephrine concentration was measured. A tissue sample was homogenized in a glass homogenizer in 300 µL 0.1 M perchloric acid, to which isopropyl–norepinephrine (100 ng/mL) (Sigma, United States) was added as an internal standard. The homogenate was centrifuged for 15 min ($12,000 \times g$). The supernatant was transferred to a separate tube. High performance liquid chromatography with two-electrode electrochemical detection was used for the analysis of norepinephrine in the supernatant [54]. The sensitivity of the measurement was 2 pg/mL. Norepinephrine concentration was measured in ng/mg of tissue.

4.3. QTL (Quantitative Trait Locus) Analysis

QTL analysis was performed on male F2 hybrids (ISIAHxWAG) at the age of 6 months (n = 126) using 149 polymorphic microsatellite markers. Their list and primer sequences are given on the website of the Institute of Cytology and Genetics SB RAS (http://icg.nsc.ru/isiah/en/category/qtl/). The position of microsatellite markers on chromosomes was determined using the RGSC Genome Assembly v 5.0. and expressed in millions of nucleotides (megabases, Mb) from the start of the chromosome. The genotyping was performed as described previously [26].

Linkage analysis was performed using the programs MAPMAKER/EXP 3.0 and MAPMAKER/QTL 1.1 [55]. The concentration of norepinephrine in the hypothalamus was transformed using the natural logarithm (ln) to reduce the asymmetry and excess (skewness and kurtosis) in the distribution of the values of the trait. A one-LOD drop-off was used to obtain an approximate 95% confidence interval for QTL position. QTL Cartographer Version 1.17, JZmapqtl [56] was used to map loci that are common for pairs of traits (bivariate analysis), and to calculate the LOD score significance thresholds. The level of statistical significance was calculated by random permutation of experimental data with replication 1000 times (permutation test) [57]. The linkage was considered significant if the experimentally obtained LOD score exceeded 5% of the threshold value in the analysis of the genome (experiment-wise threshold) [58], linkage was considered probable if the experimentally obtained LOD score exceeded 5% of the threshold value during a permutation test for a single chromosome (chromosome-wise threshold). Statistical processing of the results was carried out using Statistica 6.0 (StatSoft, Tulsa, OK, USA). The significance of differences between the mean values was evaluated using Student's t-test. The degree of dominance was calculated by the standard method [59], assuming that the complete dominance of ISIAH rat alleles is +1, and the complete dominance of WAG rat alleles is -1.

The Rat Genome Database (RGD, http://rgd.mcw.edu/) was used to compare the genetic loci found in this work with the results of studies on other model animals.

4.4. Tissue Collection for SNP Analysis

To analyze SNPs, male ISIAH/Icgn and WAG/GSto-Icgn rats were used. Each experimental group consisted of 6 rats. Samples of five tissues were taken from each animal for analysis of the transcriptome (brainstem, hypothalamus, adrenal gland, cortex and medulla of the kidney). Sequencing of transcriptomes was performed at JSC Genoanalytica (Moscow, Russia).

4.5. RNA Sequencing

Over 10 million single-end reads of 50-bp length were obtained for each sample in accordance with standard Illumina protocols as described previously [29]. All samples were analyzed as biological replicates.

Mapping was performed for the reference genome (Rnor_5.0\rn5) using the TopHat2 software [60]. The quality of the mapped data was assessed using the "CollectRnaSeqMetrics" module in the Picard software package (http://broadinstitute.github.io/picard/). Potential PCR duplicates were removed from the mapped bam data obtained for 5 different tissues of each animal (hypothalamus, brainstem, adrenal gland, renal medulla and cortex), after which they were combined into one pool for each animal with the Picard "MergeSamFiles" module for further analysis.

4.6. Polymorphism Detection

The initial set of polymorphisms was determined using the Genome Analysis Toolkit (GATK) [61] using the "HaplotypeCaller" module in the "GVCF" mode and the "GenotypeGVCFs" module for combined genotyping, using the settings for variant calling and hard filtering recommended by the GATK developers. The details were described in [29].

Determination of polymorphisms in transcriptome data of ISIAH and WAG rats was carried out relative to the reference genome sequence of BN/NhsdMcwi rats in the assembly version RGSC5.0 [62]. Further analysis of the list of polymorphic variants of ISIAH rats was carried out using the Rat Genome Sequencing Consortium data for the genome sequences of 42 rat strains and substrains including 11 hypertesive rat strains and substrains: FHH/EurMcwi, LH/MavRrrc, MHS/Gib, SBH/Ygl, SHR/OlaIpcv, SHRSP/Gla, SHR/NCrlPrin, SHR/NHsd, SHR/OlaIpcvPrin, SS/Jr, SS/JrHsdMcwi; 10 rat strains and substrains that usually serve as a normotensive control: FHL/EurMcwi, LN/MavRrrc, LL/MavRrrc, MNS/Gib, SBN/Ygl, SR/Jr, WKY/N, WKY/Gla, WKY/NCrl, WKY/NHsd; and 21 other rat strains and substrains that are used in experiments not related to hypertension: ACI/N, ACI/EurMcwi, BBDP/Wor, BN-Lx/Cub, BN-Lx/CubPrin, BN/SsN, BUF/N, DA/BklArbNsi, F334/N, F344/NHsd, F344/NCrl, SUO_F344, GK/Ox, LE/Stm (SOLiD), LEW/Crl, LEW/NCrlBR, LE/Stm (Illumina), M520/N, MR/N, WAG/Rij, WN/N [63]. Comparison of single nucleotide polymorphisms of ISIAH/Icgn and WAG/Gsto-Icgn strains with genotypes of 42 rat strains and substrains was carried out only for genomic loci sequenced in transcriptomic analysis.

4.7. Prediction of the SNP Effects

The classification of the found polymorphisms and their effects are given according to the description in the SnpEff program (http://snpeff.sourceforge.net/SnpEff_manual.html). To determine the possible effect of amino acid substitution on protein function, the Sorting Intolerant From Tolerant (SIFT) program [64] was used.

Supplementary Materials: The following are available online at https://www.mdpi.com/2075-4426/11/2/67/s1, Supplementary Table: SNPs in QTL.

Author Contributions: Conceptualization, O.E.R. and A.L.M.; data curation, O.E.R., S.E.S., Y.K.P. and M.A.G.; formal analysis, O.E.R., S.E.S. and N.I.E.; funding acquisition, O.E.R.; investigation, O.E.R., S.E.S., N.I.E., Y.K.P., M.A.G. and A.L.M.; methodology, O.E.R. and A.L.M.; supervision, O.E.R. and A.L.M.; writing—original draft, O.E.R.; writing—review and editing, O.E.R., S.E.S., N.I.E., Y.K.P., M.A.G. and A.L.M. All authors have read and agreed to the published version of the manuscript.

Funding: Genotyping was supported by budget project No. 0259-2021-0015. SNPs analysis was supported by budget project No. 0259-2021-0013. The mathematical processing of the obtained data and the preparation of the results for publication was supported by the Russian Foundation for Basic Research, grant No. 20-04-00119a.

Institutional Review Board Statement: All manipulations with animals were carried out in accordance with the European Convention for the protection of Vertebrate Animals Used for experimental and Other Scientific Purposes (ETS 123), Strasbourg, March 18, 1986 and in compliance with the rules of the Animal Care and Use Committee of Institute of Cytology and Genetics SB RAS, and approved by the Bioethical Committee of the Scientific Research Institute of Physiology and Basic Medicine (protocol No. 7 of 9 October 2015), Novosibirsk, Russia.

Informed Consent Statement: Not applicable.

Data Availability Statement: Not applicable.

Acknowledgments: The authors are grateful to JSC Genoanalytica (Moscow, Russia) for conducting the technological part of the RNA-Seq analysis. The Siberian Branch of the Russian Academy of Sciences (SB RAS) Siberian Supercomputer Center is gratefully acknowledged for providing supercomputer facilities.

Conflicts of Interest: The authors declare no conflict of interest.

References

1. Morgan, H.E.; Baker, K.M. Cardiac hypertrophy. Mechanical, neural, and endocrine dependence. *Circulation* **1991**, *83*, 13–25. [CrossRef] [PubMed]
2. Sen, S.; Tarazi, R.C.; Khairallah, P.A.; Bumpus, F.M. Cardiac hypertrophy in spontaneously hypertensive rats. *Circ. Res.* **1974**, *35*, 775–781. [CrossRef] [PubMed]
3. Kamide, K.; Rakugi, H.; Higaki, J.; Okamura, A.; Nagai, M.; Moriguchi, K.; Ohishi, M.; Satoh, N.; Tuck, M.L.; Ogihara, T. The renin-angiotensin and adrenergic nervous system in cardiac hypertrophy in fructose-fed rats. *Am. J. Hypertens.* **2002**, *15*, 66–71. [CrossRef]
4. Simpson, P.C.; Kariya, K.; Karns, L.R.; Long, C.S.; Karliner, J.S. Adrenergic hormones and control of cardiac myocyte growth. *Mol. Cell. Biochem.* **1991**, *104*, 35–43. [CrossRef] [PubMed]
5. DeLalio, L.J.; Sved, A.F.; Stocker, S.D. Sympathetic Nervous System Contributions to Hypertension: Updates and Therapeutic Relevance. *Can. J. Cardiol.* **2020**, *36*, 712–720. [CrossRef] [PubMed]
6. Macefield, V.G.; Henderson, L.A. Identification of the human sympathetic connectome involved in blood pressure regulation. *Neuroimage* **2019**, *202*, 116119. [CrossRef]
7. Bear, M.H.; Reddy, V.; Bollu, P.C. *Neuroanatomy, Hypothalamus*; StatPearls Publishing LLC: Treasure Island, FL, USA, 2020.
8. Atzori, M.; Cuevas-Olguin, R.; Esquivel-Rendon, E.; Garcia-Oscos, F.; Salgado-Delgado, R.C.; Saderi, N.; Miranda-Morales, M.; Trevino, M.; Pineda, J.C.; Salgado, H. Locus Ceruleus Norepinephrine Release: A Central Regulator of CNS Spatio-Temporal Activation? *Front. Synaptic. Neurosci.* **2016**, *8*, 25. [CrossRef]
9. Pacak, K.; Palkovits, M.; Kopin, I.J.; Goldstein, D.S. Stress-induced norepinephrine release in the hypothalamic paraventricular nucleus and pituitary-adrenocortical and sympathoadrenal activity: In vivo microdialysis studies. *Front. Neuroendocrinol.* **1995**, *16*, 89–150. [CrossRef]
10. Jiang, Z.; Chen, C.; Weiss, G.L.; Fu, X.; Fisher, M.O.; Begley, J.C.; Stevens, C.R.; Harrison, L.M.; Tasker, J.G. Acute stress desensitizes hypothalamic CRH neurons to norepinephrine and physiological stress. *bioRxiv* **2020**. [CrossRef]
11. Selvetella, G.; Lembo, G. Mechanisms of cardiac hypertrophy. *Heart Fail. Clin.* **2005**, *1*, 263–273. [CrossRef]
12. Morris, M.; Ross, J.; Sundberg, D.K. Catecholamine biosynthesis and vasopressin and oxytocin secretion in the spontaneously hypertensive rat: An in vitro study of localized brain regions. *Peptides* **1985**, *6*, 949–955. [CrossRef]
13. Oparil, S.; Chen, Y.F.; Peng, N.; Wyss, J.M. Anterior hypothalamic norepinephrine, atrial natriuretic peptide, and hypertension. *Front. Neuroendocrinol.* **1996**, *17*, 212–246. [CrossRef] [PubMed]
14. McCrossan, Z.A.; Billeter, R.; White, E. Transmural changes in size, contractile and electrical properties of SHR left ventricular myocytes during compensated hypertrophy. *Cardiovasc. Res.* **2004**, *63*, 283–292. [CrossRef] [PubMed]
15. Pacak, K.; Yadid, G.; Jakab, G.; Lenders, J.W.; Kopin, I.J.; Goldstein, D.S. In vivo hypothalamic release and synthesis of catecholamines in spontaneously hypertensive rats. *Hypertension* **1993**, *22*, 467–478. [CrossRef] [PubMed]
16. Woo, N.D.; Mukherjee, K.; Ganguly, P.K. Norepinephrine levels in paraventricular nucleus of spontaneously hypertensive rats: Role of neuropeptide Y. *Am. J. Physiol.* **1993**, *265*, H893–H898. [CrossRef]
17. Arabia, A.M.; Catapano, L.; Storini, C.; Perego, C.; De Luigi, A.; Head, G.A.; De Simoni, M.G. Impaired central stress-induced release of noradrenaline in rats with heart failure: A microdialysis study. *Neuroscience* **2002**, *114*, 591–599. [CrossRef]
18. Buzueva, I.I.; Filyushina, E.E.; Shmerling, M.D.; Markel, A.L.; Yakobson, G.S. Chromogranin location in the adrenal glands of ISIAH rats. *Bull. Exp. Biol. Med.* **2013**, *154*, 393–395. [CrossRef]

19. Bilek, R.; Safarik, L.; Ciprova, V.; Vlcek, P.; Lisa, L. Chromogranin A, a member of neuroendocrine secretory proteins as a selective marker for laboratory diagnosis of pheochromocytoma. *Physiol Res.* **2008**, *57* (Suppl. 1), S171–S179.
20. Markel, A.L.; Redina, O.E.; Gilinsky, M.A.; Dymshits, G.M.; Kalashnikova, E.V.; Khvorostova, Y.V.; Fedoseeva, L.A.; Jacobson, G.S. Neuroendocrine profiling in inherited stress-induced arterial hypertension rat strain with stress-sensitive arterial hypertension. *J. Endocrinol.* **2007**, *195*, 439–450. [CrossRef]
21. Suslonova, O.V.; Roshchevskaya, I.M.; Rasputina, A.A. Morphometry of the heart ventricles in NISAG rats during the early postnatal ontogenesis. *Isvestiia Komi Nauchnogo Cent. URO RAN* **2016**, *1*, 45–50.
22. Shmerling, M.D.; Buzueva, I.I.; Korostyshevskaia, I.M.; Lazarev, V.A.; Maksimov, V.F.; Filiushina, E.E.; Markel, A.L.; Iakobson, G.S. Stereomorphometric study of target organs in rats with hereditary stress-induced arterial hypertension at different periods of postnatal ontogenesis under changed conditions of nursing. *Morfologiia* **2005**, *128*, 85–90. [PubMed]
23. Esler, M. The sympathetic system and hypertension. *Am. J. Hypertens* **2000**, *13*, 99S–105S. [CrossRef]
24. Ryazanova, M.; Klimov, L.; Seryapina, A.; Zarytova, V.; Repkova, M.; Levina, A.; Markel, A. Nanocomposite (Si-ODN-II), containing antisense oligonucleotides targeted to mRNA of the beta-1-adrenoreceptors for hypertension therapy in rats with stress-sensitive arterial hypertension (ISIAH rats). *J. Hypertens.* **2018**, *36* (Suppl. 3), e81–e82. [CrossRef]
25. Redina, O.E.; Machanova, N.A.; Efimov, V.M.; Markel, A.L. Rats with inherited stress-induced arterial hypertension (ISIAH strain) display specific quantitative trait loci for blood pressure and for body and kidney weight on chromosome 1. *Clin. Exp. Pharmacol. Physiol.* **2006**, *33*, 456–464. [CrossRef] [PubMed]
26. Redina, O.E.; Smolenskaya, S.E.; Maslova, L.N.; Markel, A.L. The genetic control of blood pressure and body composition in rats with stress-sensitive hypertension. *Clin. Exp. Hypertens.* **2013**, *35*, 484–495. [CrossRef]
27. Redina, O.E.; Smolenskaya, S.E.; Maslova, L.N.; Markel, A.L. Genetic Control of the Corticosterone Level at Rest and Under Emotional Stress in ISIAH Rats with Inherited Stress-Induced Arterial Hypertension. *Clin. Exp. Hypertens.* **2010**, *32*, 364–371. [CrossRef]
28. Redina, O.E.; Smolenskaya, S.E.; Jacobson, G.S.; Markel, A.L. Norepinephrine content in the hypothalamus and medulla oblongata of ISIAH rats is regulated by several genetic loci. *Bull. Exp. Biol. Med.* **2009**, *148*, 223–226. [CrossRef]
29. Ershov, N.I.; Markel, A.L.; Redina, O.E. Strain-Specific Single-Nucleotide Polymorphisms in Hypertensive ISIAH Rats. *Biochemistry* **2017**, *82*, 224–235. [CrossRef]
30. Duong, C.; Charron, S.; Xiao, C.; Hamet, P.; Ménard, A.; Roy, J.; Deng, A.Y. Distinct quantitative trait loci for kidney, cardiac, and aortic mass dissociated from and associated with blood pressure in Dahl congenic rats. *Mamm Genome* **2006**, *17*, 1147–1161. [CrossRef]
31. Hirooka, Y. Sympathetic Activation in Hypertension: Importance of the Central Nervous System. *Am. J. Hypertens.* **2020**, *33*, 914–926. [CrossRef]
32. Stoll, M.; Cowley, A.W.J.; Tonellato, P.J.; Greene, A.S.; Kaldunski, M.L.; Roman, R.J.; Dumas, P.; Schork, N.J.; Wang, Z.; Jacob, H.J. A genomic-systems biology map for cardiovascular function. *Science* **2001**, *294*, 1723–1726. [CrossRef] [PubMed]
33. Charron, S.; Lambert, R.; Eliopoulos, V.; Duong, C.; Menard, A.; Roy, J.; Deng, A.Y. A loss of genome buffering capacity of Dahl salt-sensitive model to modulate blood pressure as a cause of hypertension. *Hum. Mol. Genet.* **2005**, *14*, 3877–3884. [CrossRef] [PubMed]
34. Deng, A.Y.; Nattel, S.; Shi, Y.; L'Heureux, N.; Cardin, S.; Menard, A.; Roy, J.; Tardif, J.C. Distinct genomic replacements from Lewis correct diastolic dysfunction, attenuate hypertension, and reduce left ventricular hypertrophy in Dahl salt-sensitive rats. *J. Hypertens.* **2008**, *26*, 1935–1943. [CrossRef] [PubMed]
35. Kovacs, P.; Voigt, B.; Kloting, I. Novel quantitative trait loci for blood pressure and related traits on rat chromosomes 1, 10, and 18. *Biochem. Biophys. Res. Commun.* **1997**, *235*, 343–348. [CrossRef]
36. Fisher, J.P.; Paton, J.F. The sympathetic nervous system and blood pressure in humans: Implications for hypertension. *J. Hum. Hypertens.* **2012**, *26*, 463–475. [CrossRef]
37. Gurgerian, S.V.; Vatinian, S. The multifactorial genesis of left ventricle remodeling in patients with essential arterial hypertension. *Kardiologiia* **2013**, *53*, 38–42.
38. Cohen, J.D.; Egan, B.M. The role of sympathetic activation in cardiovascular disease. *Postgrad. Med.* **2003**, *114*, 4–10. [CrossRef]
39. Saxena, A.; Moshynska, O.; Sankaran, K.; Viswanathan, S.; Sheridan, D.P. Association of a novel single nucleotide polymorphism, G(-248)A, in the 5'-UTR of BAX gene in chronic lymphocytic leukemia with disease progression and treatment resistance. *Cancer Lett.* **2002**, *187*, 199–205. [CrossRef]
40. Danckwardt, S.; Hentze, M.W.; Kulozik, A.E. 3' end mRNA processing: Molecular mechanisms and implications for health and disease. *EMBO J.* **2008**, *27*, 482–498. [CrossRef]
41. Greenbaum, L.; Smith, R.C.; Rigbi, A.; Strous, R.; Teltsh, O.; Kanyas, K.; Korner, M.; Lancet, D.; Ben-Asher, E.; Lerer, B. Further evidence for association of the RGS2 gene with antipsychotic-induced parkinsonism: Protective role of a functional polymorphism in the 3'-untranslated region. *Pharm. J.* **2009**, *9*, 103–110. [CrossRef]
42. Mendelova, A.; Holubekova, V.; Grendar, M.; Zubor, P.; Svecova, I.; Loderer, D.; Snahnicanova, Z.; Biringer, K.; Danko, J.; Lasabova, Z. Association between 3'UTR polymorphisms in genes ACVR2A, AGTR1 and RGS2 and preeclampsia. *Gen. Physiol. Biophys.* **2018**, *37*, 185–192. [CrossRef]

43. Han, Y.J.; Ma, S.F.; Wade, M.S.; Flores, C.; Garcia, J.G. An intronic MYLK variant associated with inflammatory lung disease regulates promoter activity of the smooth muscle myosin light chain kinase isoform. *J. Mol. Med.* **2012**, *90*, 299–308. [CrossRef] [PubMed]
44. Hong, M.J.; Lee, S.Y.; Choi, J.E.; Kang, H.G.; Do, S.K.; Lee, J.H.; Yoo, S.S.; Lee, E.B.; Seok, Y.; Cho, S.; et al. Intronic variant of EGFR is associated with GBAS expression and survival outcome of early-stage non-small cell lung cancer. *Thorac. Cancer* **2018**, *9*, 916–923. [CrossRef] [PubMed]
45. Ng, P.C.; Henikoff, S. Predicting the effects of amino acid substitutions on protein function. *Annu. Rev. Genomics Hum. Genet.* **2006**, *7*, 61–80. [CrossRef] [PubMed]
46. Yu, Y.; Fuscoe, J.C.; Zhao, C.; Guo, C.; Jia, M.; Qing, T.; Bannon, D.I.; Lancashire, L.; Bao, W.; Du, T.; et al. A rat RNA-Seq transcriptomic BodyMap across 11 organs and 4 developmental stages. *Nat. Commun.* **2014**, *5*, 3230. [CrossRef] [PubMed]
47. Valdez, B.C.; Henning, D.; So, R.B.; Dixon, J.; Dixon, M.J. The Treacher Collins syndrome (TCOF1) gene product is involved in ribosomal DNA gene transcription by interacting with upstream binding factor. *Proc. Natl. Acad. Sci. USA* **2004**, *101*, 10709–10714. [CrossRef]
48. Chauvet, C.; Menard, A.; Deng, A.Y. Two candidate genes for two quantitative trait loci epistatically attenuate hypertension in a novel pathway. *J. Hypertens.* **2015**, *33*, 1791–1801. [CrossRef]
49. Jacob, H.J.; Lindpaintner, K.; Lincoln, S.E.; Kusumi, K.; Bunker, R.K.; Mao, Y.P.; Ganten, D.; Dzau, V.J.; Lander, E.S. Genetic mapping of a gene causing hypertension in the stroke-prone spontaneously hypertensive rat. *Cell* **1991**, *67*, 213–224. [CrossRef]
50. Brown, D.M.; Provoost, A.P.; Daly, M.J.; Lander, E.S.; Jacob, H.J. Renal disease susceptibility and hypertension are under independent genetic control in the fawn-hooded rat. *Nat. Genet.* **1996**, *12*, 44–51. [CrossRef]
51. Yagil, C.; Sapojnikov, M.; Kreutz, R.; Katni, G.; Lindpaintner, K.; Ganten, D.; Yagil, Y. Salt susceptibility maps to chromosomes 1 and 17 with sex specificity in the Sabra rat model of hypertension. *Hypertension* **1998**, *31*, 119–124. [CrossRef]
52. Chauvet, C.; Crespo, K.; Menard, A.; Roy, J.; Deng, A.Y. Modularization and epistatic hierarchy determine homeostatic actions of multiple blood pressure quantitative trait loci. *Hum. Mol. Genet.* **2013**, *22*, 4451–4459. [CrossRef]
53. Te Pas, M.F.; Madsen, O.; Calus, M.P.; Smits, M.A. The Importance of Endophenotypes to Evaluate the Relationship between Genotype and External Phenotype. *Int. J. Mol. Sci.* **2017**, *18*, 472. [CrossRef] [PubMed]
54. Bergquist, J.; Sciubisz, A.; Kaczor, A.; Silberring, J. Catecholamines and methods for their identification and quantitation in biological tissues and fluids. *J. Neurosci. Methods* **2002**, *113*, 1–13. [CrossRef]
55. Lander, E.S.; Green, P.; Abrahamson, J.; Barlow, A.; Daly, M.J.; Lincoln, S.E.; Newburg, L. MAPMAKER: An interactive computer package for constructing primary genetic linkage maps of experimental and natural populations. *Genomics* **1987**, *1*, 174–181. [CrossRef]
56. Basten, C.J.; Weir, B.S.; Zeng, Z.-B. *QTL Cartographer, Version 1.17*; Department of Statistics, North. Carolina State University: Raleigh, NC, USA, 2004.
57. Churchill, G.A.; Doerge, R.W. Empirical Threshold Values for Quantitative Trait Mapping. *Genetics* **1994**, *138*, 963–971. [CrossRef]
58. Lander, E.; Kruglyak, L. Genetic dissection of complex traits: Guidelines for interpreting and reporting linkage results. *Nat. Genet.* **1995**, *11*, 241–247. [CrossRef] [PubMed]
59. Mather, K.; Jinks, J.L. *Introduction to Biometrical Genetics*; Chapman & Hall: London, UK, 1977; p. 231.
60. Kim, D.; Pertea, G.; Trapnell, C.; Pimentel, H.; Kelley, R.; Salzberg, S.L. TopHat2: Accurate alignment of transcriptomes in the presence of insertions, deletions and gene fusions. *Genome Biol.* **2013**, *14*, R36. [CrossRef] [PubMed]
61. McKenna, A.; Hanna, M.; Banks, E.; Sivachenko, A.; Cibulskis, K.; Kernytsky, A.; Garimella, K.; Altshuler, D.; Gabriel, S.; Daly, M.; et al. The Genome Analysis Toolkit: A MapReduce framework for analyzing next-generation DNA sequencing data. *Genome Res.* **2010**, *20*, 1297–1303. [CrossRef]
62. Gibbs, R.A.; Weinstock, G.M.; Metzker, M.L.; Muzny, D.M.; Sodergren, E.J.; Scherer, S.; Scott, G.; Steffen, D.; Worley, K.C.; Burch, P.E.; et al. Genome sequence of the Brown Norway rat yields insights into mammalian evolution. *Nature* **2004**, *428*, 493–521. [CrossRef]
63. Hermsen, R.; de Ligt, J.; Spee, W.; Blokzijl, F.; Schafer, S.; Adami, E.; Boymans, S.; Flink, S.; van Boxtel, R.; van der Weide, R.H.; et al. Genomic landscape of rat strain and substrain variation. *BMC Genom.* **2015**, *16*, 357. [CrossRef]
64. Kumar, P.; Henikoff, S.; Ng, P.C. Predicting the effects of coding non-synonymous variants on protein function using the SIFT algorithm. *Nat. Protoc.* **2009**, *4*, 1073–1081. [CrossRef] [PubMed]

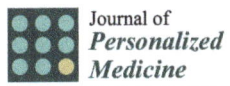

Article

Does Proteomic Mirror Reflect Clinical Characteristics of Obesity?

Olga I. Kiseleva [1,*], Viktoriia A. Arzumanian [1], Ekaterina V. Poverennaya [1], Mikhail A. Pyatnitskiy [1], Ekaterina V. Ilgisonis [1], Victor G. Zgoda [1], Oksana A. Plotnikova [2], Khaider K. Sharafetdinov [2,3,4], Andrey V. Lisitsa [1], Victor A. Tutelyan [2,4], Dmitry B. Nikityuk [2,4], Alexander I. Archakov [1] and Elena A. Ponomarenko [1]

1 Institute of Biomedical Chemistry, Pogodinskaya Street 10/8, 119121 Moscow, Russia; viktoriia.arzumanian@ibmc.msk.ru (V.A.A.); k.poverennaya@ibmc.msk.ru (E.V.P.); mpyat@ibmc.msk.ru (M.A.P.); ilgisonis@ibmc.msk.ru (E.V.I.); vic@ibmh.msk.su (V.G.Z.); fox@ibmh.msk.su (A.V.L.); alexander.archakov@ibmc.msk.ru (A.I.A.); elena.ponomarenko@ibmc.msk.ru (E.A.P.)
2 Federal Research Centre of Nutrition, Biotechnology and Food Safety, Russian Academy of Sciences, Ustinsky Passage 2/14, 109240 Moscow, Russia; plotnikova@ion.ru (O.A.P.); sharafetdinov@ion.ru (K.K.S.); tutelyan@ion.ru (V.A.T.); nikitjuk@ion.ru (D.B.N.)
3 Russian Medical Academy of Continuing Professional Education, Ministry of Health of the Russian Federation, Barrikadnaya Street 2/1, 125993 Moscow, Russia
4 I.M. Sechenov First Moscow State Medical University (Sechenov University), Ministry of Health of the Russian Federation, Trubetskaya Street 8/2, 119991 Moscow, Russia
* Correspondence: okiseleva@ibmc.msk.ru; Tel.: +7-962-999-2460

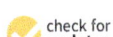

Citation: Kiseleva, O.I.; Arzumanian, V.A.; Poverennaya, E.V.; Pyatnitskiy, M.A.; Ilgisonis, E.V.; Zgoda, V.G.; Plotnikova, O.A.; Sharafetdinov, K.K.; Lisitsa, A.V.; Tutelyan, V.A.; et al. Does Proteomic Mirror Reflect Clinical Characteristics of Obesity? *J. Pers. Med.* **2021**, *11*, 64. https://doi.org/10.3390/jpm11020064

Academic Editor: Mikhail Ivanovich Voevoda

Received: 10 December 2020
Accepted: 15 January 2021
Published: 21 January 2021

Publisher's Note: MDPI stays neutral with regard to jurisdictional claims in published maps and institutional affiliations.

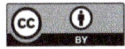

Copyright: © 2021 by the authors. Licensee MDPI, Basel, Switzerland. This article is an open access article distributed under the terms and conditions of the Creative Commons Attribution (CC BY) license (https://creativecommons.org/licenses/by/4.0/).

Abstract: Obesity is a frightening chronic disease, which has tripled since 1975. It is not expected to slow down staying one of the leading cases of preventable death and resulting in an increased clinical and economic burden. Poor lifestyle choices and excessive intake of "cheap calories" are major contributors to obesity, triggering type 2 diabetes, cardiovascular diseases, and other comorbidities. Understanding the molecular mechanisms responsible for development of obesity is essential as it might result in the introducing of anti-obesity targets and early-stage obesity biomarkers, allowing the distinction between metabolic syndromes. The complex nature of this disease, coupled with the phenomenon of metabolically healthy obesity, inspired us to perform data-centric, hypothesis-generating pilot research, aimed to find correlations between parameters of classic clinical blood tests and proteomic profiles of 104 lean and obese subjects. As the result, we assembled patterns of proteins, which presence or absence allows predicting the weight of the patient fairly well. We believe that such proteomic patterns with high prediction power should facilitate the translation of potential candidates into biomarkers of clinical use for early-stage stratification of obesity therapy.

Keywords: obesity; BMI; blood tests; proteomics; mass spectrometry

1. Introduction

Obesity in most cases is blatantly visible by the unaided eye. Paradoxically, at the same time both clinicians and citizens tend to ignore this pathology, acquiring the scale of "globesity" [1,2]. Being a generally preventable disease, obesity, resulting from the excess of body fat, often entails the development of 50+ various pathologies, significant disability, and premature death [3].

The pathogenesis of obesity involves the interaction of genetic, environmental, and behavioral factors [4]. Each time, figuring out the characteristic features in the biomedical portrait of obesity, scientists are trying to resolve the nature vs nurture debate [5]. The multifactorial nature and high comorbidity of obesity make it difficult to understand the clear molecular nature of this disease. Moreover, about a third of obese patients are "metabolically healthy" with little or no evidence of metabolic syndrome. There are four central features (insulin resistance, increased visceral fat, atherogenic dyslipidemia, and endothelial dysfunction), which make up the essential definition for metabolic syndrome. Among them, only the first two are obligatory [6].

However, metabolic syndrome is not the one and only way to identify individuals with increased risk of cardiovascular diseases and diabetes, as well as other comorbidities. Reliable identification of individuals with a significant risk of endocrine or cardiovascular complications requires assessment methods taking into account orthogonal factors (e.g., family history, age, sex, smoking, and other crucial parameters) [6].

Importantly, the "healthy" phenotype of an obese individual with no metabolic aberrations is not constant. Thus, the metabolism of half of such patients ceases being "healthy" in ca. 10 years [7]. It means that early diagnostics and intervening even for "metabolically healthy obesity" is crucial. The dynamic nature of obesity makes it even more difficult to find out meaningful differences between normal state, metabolically healthy, and unhealthy obesity.

Despite the apparent obviousness of strategies for treatment and prevention of obesity, unfortunately, in the long term, they demonstrate low efficiency, primarily because standard pharmacological solutions and significant behavioral changes regarding nutrition and activity, in most cases, do not take root in the modus vivendi of the patients.

A major diagnostic criterion of obesity is body mass index (BMI), expressed by a person's weight divided by the square of his or her height. BMI reliably indicates the anthropometric condition for the overwhelming majority of cases; however, it does not accurately reflect the severity of the health risks [8,9]. The same could be stated for traditional laboratory tests, including monitoring of triglycerides and lipid profiles [10].

The dynamic and multifactorial nature of obesity may be the reason why there are still no biomarkers approved by the FDA or other reputable organizations that could be effectively used to diagnose this disease in personalized—not "one size fits all"—mode.

High-throughput technologies accelerated life science dramatically: the speed of reading the sequences of biological macromolecules is no longer a bottleneck for unraveling the mechanisms of health and disease [11]. Since the sequencing of DNA emerged, a wide range of projects aimed at establishing genetic markers of various medical conditions were performed, and obesity is no exception. Several large-scale genomic studies (e.g., DiOGenes, which explored biological samples from 350 European families [12,13]) paved the way for a further selection of nutritional recommendations through understanding the dynamics of weight maintenance based on the uniqueness of a particular patient [14].

Technical progress in the exploration of the proteome, the final level of transmission of biological information and predecessor of the metabolome, achieved during the last decade has provided a base for illuminating risks and improving current therapeutic strategies [15]. Proteomics allows the development of a personalized molecular profile that takes into account the pattern of biomarkers. This "molecular mirror" reflects all significant processes in the body, including systemic chronic inflammation, associated with obesity [16–18].

In the study, we used a proteomics approach to get a panoramic picture of the proteome of patients with respect to their weight status. To the best of our knowledge, we provide the first evidence that qualitative plasma protein landscape significantly differs from classic clinical parameters on an issue of obesity. We highlighted proteins, which could play a significant role in the development of obesity and obesity-associated disease and should be additionally explored as a prominent tool to improve risk stratification.

2. Materials and Methods
2.1. Sample Collection

One hundred and four human plasma samples were obtained from the patients of the Clinic of "Federal Research Centre of Nutrition, Biotechnology and Food Safety" (Moscow, Russia).

All study participants gave informed consent confirming their willingness to participate in the research. All procedures performed in studies involving human participants were under the ethical standards of the institutional or national research committee and with the 1964 Helsinki declaration and its later amendments or comparable ethical standards. The study was approved by the relevant ethical review committee of the Federal Research Centre of Nutrition, Biotechnology and Food Safety (protocol #4 from 15 June 2018).

The present study included 104 individuals in accordance with the inclusion and exclusion criteria. The inclusion criteria were the age of the study participants from 18 to 45 years, BMI from 18.5, absence of diagnosed somatic and mental disorders.

Individuals younger than 18 and older than 45 years were excluded from the study, as well as pregnant/breastfeeding patients, patients with mental disorders, identified cancer, cardiovascular and any gastrointestinal diseases, other somatic disorders, and recent (6 months) weight loss.

The patients were divided into groups according to their body mass indexes. BMI, calculated as the mass of the individual in kilograms divided by his/her height in meters squared, is one of the most popular metrics to characterize body condition [19].

Five groups of patients (Table 1) were enrolled for this study: controls (NORM, BMI = 18.5–24.9), overweight patients (OW, BMI = 25.0–29.9), and patients with obesity stage 1 (OB1, BMI = 30.0–34.9), 2 (OB2, BMI = 35.0–39.9), and 3 (OB3, BMI > 40.0).

Table 1. Characteristics of patients enrolled in the study.

	NORM	OW	OB1	OB2	OB3	p-Value [1]
Number of patients	22 13/9 (f/m)	21 10/11 (f/m)	19 10/9 (f/m)	21 10/11 (f/m)	21 11/10 (f/m)	-
Age (years, mean ± std. deviation)	30.54 ± 5.34	32.90 ± 6.66	29.89 ± 8.16	32.62 ± 7.92	34.05 ± 6.64	0.4
Height (cm ± std. deviation)	172.65 ± 7.31	171.99 ± 11.81	170.15 ± 11.99	172.26 ± 9.74	172.08 ± 9.72	0.7
Weight (kg ± std. deviation)	64.93 ± 8.12	81.80 ± 12.24	94.44 ± 13.23	109.62 ± 13.67	140.33 ± 27.76	<0.001
BMI (kg/m^2 ± std. deviation)	21.73 ± 1.90	27.52 ± 1.35	32.51 ± 1.69	36.81 ± 1.39	46.99 ± 5.81	<0.001

[1] To refute the theory that the group characteristics do not differ significantly, a p-value < 0.05 was used. p-value, calculated for age and height characteristics of groups under study, provides evidence, that differences of age and height groups are statistically insignificant. NORM—individuals with BMI = 18.5–24.9; OW—overweight patients with BMI = 25.0–29.9; OB1—patients with obesity stage 1 and BMI = 30.0–34.9; OB2—patients with obesity stage 2 and BMI = 35.0–39.9; OB3—patients with obesity stage 3 and BMI > 40.0.

Venous blood samples were collected into EDTA tubes after overnight fasting and centrifuged at $1500\times g$, for 10 min at room temperature. Plasma fractions were stored at −80 °C in cryotubes until processing. Samples were randomized prior to proteomic investigation to avoid potential batch effects.

2.2. Anthropometric and Clinical Tests

2.2.1. Anthropometric Tests

The BMIs of the patients were evaluated according to the standard formula [19]. The weight distributions were measured using the bioelectrical impedance analysis method.

2.2.2. Biochemical Blood Test and Complete Blood Count

Serum levels of fasting plasma glucose, triglycerides, high-density lipoprotein, low-density lipoprotein, cholesterol, alanine aminotransferase, aspartate aminotransferase, γ-glutamyl transpeptidase, alkaline phosphatase, uric acid, urea, creatinine, albumin, bilirubin, etc. were determined according to standard protocols. Blood levels of hemoglobin, hematocrit, and blood cell indexes were established according to standard protocols [20].

Results of anthropometric and blood tests are provided in Supplementary Table S1.

2.3. Sample Preparation

2.3.1. The Depletion of Blood Plasma

The immunoaffinity depletion of the high abundance plasma proteins (albumin and IgG) was used to enhance the detection of lower abundance but more insightful proteins in further shotgun proteomic analysis. For plasma depletion, we used ProteoPrep Kit (Sigma-Aldrich, St. Louis, MO, USA). The depletion was carried out following the manufacturer's instructions [21].

2.3.2. Trypsinolysis of Depleted Plasma

The depleted blood plasma samples (175 µg of total protein) were in-solution digested in accordance with a standard protocol [22]. In brief, proteins were denatured and reduced with a solution containing sodium deoxycholate, tris-2-carboxyethyl-phosphine hydrochloride, and 1,4-dithiothreitol, and further alkylated with vinylpyridine. Trypsin was added to the sample (trypsin/total protein = 1/100) and then incubated within 2 h at a temperature of 44 °C. After 2 h, an aliquot of trypsin was added and then incubated for 2 h at 37 °C. Trypsinolysis was quenched by adding formic acid to each sample to a final concentration of 5%, then a mixture of peptides was centrifuged at 10,000 rpm within 15 min. The supernatant was collected and subjected to further chromatography-mass spectrometric analysis.

2.4. HPLC-MS/MS Analysis

Separation and identification of the peptides were performed on an Ultimate 3000 nano-flow HPLC (Thermo Fisher Scientific, Cleveland, OH, USA) connected to Orbitrap Exactive (Thermo Fisher Scientific, Cleveland, OH, USA) mass spectrometer equipped with a Nanospray Flex NG ion source (Thermo Fisher Scientific, Cleveland, OH, USA). Peptide separation was carried out on an RP-HPLC column Zorbax 300SB-C18 (C18 particle size of 3.5 µm, inner diameter of 75 µm and length of 150 mm, Acclaim® PepMap™ RSLC, Thermo Fisher Scientific, Cleveland, OH, USA) using a linear 90-min gradient from 95% solvent A (0.1% formic acid) and 5% solvent B (0.1% formic acid, 80% acetonitrile) to 60% solvent B over 95 min at a flow rate of 0.3 µL/min.

Mass spectra were registered in the positive ion mode. Data was acquired in the Orbitrap Exactive analyzer with a resolution of 70,000 (at m/z 400) for MS and 15,000 (m/z 400) for MS/MS scans. For peptide fragmentation higher energy collisional dissociation (HCD) was used, the signal threshold was set to 17,500 for an isolation window of 1 m/z and the first mass of HCD spectra was set to 100 m/z. The collision energy was set to 35%. Fragmented precursors were dynamically excluded from targeting for 10 s. Singly charged ions and ions with not defined charge states were excluded from triggering MS/MS scans. Three LC-MS/MS repetitions were performed for each plasma sample.

2.5. Interpretation of Experimental Data

Raw files were converted into .mgf files by MSConvert (v. 3.0). Each of the 312 mgf files containing the feature list for protein identification was processed by SearchGUI software (v. 4.0.4 [23]) using three search engines (X!Tandem, MS-GF+, OMMSA) against SwissProt library of human canonical and alternatively spliced protein sequences in automatic mode [24]. Trypsin was specified as the proteolytic enzyme; maximum of 2 missing cleavages were allowed. Pyridylethylation (C) was used as a constant modification, and oxidation of methionine was set as a variable one. Charge states of +2, +3, and +4 were selected as parent ions. Mass tolerance was set to ±15 ppm for precursor ions and ±0.01 Da for fragment ions. The cut-off of false discovery rates for peptide-spectra matches, peptides, and proteins was ≤1%. Results were visualized in PeptideShaker (v. 2.0.5 [25]). The MS data were deposited to the ProteomeXchange Consortium via the PRIDE partner repository [26] with the dataset identifier PXD023526.

2.6. Statistical Analysis

Clustering analysis of clinical and anthropometric tests was performed using Ward's method and Euclidean distance for normalized data. Clustering patterns of protein presence/absence were done using Ward's method and Jaccard distance metric. All statistical analyses and graphics were performed using R version 4.0 [27].

Each protein of interest was annotated with its GO-terms from UniProt using ViSEAGO package [28]. We used the "2020-03" GO release and "2020_01" UniProt release.

When comparing the results of proteomic and clinical analysis, we explored publicly available data on the relationship between proteins and parameters of clinical analysis. The automatic analysis of the texts of scientific publications was performed by Scanbious platform [29,30], which visualizes semantic networks between objects of various types (names of proteins, pathological processes, etc.).

We predicted the BMI of the patient based on the pattern of presence/absence of certain proteins in his/her blood plasma using the Least Absolute Shrinkage and Selection Operator (LASSO) regression implemented in glmnet package [31]. We performed 10 iterations, each time randomly selecting 90% of the samples. For each iteration we needed to select the optimum value of LASSO tuning parameter lambda, which penalizes the sum of the absolute values of the coefficient. Optimum value of lambda was also selected by performing cross-validation (10 runs of 10-fold cross-validation cycle). The lambda with the minimum average error was selected as a lambda for the current iteration. Final model included only proteins, which were selected at every iteration (10 out of 10 times). Model performance was estimated as the median absolute error which was defined as the median of absolute differences between the true BMI and the predicted BMI.

3. Results and Discussion

3.1. Clinical Component

Much attention has been riveted on the phenomenon of metabolically healthy obesity (MHO), characterized by the absence of the metabolic abnormalities that traditionally accompany excess adiposity [32]. Thus, a substantial proportion of the obese subjects does not seem to be at an (at least temporarily, [33]) increased risk of mortality and metabolic complications of obesity. MHO is characterized by the absence of dyslipidemia, hypertension, insulin resistance, and chronic inflammation.

Moreover, lean subjects may possess abnormal metabolic parameters (exhibiting metabolically unhealthy non-obesity, MUNO) [34]. A gradient of metabolically healthy and unhealthy obese and lean phenotypes makes the revealing of abnormalities as well as relevant prevention of risks more difficult even for non-obese individuals.

To elucidate whether there is a bias to any of the selected extremes (four combinations of metabolic status and BMI) in our sample collection, we selected the monitored parameters of blood and anthropometric tests (Supplementary Table S1), which significantly differed between groups under study (NORM, OW, OB1, OB2, OB3). For these differed parameters, we performed a principal components analysis (Supplementary File S1) and hierarchical cluster analysis (Figure 1) using Ward's minimum variance. The results of cluster analysis were evaluated with the Adjusted Rand Index (ARI), which reflects an agreement between two partitions: one given by the clustering process and the other defined by external criteria.

In our case, ARI was equal to 0.051, which indicates a low similarity between resulting and expected clustering. According to the obtained result, it is not possible to explicitly define the boundaries between groups of subjects with different weight conditions under study.

The impossibility to unambiguously divide patients according to their weight conditions based only on the results of clinical tests once again emphasizes the controversial and considerably challenging nature of obesity and indicates the need for orthogonal data.

In our opinion, the most promising for solving this problem will be the transition to the proteome level and multiplex assessment of the patient's proteome landscape.

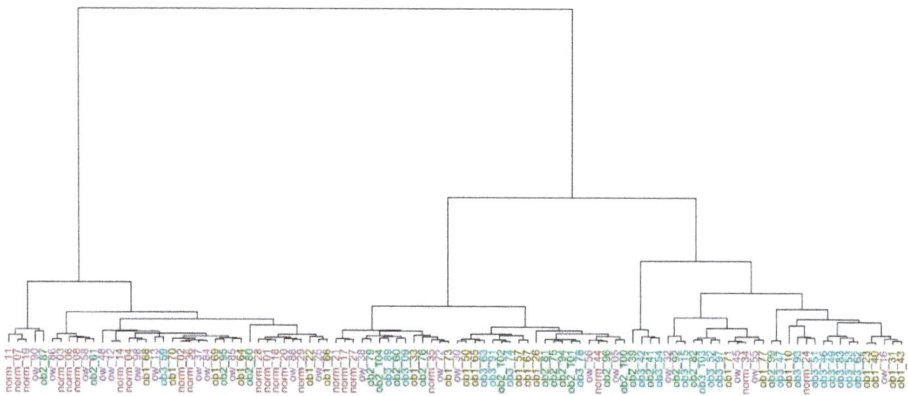

Figure 1. Visualization of the results of hierarchical cluster analysis of significantly different parameters of clinical and anthropometric tests performed for patients with different weight conditions. Sample IDs are presented as follows: group_number of the sample (NORM—normal weight, OW—overweight, OB1, 2, 3—obesity stage 1, 2, and 3, correspondingly).

3.2. Proteomic Component

In total, 154 proteins were reliably identified in the entire collection of plasma samples. These proteins are predominantly associated with peptidase activity, receptor binding, and lipid transporter activity. Most of the proteins are localized in blood microparticles or plasma lipoprotein particles and vesicles, and therefore we expect stable detection of them under various mass spectrometric protocols. Of those, 36 proteins were consistently found in all plasma samples under study. A total of 138 proteins were identified in the NORM group of lean subjects. A total of 148 proteins were identified in the integrated group of overweight (OW) and obese (OB1, OB2, OB3) samples.

Next, we performed a principal components analysis (Supplementary File S1) and studied possible relationships between the pattern of presence/absence of proteins in blood plasma and the patient's BMI using cluster analysis.

Preliminarily, unrepresentative proteins (identified in a single sample in the collection) and non-specific proteins (identified in all samples) were excluded from the calculations. The data matrix consisted of 104 rows (samples) and 101 columns (proteins).

The pattern of 15 proteins (namely, P07225, P00748, P07357, P07358, P09871, P01591, P01861, O43866, P00736, P02654, P13671, P25311, P01619, P01859, and P29622) allows to distinguish (Figure 2a) a group of 14 samples with increased BMI (mean 39 vs 33, p-value = 0.002). Moreover, 11 of them belong to the OB2 and OB3 groups, and three samples were obtained from overweight individuals. It should be noted that these three patients from OW were diagnosed with blood lipids disorder (there are seven samples with such a diagnosis in the whole OW group). Half of the samples from the OB2 and OB3 groups were also characterized by this diagnosis. As part of a pattern of 15 proteins for 5 (P07225 [35], O43866 [36,37], P02654 [38], P25311 [39–41], P29622 [42]) the association with the obesity was shown. It is noteworthy that five of these 15 proteins are complement components, included in two complexes: P07358, P07357, and P13671 organize membrane attack complex (MAC), that plays a key role in the innate and adaptive immune response, and P09871 and P00736 combine with serine protease to form the first component of the classical and less variable pathway of the complement system, also associated with obesity [43,44].

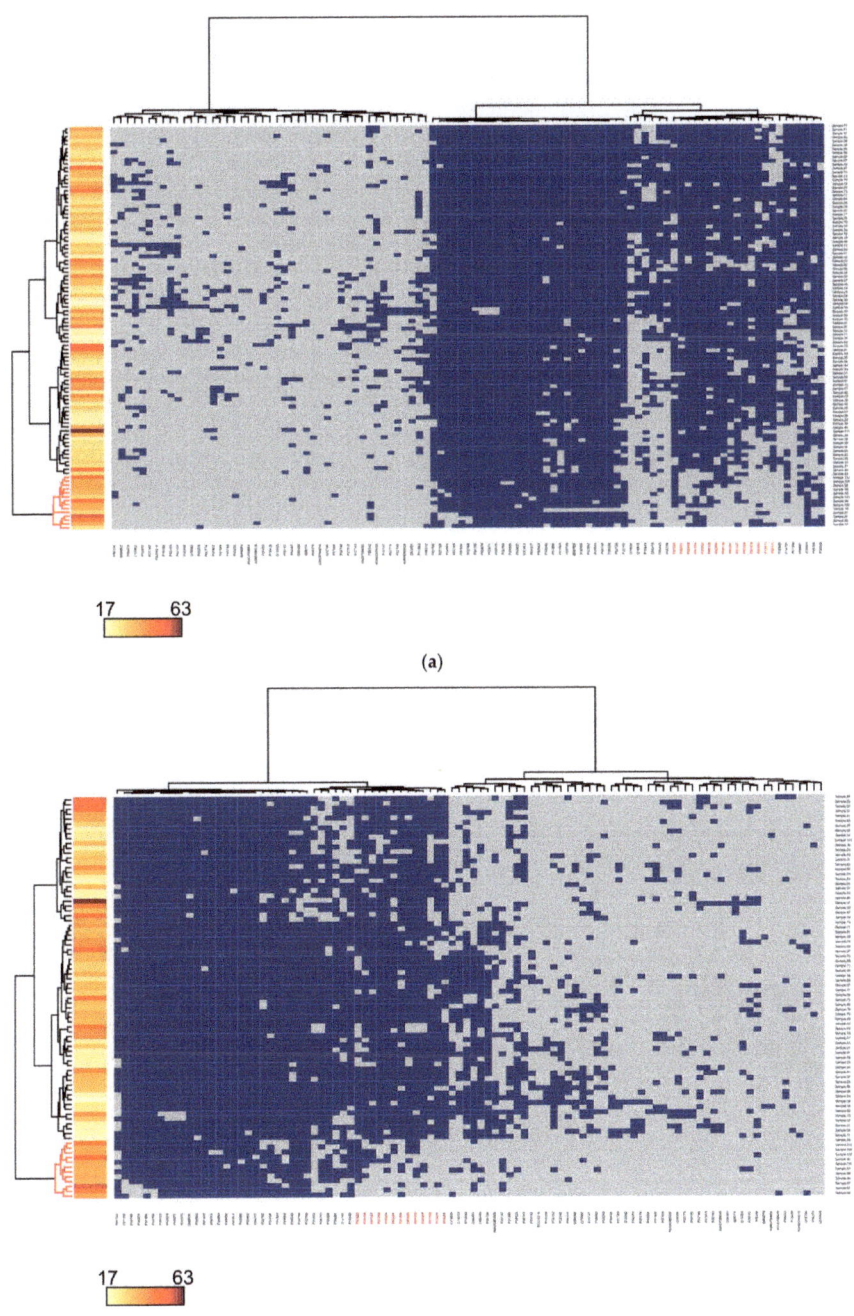

Figure 2. Cluster analysis of the presence/absence patterns of (**a**) 101 proteins (columns) in 104 blood plasma samples (rows) for all 104 samples under study (rows) and (**b**) 98 proteins (columns) in 83 samples, excluding plasma samples obtained from overweight individuals. The color bar indicates BMI.

The collection of the samples under study contains blood plasma from overweight patients with an increased body mass index (OW), but not exceeding the threshold values required for the diagnosis of obesity, which could affect the results of cluster analysis. In this respect, we removed from consideration 21 samples from the borderline OW group, as a result, the total number of identified proteins remained practically unchanged, as well as the set of proteins common for the two—NORM and OB—groups. The updated matrix consisted of 83 rows (samples) and 98 columns (proteins) plotted with the same parameters. Clustering indices improved slightly, so for the group with high BMI its mean value was 42, and for the rest—32 (p-value = 0.002, Figure 2b).

The composition of the cluster with high BMI practically did not change—three samples from the OW group left, and one image from the OB2 group was added. Accordingly, the pattern of specific proteins did not change significantly, it included 13 proteins, where 12, except two immunoglobulins (P01619 and P01859) and serpin (P29622), coincide with the results of the pattern of proteins according to the all-samples clustering. New in the resulting pattern is the component of the above MAC complex—P07360.

3.3. BMI Prediction

To assess the contribution of proteins to obesity, an attempt to predict the BMI of the sample based on proteomic data was performed. For this, using the LASSO method, we built a regression model predicting the BMI of a sample according to the pattern of presence/absence of proteins in blood plasma. The model based on all data consisted of five proteins (P08185, P0DJI8, P10643, P25311, and P35858), and the median absolute error (MAE) was 5.1 kg/m^2 (Figure 3a). At the same time, the model obtained on the basis of processing data excluding samples from the OW group showed a higher accuracy, MAE = 3.2 kg/m^2 (Figure 3b), and the number of proteins required to build the model was 18.

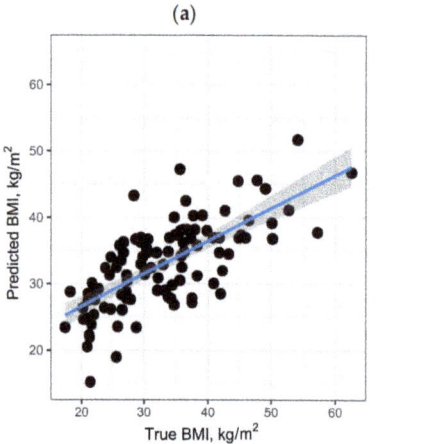
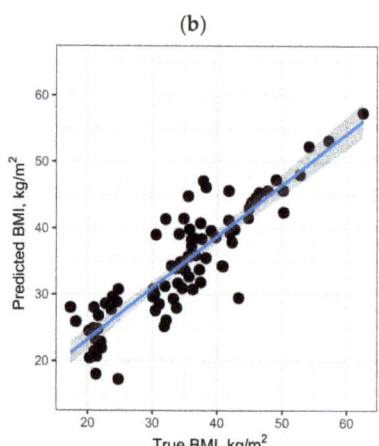

Figure 3. BMI prediction based on pattern of presence/absence of proteins for (**a**) all samples and for (**b**) collection without plasma samples obtained from overweight individuals.

It is noteworthy that the pattern of 18 proteins includes five proteins from the model with lower predictive power, as well as three previously considered proteins of the complement system (P00736, P07358, P07360) included in the MAC complex, which is indirectly associated with obesity [45].

Text-mining [29,30] performed for these proteins and their relations with pathological processes showed that 15 out of 18 proteins (Table 2) are associated to varying degrees with metabolic disorders, including obesity. For example, according to our model, the absence of sex hormone-binding globulin (P04278) correlates with increased BMI, which is confirmed by studies on its expression, where it was shown that inhibition of the corresponding gene leads to the development of obesity [46].

Table 2. Proteins included into predicting pattern and their association with obesity.

#	UniProt ID	Gene Name	References	Comment on the Association with Obesity
1	A0A0C4DH25	IGKV3D-20	-	-
2	P00736	C1R	[43,47]	High expression of complement components in omental adipose tissue
3	P00742	F10	[48,49]	Chronic low-grade inflammation, but is likely also due to direct effects of adipose tissue on mediators of coagulation
4	P01700	IGLV1-47	[50]	Differentially expressed gene in normal individuals and obese patients with breast cancer
5	P02655	APOC2	[51,52]	Cofactor for lipoprotein lipase, a plasma enzyme that hydrolyzes triglycerides/agent for obesity
6	P04278	SHBG	[46,53]	Decreased SHBG levels may be one of the components of the metabolic syndrome
7	P07358	C8B	[54]	Protein encoded by C8B gene and associated with complement activation was shared across diets indicating that a core set of proteins participate in tissue response to high-fat diet
8	P07360	C8G	[54]	Protein encoded by C8G gene and associated with complement activation was shared across diets indicating that a core set of proteins participate in tissue response to high-fat diet
9	P08185	SERPINA6	[55–59]	Corticosteroid-binding globulin polymorphism could influence obesity, metabolic, or hypothalamo-pituitary adrenal axis activity parameters
10	P0DJI8	SAA1	[60,61]	Major acute phase protein, correlating with obesity and insulin resistance in human
11	P10643	C7	[47]	Constituent of the membrane attack complex (MAC) that plays a key role in the innate and adaptive immune response by forming pores in the plasma membrane of target cells
12	P20742	PZP	-	PZP levels are individual-specific, do not correlate strongly with obesity
13	P22352	GPX3	[62–66]	GPX3 expression is significantly higher in lean compared to obese as well as in insulin-sensitive compared insulin-resistant individuals with obesity
14	P25311	AZGP1	[39–41,67–71]	AZGP1 stimulates lipid degradation in adipocytes and causes the extensive fat losses associated with some advanced cancers. May bind polyunsaturated fatty acids. Can promote the browning of white adipose tissue and can serve as a potential therapeutic target for treating metabolic diseases such as obesity. It is reduced in obesity, with a trend to further decrease with prediabetes and type 2 diabetes
15	P35858	IGFALS	[72]	IGFALS is involved in protein-protein interactions that result in protein complexes, receptor-ligand binding or cell adhesion. Children and adolescents with a variety of illnesses and metabolic disorders have altered circulating IGF-I and IGFBP levels. Circulating IGF and IGFBP levels overlap with normal values
16	P51884	LUM	[73]	LUM over-expression in visceral fat and liver resulted in improved insulin sensitivity and glucose clearance. Over-expression of LUM increases insulin sensitivity
17	Q06033	ITIH3	[43,74]	ITIH3 negatively correlated with obesity
18	Q96KN2	CNDP1	[75]	An increased risk for obesity/overweight due to genotypes of CNDP1 was observed only in the group with a low carotene/carbohydrate intake ratio. In the high carotene/carbohydrate intake group, the genotype of CNDP1 was no risk factor for obesity/overweight

Summarizing the above said, we can conclude that among the reliably and reliably detected proteins [76] in blood plasma, there is a pattern that has predictive power in the issue of obesity. The minimum pattern size is five proteins. Expanding the panel increases the level of BMI prediction accuracy, which can be critical in examining borderline states in metabolically healthy obese and unhealthy lean, and also provide researchers with additional information about body composition status even when exploring protein profiles from the patients with non-obesity disorders.

We would like to stress that our intention was not to build the perfect BMI prediction model (the dataset is quite limited for this task) but rather to point to some plasma proteins likely associated with obesity when analyzed together. We suppose that the further studies needed to elaborate on this issue will also allow detection of the transition from a "metabolically healthy" phenotype of the patient with a high BMI to an "unhealthy" one.

4. Conclusions

According to the authors' knowledge, no approved omics pattern has been developed to distinguish individuals at increased risk of obesity and its comorbidities. In the present study, we analyzed clinical and anthropometrical parameters of 104 subjects with different weight conditions. Each individual was also characterized by the profile of core proteins circulating through his/her blood plasma.

Our main conclusions were two-fold:

1. We demonstrated the impossibility to divide patients according to their weight conditions based only on the results of standard blood tests. Orthogonal, in our case—proteomic, data upgrades the level of understanding of the controversial nature of obesity.
2. Our overall results indicate that studies of proteins circulating in blood have the prediction power of the weight status of the patient under study. We composed two proteomic patterns (including 5 and 18 proteins, respectively), which provide additional information about the patient's phenotype for more personalized treatment.

We strongly believe that such proteomic patterns have great potential as warning labels, signaling about obesity-associated alterations, and, thus, improving early-stage therapy of both metabolically unhealthy obese and lean individuals.

Supplementary Materials: The following are available online at https://www.mdpi.com/2075-4426/11/2/64/s1, Table S1: Anthropometrical and clinical characteristic of individuals under study; File S1: Principal Components Analysis of clinical parameters and proteins identified in the samples of blood plasma.

Author Contributions: Conceptualization, E.A.P. and K.K.S.; sample collection, O.A.P., E.A.P. and E.V.I.; methodology, V.G.Z., V.A.A. and O.I.K.; data curation, V.A.A., O.I.K., E.V.P. and E.V.I.; writing, O.I.K., E.V.P., M.A.P. and V.A.A.; visualization, V.A.A. and M.A.P.; revision, O.I.K., V.A.A., E.V.P., M.A.P., K.K.S., D.B.N.; project administration and funding acquisition, E.A.P., A.V.L., V.A.T., D.B.N., A.I.A. All authors have read and agreed to the published version of the manuscript.

Funding: This research was funded by the Ministry of Science and Higher Education of the Russian Federation within the framework of state support for the creation and development of World-Class Research Centers "Digital biodesign and personalized healthcare" No. 075-15-2020-913.

Institutional Review Board Statement: The study was conducted according to the guidelines of the Declaration of Helsinki, and approved by the Institutional Ethics Committee of the Federal Research Centre of Nutrition, Biotechnology and Food Safety (protocol #4 from 15.06.2018).

Informed Consent Statement: Informed consent was obtained from all subjects involved in the study.

Data Availability Statement: The data presented in this study are available in PRIDE repository (dataset identifier PXD023526); Supplementary Materials are available via link https://zenodo.org/record/4432333#.YAbOw1X7QuU.

Acknowledgments: We would like to thank Alexandra M. Nazarova for her help in sample collection and annotation. We acknowledge the IBMC "Human Proteome" Core Facility for access to the computer cluster and assistance with the generation of mass spectrometry data.

Conflicts of Interest: The authors declare no conflict of interest.

References

1. Lifshitz, F.; Lifshitz, J.Z. Globesity: The root causes of the obesity epidemic in the USA and now worldwide. *Pediatr. Endocrinol. Rev.* **2014**, *12*, 17–34. [PubMed]
2. Obesity and Overweight. Available online: https://www.who.int/news-room/fact-sheets/detail/obesity-and-overweight (accessed on 9 December 2020).
3. Mechanick, J.I.; Apovian, C.; Brethauer, S.; Garvey, W.T.; Joffe, A.M.; Kim, J.; Kushner, R.F.; Lindquist, R.; Pessah-Pollack, R.; Seger, J.; et al. Clinical Practice Guidelines for the Perioperative Nutrition, Metabolic, and Nonsurgical Support of Patients Undergoing Bariatric Procedures—2019 Update: Cosponsored by American Association of Clinical Endocrinologists/American College of Endocrinology. *Endocr. Pract.* **2019**, *25*, 1346–1359. [CrossRef] [PubMed]
4. Srensen, T.I.A. Challenges in the study of causation of obesity. *Proc. Nutr. Soc.* **2009**, *68*, 43–54. [CrossRef] [PubMed]
5. Jackson, S.E.; Llewellyn, C.H.; Smith, L. The obesity epidemic—Nature via nurture: A narrative review of high-income countries. *SAGE Open Med.* **2020**, *8*, 205031212091826. [CrossRef] [PubMed]
6. Huang, P.L. A comprehensive definition for metabolic syndrome. *Dis. Model. Mech.* **2009**, *2*, 231–237. [CrossRef]
7. Magkos, F. Metabolically healthy obesity: What's in a name? *Am. J. Clin. Nutr.* **2019**, *110*, 533–537. [CrossRef]
8. Parente, E.B. Is body mass index still a good tool for obesity evaluation? *Arch. Endocrinol. Metab.* **2016**, *60*, 507–509. [CrossRef]
9. Poirier, P. Adiposity and cardiovascular disease: Are we using the right definition of obesity? *Eur. Heart J.* **2007**, *28*, 2047–2048. [CrossRef]
10. Kushner, R.F. Clinical assessment and management of adult obesity. *Circulation* **2012**, *126*, 2870–2877. [CrossRef]
11. Karahalil, B. Overview of Systems Biology and Omics Technologies. *Curr. Med. Chem.* **2016**, *23*, 4221–4230. [CrossRef]
12. Feskens, E.J.M.; Sluik, D.; Du, H. The Association Between Diet and Obesity in Specific European Cohorts: DiOGenes and EPIC-PANACEA. *Curr. Obes. Rep.* **2014**, *3*, 67–78. [CrossRef]
13. Larsen, T.M.; Dalskov, S.; Van Baak, M.; Jebb, S.; Kafatos, A.; Pfeiffer, A.; Martinez, J.A.; Handjieva-Darlenska, T.; Kunešová, M.; Holst, C.; et al. The diet, obesity and genes (diogenes) dietary study in eight European countries—A comprehensive design for long-term intervention. *Obes. Rev.* **2010**, *11*, 76–91. [CrossRef]
14. Goodarzi, M.O. Genetics of obesity: What genetic association studies have taught us about the biology of obesity and its complications. *Lancet Diabetes Endocrinol.* **2018**, *6*, 223–236. [CrossRef]
15. López-Villar, E.; Martos-Moreno, G.; Chowen, J.A.; Okada, S.; Kopchick, J.J.; Argente, J. A proteomic approach to obesity and type 2 diabetes. *J. Cell. Mol. Med.* **2015**, *19*, 1455–1470. [CrossRef] [PubMed]
16. Karczewski, J.; Śledzińska, E.; Baturo, A.; Jończyk, I.; Maleszko, A.; Samborski, P.; Begier-Krasińska, B.; Dobrowolska, A. Obesity and inflammation. *Eur. Cytokine Netw.* **2018**, *29*, 83–94. [CrossRef] [PubMed]
17. Cottam, D.R.; Mattar, S.G.; Barinas-Mitchell, E.; Eid, G.; Kuller, L.; Kelley, D.E.; Schauer, P.R. The chronic inflammatory hypothesis for the morbidity associated with morbid obesity: Implications and effects of weight loss. *Obes. Surg.* **2004**, *14*, 589–600. [CrossRef]
18. Kim, S.W.; Choi, J.W.; Yun, J.W.; Chung, I.S.; Cho, H.C.; Song, S.E.; Im, S.S.; Song, D.K. Proteomics approach to identify serum biomarkers associated with the progression of diabetes in Korean patients with abdominal obesity. *PLoS ONE* **2019**, *14*. [CrossRef]
19. Flegal, K.M. Body-mass index and all-cause mortality. *Lancet* **2017**, *389*, 2284–2285. [CrossRef]
20. The WHO STEPwise Approach to Noncommunicable Disease Risk Factor Surveillance. Available online: https://www.who.int/ncds/surveillance/steps/STEPS_Manual.pdf (accessed on 19 December 2020).
21. ProteoPrep®Immunoaffinity Albumin and IgG Depletion Kit. Available online: https://www.sigmaaldrich.com/content/dam/sigma-aldrich/docs/Sigma/Bulletin/protiabul.pdf (accessed on 9 December 2020).
22. Petushkova, N.A.; Zgoda, V.G.; Pyatnitskiy, M.A.; Larina, O.V.; Teryaeva, N.B.; Potapov, A.A.; Lisitsa, A. V Post-translational modifications of FDA-approved plasma biomarkers in glioblastoma samples. *PLoS ONE* **2017**, *12*, e0177427. [CrossRef]
23. Barsnes, H.; Vaudel, M. SearchGUI: A Highly Adaptable Common Interface for Proteomics Search and de Novo Engines. *J. Proteome Res.* **2018**, *17*, 2552–2555. [CrossRef]
24. Kiseleva, O.; Poverennaya, E.; Shargunov, A.; Lisitsa, A. Proteomic Cinderella: Customized analysis of bulky MS/MS data in one night. *J. Bioinform. Comput. Biol.* **2017**. [CrossRef] [PubMed]
25. Vaudel, M.; Burkhart, J.M.; Zahedi, R.P.; Oveland, E.; Berven, F.S.; Sickmann, A.; Martens, L.; Barsnes, H. PeptideShaker enables reanalysis of MS-derived proteomics data sets. *Nat. Biotechnol.* **2015**, *33*, 22–24. [CrossRef] [PubMed]
26. Perez-Riverol, Y.; Csordas, A.; Bai, J.; Bernal-Llinares, M.; Hewapathirana, S.; Kundu, D.J.; Inuganti, A.; Griss, J.; Mayer, G.; Eisenacher, M.; et al. The PRIDE database and related tools and resources in 2019: Improving support for quantification data. *Nucleic Acids Res.* **2019**, *47*, D442–D450. [CrossRef] [PubMed]
27. R Core Team. R: The R Project for Statistical Computing. Available online: https://www.r-project.org/ (accessed on 25 March 2020).
28. Brionne, A.; Juanchich, A.; Hennequet-Antier, C. ViSEAGO: A Bioconductor package for clustering biological functions using Gene Ontology and semantic similarity. *BioData Min.* **2019**, *12*, 16. [CrossRef] [PubMed]

29. Ponomarenko, E.; Lisitsa, A.; Ilgisonis, E.; Archakov, A. Construction of protein semantic networks using PubMed/MEDLINE. *Mol Biol.* **2010**, *44*, 152–161. [CrossRef]
30. Ilgisonis, E.; Lisitsa, A.; Kudryavtseva, V.; Ponomarenko, E. Creation of Individual Scientific Concept-Centered Semantic Maps Based on Automated Text-Mining Analysis of PubMed. *Adv. Bioinform.* **2018**, *2018*, 4625394. [CrossRef]
31. Friedman, J.; Hastie, T.; Tibshirani, R. Regularization paths for generalized linear models via coordinate descent. *J. Stat. Softw.* **2010**, *33*, 1–22. [CrossRef] [PubMed]
32. Blüher, M. Mechanisms in endocrinology: Are metabolically healthy obese individuals really healthy? *Eur. J. Endocrinol.* **2014**, *171*, R209–R219. [CrossRef]
33. Soriguer, F.; Gutiérrez-Repiso, C.; Rubio-Martín, E.; García-Fuentes, E.; Almaraz, M.C.; Colomo, N.; De Antonio, I.E.; De Adana, M.S.R.; Chaves, F.J.; Morcillo, S.; et al. Metabolically healthy but obese, a matter of time? Findings from the prospective pizarra study. *J. Clin. Endocrinol. Metab.* **2013**, *98*, 2318–2325. [CrossRef] [PubMed]
34. Rotar, O.; Boyarinova, M.; Orlov, A.; Solntsev, V.; Zhernakova, Y.; Shalnova, S.; Deev, A.; Konradi, A.; Baranova, E.; Chazova, I.; et al. Metabolically healthy obese and metabolically unhealthy non-obese phenotypes in a Russian population. *Eur. J. Epidemiol.* **2017**, *32*, 251–254. [CrossRef]
35. Kobayashi, M.; Mizuno, T.; Yuki, H.; Kambara, T.; Betsunoh, H.; Nukui, A.; Abe, H.; Fukabori, Y.; Yashi, M.; Kamai, T. Association between serum prostate-specific antigen level and diabetes, obesity, hypertension, and the laboratory parameters related to glucose tolerance, hepatic function, and lipid profile: Implications for modification of prostate-specific antigen threshold. *Int. J. Clin. Oncol.* **2020**, *25*, 472–478. [CrossRef] [PubMed]
36. Arai, S.; Miyazaki, T. Impacts of the apoptosis inhibitor of macrophage (AIM) on obesity-associated inflammatory diseases. *Semin. Immunopathol.* **2014**, *36*, 3–12. [CrossRef] [PubMed]
37. Tomita, T.; Arai, S.; Kitada, K.; Mizuno, M.; Suzuki, Y.; Sakata, F.; Nakano, D.; Hiramoto, E.; Takei, Y.; Maruyama, S.; et al. Apoptosis inhibitor of macrophage ameliorates fungus-induced peritoneal injury model in mice. *Sci. Rep.* **2017**, *7*, 6450. [CrossRef] [PubMed]
38. Westerterp, M.; Berbée, J.F.P.; Delsing, D.J.M.; Jong, M.C.; Gijbels, M.J.J.; Dahlmans, V.E.H.; Offerman, E.H.; Romijn, J.A.; Havekes, L.M.; Rensen, P.C.N. Apolipoprotein C-I binds free fatty acids and reduces their intracellular esterification. *J. Lipid Res.* **2007**, *48*, 1353–1361. [CrossRef]
39. Fan, G.; Dang, X.; Li, Y.; Chen, J.; Zhao, R.; Yang, X. Zinc-α2-glycoprotein promotes browning of white adipose tissue in cold-exposed male mice. *Mol. Cell. Endocrinol.* **2020**, *501*, 110669. [CrossRef]
40. Severo, J.S.; Morais, J.B.S.; Beserra, J.B.; dos Santos, L.R.; de Sousa Melo, S.R.; de Sousa, G.S.; de Matos Neto, E.M.; Henriques, G.S.; do Nascimento Marreiro, D. Role of Zinc in Zinc-α2-Glycoprotein Metabolism in Obesity: A Review of Literature. *Biol. Trace Elem. Res.* **2020**, *193*, 81–88. [CrossRef]
41. Hosseinzadeh-Attar, M.J.; Mahdavi-Mazdeh, M.; Yaseri, M.; Zahed, N.S.; Alipoor, E. Comparative Assessment of Serum Adipokines Zinc-α2-glycoprotein and Adipose Triglyceride Lipase, and Cardiovascular Risk Factors Between Normal Weight and Obese Patients with Hemodialysis. *Arch. Med. Res.* **2017**, *48*, 459–466. [CrossRef]
42. Quinton, R.; Duke, V.M.; Robertson, A.; Kirk, J.M.W.; Matfin, G.; De Zoysa, P.A.; Azcona, C.; MacColl, G.S.; Jacobs, H.S.; Conway, G.S.; et al. Idiopathic gonadotrophin deficiency: Genetic questions addressed through phenotypic characterization. *Clin. Endocrinol.* **2001**, *55*, 163–174. [CrossRef]
43. Zhang, J.; Wright, W.; Bernlohr, D.A.; Cushman, S.W.; Chen, X. Alterations of the classic pathway of complement in adipose tissue of obesity and insulin resistance. *Am. J. Physiol. Endocrinol. Metab.* **2007**, *292*. [CrossRef]
44. Cominetti, O.; Núñez Galindo, A.; Corthésy, J.; Valsesia, A.; Irincheeva, I.; Kussmann, M.; Saris, W.H.M.; Astrup, A.; McPherson, R.; Harper, M.E.; et al. Obesity shows preserved plasma proteome in large independent clinical cohorts. *Sci. Rep.* **2018**, *8*, 1–13. [CrossRef]
45. Shim, K.; Begum, R.; Yang, C.; Wang, H. Complement activation in obesity, insulin resistance, and type 2 diabetes mellitus. *World J. Diabetes* **2020**, *11*, 1–12. [CrossRef] [PubMed]
46. Hautanen, A. Synthesis and regulation of sex hormone-binding globulin in obesity. *Int. J. Obes.* **2000**, *24*, S64–S70. [CrossRef] [PubMed]
47. Gabrielsson, B.G.; Johansson, J.M.; Lönn, M.; Jernås, M.; Olbers, T.; Peltonen, M.; Larsson, I.; Lönn, L.; Sjöström, L.; Carlsson, B.; et al. High expression of complement components in omental adipose tissue in obese men. *Obes. Res.* **2003**, *11*, 699–708. [CrossRef] [PubMed]
48. Kornblith, L.Z.; Howard, B.; Kunitake, R.; Redick, B.; Nelson, M.; Cohen, M.J.; Callcut, R. Obesity and clotting: Body mass index independently contributes to hypercoagulability after injury. *J. Trauma Acute Care Surg.* **2015**, *78*, 30–36. [CrossRef]
49. Kaye, S.M.; Pietiläinen, K.H.; Kotronen, A.; Joutsi-Korhonen, L.; Kaprio, J.; Yki-Järvinen, H.; Silveira, A.; Hamsten, A.; Lassila, R.; Rissanen, A. Obesity-Related Derangements of Coagulation and Fibrinolysis: A Study of Obesity-Discordant Monozygotic Twin Pairs. *Obesity* **2012**, *20*, 88–94. [CrossRef]
50. Hassan, M.A.; Al-Sakkaf, K.; Shait Mohammed, M.R.; Dallol, A.; Al-Maghrabi, J.; Aldahlawi, A.; Ashoor, S.; Maamra, M.; Ragoussis, J.; Wu, W.; et al. Integration of Transcriptome and Metabolome Provides Unique Insights to Pathways Associated With Obese Breast Cancer Patients. *Front. Oncol.* **2020**, *10*, 804. [CrossRef]

51. Sakurai, T.; Sakurai, A.; Vaisman, B.L.; Amar, M.J.; Liu, C.; Gordon, S.M.; Drake, S.K.; Pryor, M.; Sampson, M.L.; Yang, L.; et al. Creation of apolipoprotein C-II (ApoC-II) mutant mice and correction of their hypertriglyceridemia with an ApoC-II mimetic peptides. *J. Pharmacol. Exp. Ther.* **2016**, *356*, 341–353. [CrossRef]
52. Wolska, A.; Dunbar, R.L.; Freeman, L.A.; Ueda, M.; Amar, M.J.; Sviridov, D.O.; Remaley, A.T. Apolipoprotein C-II: New findings related to genetics, biochemistry, and role in triglyceride metabolism. *Atherosclerosis* **2017**, *267*, 49–60. [CrossRef]
53. Cooper, L.A.; Page, S.T.; Amory, J.K.; Anawalt, B.D.; Matsumoto, A.M. The association of obesity with sex hormone-binding globulin is stronger than the association with ageing—Implications for the interpretation of total testosterone measurements. *Clin. Endocrinol.* **2015**, *83*, 828–833. [CrossRef]
54. Plubell, D.L.; Fenton, A.M.; Wilmarth, P.A.; Bergstrom, P.; Zhao, Y.; Minnier, J.; Heinecke, J.W.; Yang, X.; Pamir, N. GM-CSF driven myeloid cells in adipose tissue link weight gain and insulin resistance via formation of 2-aminoadipate. *Sci. Rep.* **2018**, *8*, 1–12. [CrossRef]
55. England, J.; Drouin, S.; Beaulieu, P.; St-Onge, P.; Krajinovic, M.; Laverdière, C.; Levy, E.; Marcil, V.; Sinnett, D. Genomic determinants of long-term cardiometabolic complications in childhood acute lymphoblastic leukemia survivors. *BMC Cancer* **2017**, *17*, s12885-s017. [CrossRef] [PubMed]
56. Barat, P.; Corcuff, J.B.; Tauber, M.; Moisan, M.P. Associations of glucocorticoid receptor and corticosteroid-binding globulin gene polymorphisms on fat mass and fat mass distribution in prepubertal obese children. *J. Physiol. Biochem.* **2012**, *68*, 645–650. [CrossRef] [PubMed]
57. Moisan, M.P. Genotype-phenotype associations in understanding the role of corticosteroid-binding globulin in health and disease animal models. *Mol. Cell. Endocrinol.* **2010**, *316*, 35–41. [CrossRef] [PubMed]
58. Barat, P.; Duclos, M.; Gatta, B.; Roger, P.; Mormede, P.; Moisan, M.P. Corticosteroid binding globulin gene polymorphism influences cortisol driven fat distribution in obese women. *Obes. Res.* **2005**, *13*, 1485–1490. [CrossRef]
59. Joyner, J.M.; Hutley, L.J.; Bachmann, A.W.; Torpy, D.J.; Prins, J.B. Greater replication and differentiation of preadipocytes in inherited corticosteroid-binding globulin deficiency. *Am. J. Physiol. Endocrinol. Metab.* **2003**, *284*, E1049–E1054. [CrossRef] [PubMed]
60. Blank, N.; Hegenbart, U.; Dietrich, S.; Brune, M.; Beimler, J.; Röcken, C.; Müller-Tidow, C.; Lorenz, H.M.; Schönland, S.O. Obesity is a significant susceptibility factor for idiopathic AA amyloidosis. *Amyloid* **2018**, *25*, 37–45. [CrossRef] [PubMed]
61. Wang, Y.; Cao, F.; Wang, Y.; Yu, G.; Jia, B.L. Silencing of SAA1 inhibits palmitate- or high-fat diet induced insulin resistance through suppression of the NF-κB pathway. *Mol. Med.* **2019**, *25*, 17. [CrossRef] [PubMed]
62. Langhardt, J.; Flehmig, G.; Klöting, N.; Lehmann, S.; Ebert, T.; Kern, M.; Schön, M.R.; Gärtner, D.; Lohmann, T.; Dressler, M.; et al. Effects of Weight Loss on Glutathione Peroxidase 3 Serum Concentrations and Adipose Tissue Expression in Human Obesity. *Obes. Facts* **2018**, *11*, 475–490. [CrossRef]
63. Yang, X.; Deignan, J.L.; Qi, H.; Zhu, J.; Qian, S.; Zhong, J.; Torosyan, G.; Majid, S.; Falkard, B.; Kleinhanz, R.R.; et al. Validation of candidate causal genes for obesity that affect shared metabolic pathways and networks. *Nat. Genet.* **2009**, *41*, 415–423. [CrossRef]
64. Jobgen, W.; Fu, W.J.; Gao, H.; Li, P.; Meininger, C.J.; Smith, S.B.; Spencer, T.E.; Wu, G. High fat feeding and dietary L-arginine supplementation differentially regulate gene expression in rat white adipose tissue. *Amino Acids* **2009**, *37*, 187–198. [CrossRef]
65. Yun, S.L.; Kim, A.Y.; Jin, W.C.; Kim, M.; Yasue, S.; Hee, J.S.; Masuzaki, H.; Kyong, S.P.; Jae, B.K. Dysregulation of adipose glutathione peroxidase 3 in obesity contributes to local and systemic oxidative stress. *Mol. Endocrinol.* **2008**, *22*, 2176–2189. [CrossRef]
66. Asayama, K.; Nakane, T.; Dobashi, K.; Kodera, K.; Hayashibe, H.; Uchida, N.; Nakazawa, S. Effect of obesity and troglitazone on expression of two glutathione peroxidases: Cellular and extracellular types in serum, kidney and adipose tissue. *Free Radic. Res.* **2001**, *34*, 337–347. [CrossRef] [PubMed]
67. Russell, S.T.; Tisdale, M.J. Role of β-adrenergic receptors in the anti-obesity and anti-diabetic effects of zinc-α2-glycoprotien (ZAG). *Biochim. Biophys. Acta Mol. Cell Biol. Lipids* **2012**, *1821*, 590–599. [CrossRef] [PubMed]
68. Zhu, H.J.; Dong, C.X.; Pan, H.; Ping, X.C.; Li, N.S.; Dai, Y.F.; Wang, L.J.; Yang, H.B.; Zhao, W.G.; Gong, F.Y. Rs4215 SNP in zinc-α2-glycoprotein gene is associated with obesity in Chinese north Han population. *Gene* **2012**, *500*, 211–215. [CrossRef]
69. Balaz, M.; Vician, M.; Janakova, Z.; Kurdiova, T.; Surova, M.; Imrich, R.; Majercikova, Z.; Penesova, A.; Vlcek, M.; Kiss, A.; et al. Subcutaneous adipose tissue zinc-α2-glycoprotein is associated with adipose tissue and whole-body insulin sensitivity. *Obesity* **2014**, *22*, 1821–1829. [CrossRef]
70. Ge, S.; Ryan, A.S. Zinc-α2-Glycoprotein expression in adipose tissue of obese postmenopausal women before and after weight loss and exercise + weight loss. *Metabolism* **2014**, *63*, 995–999. [CrossRef]
71. Liu, M.; Zhu, H.; Dai, Y.; Pan, H.; Li, N.; Wang, L.; Yang, H.; Yan, K.; Gong, F. Zinc-α2-glycoprotein is associated with obesity in Chinese people and HFD-induced obese mice. *Front. Physiol.* **2018**, *9*, 62. [CrossRef]
72. Wang, C.; Roy-Gagnon, M.-H.; Lefebvre, J.-F.; Burkett, K.M.; Dubois, L. Modeling gene-environment interactions in longitudinal family studies: A comparison of methods and their application to the association between the IGF pathway and childhood obesity. *BMC Med. Genet.* **2019**, *20*, 9. [CrossRef]
73. Wolff, G.; Taranko, A.E.; Meln, I.; Weinmann, J.; Sijmonsma, T.; Lerch, S.; Heide, D.; Billeter, A.T.; Tews, D.; Krunic, D.; et al. Diet-dependent function of the extracellular matrix proteoglycan Lumican in obesity and glucose homeostasis. *Mol. Metab.* **2019**, *19*, 97–106. [CrossRef]

74. Geyer, P.E.; Wewer Albrechtsen, N.J.; Tyanova, S.; Grassl, N.; Iepsen, E.W.; Lundgren, J.; Madsbad, S.; Holst, J.J.; Torekov, S.S.; Mann, M. Proteomics reveals the effects of sustained weight loss on the human plasma proteome. *Mol. Syst. Biol.* **2016**, *12*, 901. [CrossRef]
75. Albrecht, T.; Schilperoort, M.; Zhang, S.; Braun, J.D.; Qiu, J.; Rodriguez, A.; Pastene, D.O.; Krämer, B.K.; Köppel, H.; Baelde, H.; et al. Carnosine attenuates the development of both type 2 diabetes and diabetic nephropathy in BTBR ob/ob mice. *Sci. Rep.* **2017**, *7*, srep44492. [CrossRef] [PubMed]
76. Kiseleva, O.I.; Ponomarenko, E.A.; Romashova, Y.A.; Poverennaya, E.V.; Lisitsa, A.V. Detectability of plasma proteins in SRM measurements. *Curr. Proteom.* **2019**, *16*, 74–81. [CrossRef]

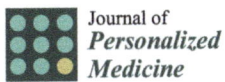

Article

The Mutation Spectrum of Maturity Onset Diabetes of the Young (MODY)-Associated Genes among Western Siberia Patients

Dinara E. Ivanoshchuk [1,2,*], Elena V. Shakhtshneider [1,2], Oksana D. Rymar [2], Alla K. Ovsyannikova [2], Svetlana V. Mikhailova [1], Veniamin S. Fishman [1], Emil S. Valeev [1], Pavel S. Orlov [1,2] and Mikhail I. Voevoda [1]

1 Federal Research Center Institute of Cytology and Genetics, Siberian Branch of Russian Academy of Sciences (SB RAS), Prospekt Lavrentyeva 10, 630090 Novosibirsk, Russia; shakhtshneyderev@bionet.nsc.ru (E.V.S.); mikhail@bionet.nsc.ru (S.V.M.); minja@bionet.nsc.ru (V.S.F.); emil@bionet.nsc.ru (E.S.V.); orlovpavel86@gmail.com (P.S.O.); mvoevoda@ya.ru (M.I.V.)
2 Institute of Internal and Preventive Medicine—Branch of Institute of Cytology and Genetics, SB RAS, Bogatkova Str. 175/1, 630004 Novosibirsk, Russia; orymar23@gmail.com (O.D.R.); aknikolaeva@bk.ru (A.K.O.)
* Correspondence: dinara@bionet.nsc.ru or dinara2084@mail.ru; Tel.: +7-(383)-363-4963; Fax: +7-(383)-333-1278

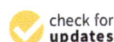

Abstract: Maturity onset diabetes of the young (MODY) is a congenital form of diabetes characterized by onset at a young age and a primary defect in pancreatic-β-cell function. Currently, 14 subtypes of MODY are known, and each is associated with mutations in a specific gene: *HNF4A*, *GCK*, *HNF1A*, *PDX1*, *HNF1B*, *NEUROD1*, *KLF11*, *CEL*, *PAX4*, *INS*, *BLK*, *KCNJ11*, *ABCC8*, and *APPL1*. The most common subtypes of MODY are associated with mutations in the genes *GCK*, *HNF1A*, *HNF4A*, and *HNF1B*. Among them, up to 70% of cases are caused by mutations in *GCK* and *HNF1A*. Here, an analysis of 14 MODY genes was performed in 178 patients with a MODY phenotype in Western Siberia. Multiplex ligation-dependent probe amplification analysis of DNA samples from 50 randomly selected patients without detectable mutations did not reveal large rearrangements in the MODY genes. In 38 patients (37% males) among the 178 subjects, mutations were identified in *HNF4A*, *GCK*, *HNF1A*, and *ABCC8*. We identified novel potentially causative mutations p.Lys142*, Leu146Val, Ala173Glnfs*30, Val181Asp, Gly261Ala, IVS7 c.864 −1G>T, Cys371*, and Glu443Lys in *GCK* and Ser6Arg, IVS 2 c.526 +1 G>T, IVS3 c.713 +2 T>A, and Arg238Lys in *HNF1A*.

Keywords: maturity onset diabetes of the young; MODY; diabetes mellitus; multiplex ligation-dependent probe amplification; next-generation sequencing; GCK; HNF1A; HNF4A; HNF1B; single-nucleotide variant; population

Citation: Ivanoshchuk, D.E.; Shakhtshneider, E.V.; Rymar, O.D.; Ovsyannikova, A.K.; Mikhailova, S.V.; Fishman, V.S.; Valeev, E.S.; Orlov, P.S.; Voevoda, M.I. The Mutation Spectrum of Maturity Onset Diabetes of the Young (MODY)-Associated Genes among Western Siberia Patients. *J. Pers. Med.* **2021**, *11*, 57. https://doi.org/10.3390/jpm11010057

Received: 10 December 2020
Accepted: 13 January 2021
Published: 18 January 2021

Publisher's Note: MDPI stays neutral with regard to jurisdictional claims in published maps and institutional affiliations.

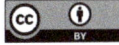

Copyright: © 2021 by the authors. Licensee MDPI, Basel, Switzerland. This article is an open access article distributed under the terms and conditions of the Creative Commons Attribution (CC BY) license (https://creativecommons.org/licenses/by/4.0/).

1. Introduction

Maturity onset diabetes of the young (MODY) is a congenital form of diabetes characterized by onset at a young age and a primary defect in pancreatic-β-cell function. This type of diabetes (OMIM # 606391) differs from classic types of diabetes mellitus (types 1 and 2, or T1DM and T2DM) in its clinical course, treatment strategies, and prognosis [1,2]. MODY is predominantly inherited in an autosomal dominant manner, but cases of spontaneous mutagenesis and germline mosaicism have been described [3,4]. MODY can be suspected [5] when hyperglycemia is detected in patients under 25–35 years of age, there is little or no need for insulin, secretion of C-peptide is intact, β-cell antibodies are absent, and dysfunction of pancreatic β-cells results in a decrease in the insulin amount. MODY patients usually have a normal body mass index. Currently, 14 subtypes of MODY are known, and each is associated with mutations in a specific gene: *HNF4A*, *GCK*, *HNF1A*, *PDX1*, *HNF1B*, *NEUROD1*, *KLF11*, *CEL*, *PAX4*, *INS*, *BLK*, *KCNJ11*, *ABCC8*, and *APPL1* [6]. The genes associated with MODY are presented in Table 1.

Table 1. The genes associated with maturity onset diabetes of the young (MODY).

MODY Type	Gene	Protein Name	Genomic Location GRCh37 (hg19)
MODY1	HNF4A	Hepatic Nuclear Factor 4 Alpha	chr20:42,984,340-43,061,485
MODY2	GCK	Glucokinase (Hexokinase 4)	chr7:44,183,870-44,237,769
MODY3	HNF1A	Hepatocyte Nuclear Factor 1-Alpha	chr12:121,416,346-121,440,315
MODY4	PDX1	Pancreatic and Duodenal Homeobox 1	chr13:28,494,157-28,500,451
MODY5	HNF1B	Hepatocyte Nuclear Factor 1-Beta	chr17:36,046,434-36,105,237
MODY6	NEUROD1	Neuronal Differentiation 1	chr2:182,537,815-182,545,603
MODY7	KLF11	Krüppel-Like Factor 11	chr2:10,182,976-10,194,963
MODY8	CEL	Carboxyl Ester Lipase	chr9:135,937,365-135,947,248
MODY9	PAX4	Paired Box 4	chr7:127,250,346-127,255,982
MODY10	INS	Insulin	chr11:2,181,009-2,182,571
MODY11	BLK	BLK Proto-Oncogene, Src Family Tyrosine Kinase	chr8:11,351,510-11,422,113
MODY12	ABCC8	ATP-Binding Cassette Subfamily C Member 8	chr11:17,414,432-17,498,449
MODY13	KCNJ11	Potassium Inwardly Rectifying Channel Subfamily J Member 11	chr11:17,406,795-17,410,878
MODY14	APPL1	Adaptor Protein, Phosphotyrosine Interacting with PH Domain and Leucine Zipper 1	chr3:57,261,765-57,307,499

The most common subtypes of MODY are associated with mutations in the genes GCK, HNF1A, HNF4A, and HNF1B [7]; among them, up to 70% of cases are caused by mutations in GCK and HNF1A [8]. Clinical manifestations of MODY are diverse and may vary even among members of the same family, i.e., carriers of identical mutations. This phenotypic variation is due to the interaction of the mutations with different genetic backgrounds and with environmental factors (e.g., the lifestyle) [9]. Identification of mutations causing MODY is important for early diagnosis of the disease in first-degree relatives of a proband. Up to 80% of MODY cases remain undetected or are misdiagnosed as T1DM or T2DM, resulting in incorrect treatment, including unjustified insulin therapy and its complications [1]. Next-generation sequencing (NGS) is most commonly used in MODY diagnostics and allows for simultaneous analysis of numerous genes and for the identification of single-nucleotide variants (SNVs) or small deletions or insertions, which constitute the majority of the known mutations causing this disease [10]. Nonetheless, large rearrangements in MODY-associated genes have been described, including heterozygosity of a complete HNF1B deletion [11,12], detected by multiplex ligation-dependent probe amplification (MLPA). This method makes it possible to detect variations in the copy number of a gene and accordingly is widely used in molecular diagnostics of diseases whose pathogenesis is associated with deletions or duplications of certain genomic regions [13]. The purpose of the present study was to determine the spectrum of genetic variants in patients with a MODY phenotype in Russia (Western Siberia) by whole-exome sequencing, targeted sequencing, and MLPA.

2. Materials and Methods

2.1. Patients

The study protocol was approved by the Ethics Committee of the Institute of Internal and Preventive Medicine- branch of the Institute of Cytology and Genetics, SB RAS, Novosibirsk, Russia, protocol number 7, 22 June 2008. Written informed consent to be examined and to participate in the study was obtained from each patient or his/her parent or legal guardian.

A total of 178 unrelated patients aged 4 to 35 years (23.4 ± 11.1 years [mean $\pm$ SD]; 41.7% males) with a MODY phenotype and 140 available family members were enrolled in this study (Figure 1).

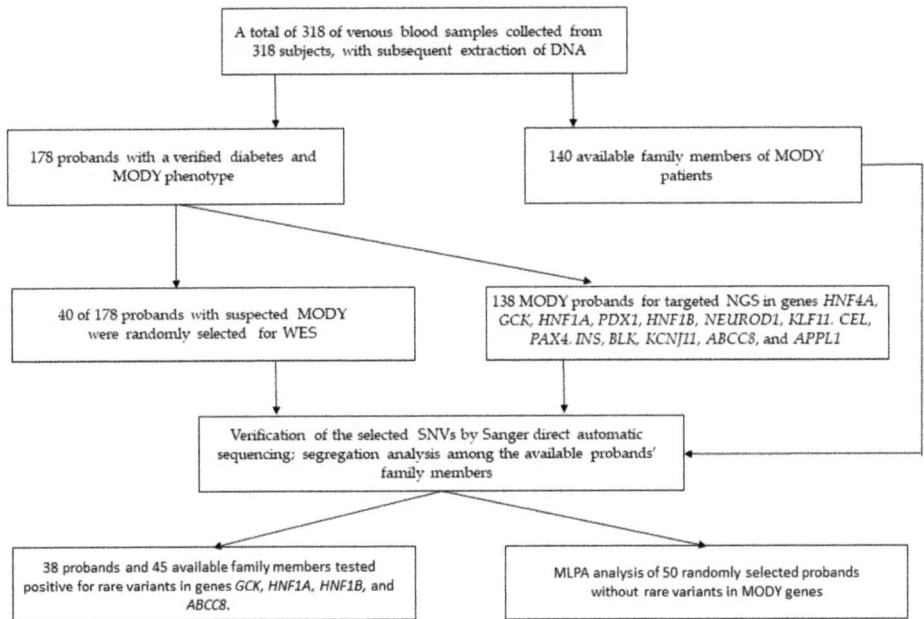

Figure 1. The study design. DNA: deoxyribonucleic acid, MLPA: multiplex ligation-dependent probe amplification, MODY: maturity onset diabetes of the young, SNV: single-nucleotide variant, WES: whole-exome sequencing.

All 178 probands were examined in the Clinical Department of the Institute of Internal and Preventive Medicine from the year 2014 to 2020. The probands were referred for molecular genetic testing if they met the following criteria: a verified diagnosis of diabetes [according to the criteria of the American Diabetes Association: HbA1C ≥6.5%, or fasting plasma glucose ≥126 mg/dL (7.0 mmol/L), or 2-h plasma glucose ≥200 mg/dL (11.1 mmol/L) during an oral glucose tolerance test (in the absence of unequivocal hyperglycemia; the result should be confirmed by repeat testing), or a patient with classic symptoms of hyperglycemia or hyperglycemic crisis with a random plasma glucose ≥200 mg/dL (11.1 mmol/L)] [14]; a debut of the disease in probands at the age of 35 years or earlier; a family history of diabetes mellitus; the absence of obesity; the absence of antibodies against pancreas islet cells and glutamic acid decarboxylase; intact secretory function of β-cells; normal or mildly reduced C-peptide levels; no need for insulin therapy; and the absence of ketoacidosis at the onset of the disease. Patients with clinical features of untypical diabetes (differing from those of T1DM and T2DM) and, in some cases, lacking a family history were included in this study because MODY can be occasionally caused by de novo mutations [3,4]. Patients with a history of tuberculosis, infection with the human immunodeficiency virus, an infectious disease caused by hepatitis B or C virus that required antiviral treatment, or substance abuse or alcoholism in the 2 years before the examination were excluded from this study. The studied MODY group may have included patients with MODY, patients with T1DM and negative test results on antibodies, and patients with early-onset T2DM.

2.2. Isolation of Genomic DNA

Genomic DNA was isolated from venous blood leukocytes by phenol–chloroform extraction [15].

2.3. Genome Library Preparation and Sequencing

At the first stage, exome sequencing was performed on 40 randomly selected probands from the MODY group. The exome sequencing was carried out on an Illumina HiSeq 1500 instrument (Illumina, San Diego, CA, USA). The enrichment and library preparation were performed using the SureSelectXT Human All Exon v.5 + UTRs Kit. Whole-exome libraries were prepared with the AmpliSeq Exome Kit (Thermo Fisher Scientific, Walthamm, MA, USA). On the DNA samples from the other patients (138 unrelated probands), we performed targeted sequencing. In the target panel, we included coding parts and adjacent splicing sites of the following MODY-associated genes: *HNF4A, GCK, HNF1A, PDX1, HNF1B, NEUROD1, KLF11, CEL, PAX4, INS, BLK, KCNJ11, ABCC8,* and *APPL1*. Oligodeoxynucleotide probes and the KAPA HyperPlus Kit (Roche, Basel, Switzerland) were used to prepare libraries at the Genomics Multi-Access Center (Institute of Cytology and Genetics, SB RAS, Novosibirsk, Russia). The quality of the analyzed DNA and of the prepared libraries was evaluated by means of a capillary electrophoresis system, the Agilent 2100 Bioanalyzer (Agilent Technologies Inc., Santa Clara, CA, USA). Analysis of each fully prepared library was conducted on the Illumina MiSeq platform (Illumina, San Diego, CA, USA).

2.4. Bioinformatic Analysis

The sequence reads were mapped to the reference human genome (GRCh37/hg19) via the Burrow–Wheeler Alignment tool (BWA v.0.7.17) [16]. Polymerase chain reaction (PCR)-generated duplicates were removed with MarkDuplicates of PicardTools (https://gatk.broadinstitute.org/hc/en-us). Base quality recalibration and searches for SNVs were conducted using Genome Analysis Toolkit (GATK) v.3.3, with BaseRecalibration and HaplotypeCaller tools, respectively; variant calling included local remapping of short insertions/deletions and correction of base quality [17].

The depth of coverage was 34× to 53×. SNVs with genotype quality scores <20 were filtered out and excluded from further analysis. In sequenced groups, we kept sequence variants if they were present in 10 or more variant reads with a quality score $\geq$20. Annotation of the SNVs was performed in the ANNOVAR (ANNOtate VARiation) software [18] with the help of populational data gnomAD [19] as a basic source and databases for several specific populations, such as The Greater Middle East (GME) Variome Project (http://igm.ucsd.edu/gme/), ABraOM: Brazilian genomic variants (http://abraom.ib.usp.br/), Korean Personal Genome Project (http://opengenome.net/Main_Page), other available data from populations and data on clinical significance (ClinVar) [20], and the Human Gene Mutation Database (HGMD) [10]; literature data were taken into account too.

Possible functional effects of SNVs were assessed in the dbNSFP database (https://sites.google.com/site/jpopgen/dbNSFP), aggregating data from 37 in silico prediction tools (SIFT, Polyphen2, MutationTaster2, PROVEAN, and others), nine conservation scores (e.g., PhyloP, phastCons, GERP++, and SiPhy), and data on population frequencies. Thresholds for prediction scores were set according to respective authors' recommendations; for the conservation ratio, we set one single threshold at 0.7, which means that a variant can be considered conserved if its predicted conservation score is greater than the scores of 70% variants.

Variants described in ClinVar, Leiden Open Variation Database (https://www.lovd.nl/), or predicted in silico as benign (B) or likely benign (LB) as well as variants with minor allele frequency higher than 0.01% in any of the population databases listed above were excluded from the analysis. The pathogenicity of each novel candidate mutation was assessed according to the recommendations of the American College of Medical Genetics and Genomics (ACMG) and the Association for Molecular Pathology [21]. Using these criteria, we also assessed two variants (p.Val590Met in the *HNF1A* gene in proband P81 and p.Ala173Thr in the *GCK* gene in P90) previously reported without any description of a phenotype (Table 2).

Table 2. The genetic variants identified in Western Siberia patients with a phenotype of maturity onset diabetes of the young (MODY).

Patient ID, Gender	Gene	Variant Status	Nucleotide Changes *	Amino Acid Changes	Location	Genotype	Minor Allele Frequency (gnomAD)	dbSNP ID	ClinVar Variation ID	HGMD	Pathogenicity According to ACMG [21], Evidence	LOVD Database ID	Segregation with Phenotype in Family
P6, Female P50, Male	GCK	Known	c.106C>T	p.Arg36Trp	Exon 2	Heterozygous Heterozygous	0.000014	rs762263694	431973	CM940823	PR	GCK_000007	Yes Yes
P59, Female	GCK	Known	c.110T>C	p.Met37Thr	Exon 2	Heterozygous	NA	NA	NA	NA	PR	GCK_000100	Yes
P17, Female	GCK	Known	c.130G>A	p.Gly44Ser	Exon 2	Heterozygous	NA	rs267601516	76898	CM013265	PR	GCK_000029	Yes
P74, Female	GCK	Known	c.238G>A	p.Gly80Ser	Exon 3	Heterozygous	NA	rs1554335761	449415	CM970630	PR	NA	Yes
P51, Male	GCK	Novel	c.424A>T	p.Lys142*	Exon 4	Heterozygous	NA	NA	NA	NA	Pathogenic, PVS1, PM2, PM1, PP1	NA	Yes
P4, Male	GCK	Novel	c.436C>G	p. Leu146Val	Exon 4	Heterozygous	NA	NA	NA	NA	Pathogenic, PS1, PS3, PM2, PP1	NA	Yes
P10, Male	GCK	Known	c.449T>A	p. Phe150Tyr	Exon 4	Heterozygous	NA	rs193922297	129142	CM097114	PR	NA	Yes
P86, Female	GCK	Novel	c.517_520del	p.Ala173Glnfs*30	Exon 5	Heterozygous	NA	NA	NA	NA	Pathogenic, PVS1, PS1, PM2, PM4, PP1, PP3	NA	Yes
P90, Male	GCK	Known	c.517G>A	p.Ala173Thr	Exon 5	Heterozygous	NA	NA	NA	NA	Pathogenic, PS1, PM2, PM5, PP1, PP3	GCK_000217	Yes
P80, Female P46, Female	GCK	Novel	c.542T>A	Val181Asp	Exon 5	Heterozygous Heterozygous	NA	NA	NA	NA	Pathogenic, PS1, PM2, PM5, PP1, PP3	NA	Yes Yes
P14, Female	GCK	Known	c.580-1G>A	-	Intron 5	Heterozygous	NA	rs1554335421	449414	CS052048	PR	NA	Yes
P30, Female	GCK	Known	c.660C>A	p.Cys220*	Exon 6	Heterozygous	NA	NA	NA	CM020443	PR	NA	Yes
P68, Female	GCK	Known	c.700T>C	p.Tyr234His	Exon 7	Heterozygous	NA	NA	NA	CM096864	PR	NA	Yes
P40, Female	GCK	Known	c.752T>C	p. et251hr	Exon 7	Heterozygous	NA	rs193922326	36251	CM096876	PR	NA	Yes
P67, Male	GCK	Known	c.755G>A	p.Cys252Tyr	Exon 7	Heterozygous	NA	NA	NA	CM021266	PR	NA	NA
P83, Male	GCK	Known	c.771G>A	p.Trp257*	Exon7	Heterozygous	NA	NA	NA	NA	Reported in [22]	NA	NA
P3, Male P77, Female	GCK	Known	c.772G>T	p.Gly258Cys	Exon 7	Heterozygous	NA	rs1583596378	804857	CM032578	PR	NA	NA Yes
P88, Female	GCK	Novel	.782G>C	p.Gly261Ala	Exon 7	Heterozygous	NA	NA	NA	NA	Pathogenic, PVS1, PM5, PP3	NA	Yes
P54, Male	GCK	Novel	c.864-1G>T	-	Intron 7	Heterozygous	NA	NA	NA	NA	Pathogenic, PVS1, PM2, PP1, PP3	NA	Yes
P57, Male	GCK	Novel	c.1113C>A	p.Cys371*	Exon 9	Heterozygous	NA	NA	NA	NA	Pathogenic, PVS1, PS1, PM1, PM2, PM5, PP1	NA	Yes
P70, Female	GCK	Known	c.1120G>A	p.Val374Met	Exon 9	Heterozygous	NA	rs1415041911	447380	CM096927	PR	NA	Yes
P61, Female	GCK	Known	c.1148C>A	p.Ser383*	Exon 9	Heterozygous	0.0000042	rs777870079	NA	CM032579	PR	NA	Yes

Table 2. Cont.

Patient ID, Gender	Gene	Variant Status	Nucleotide Changes *	Amino Acid Changes	Location	Genotype	Minor Allele Frequency (gnomAD)	dbSNP ID	ClinVar Variation ID	HGMD	Pathogenicity According to ACMG [21], Evidence	LOVD Database ID	Segregation with Phenotype in Family
P87, Male	GCK	Novel	c.1327G>A	p.Glu443Lys	Exon 10	Heterozygous	NA	NA	NA	NA	Likely pathogenic, PM1, PM2, PP2, PP3	NA	NA
P19, Female	HNF1A	Novel	c.18C>G	p.Ser6Arg	Exon 1	Heterozygous	NA	NA	NA	NA	Likely pathogenic, PS4, PM2, PP1, PP2, PP3	NA	Yes
P11, Female	HNF1A	Known	c.185A>G	p.Asn62Ser	Exon 1	Heterozygous	0.00012	rs3771129682	447485	CM064300	PR	HNF1A_000235	NA
P34, Female	HNF1A	Novel	c.526 +1G>T	-	Intron 2	Heterozygous	NA	NA	NA	NA	Pathogenic, PVS1, PM2, PP1, PP2, PP3	NA	Yes
P65, Female	HNF1A	Known	c.608G>A	p.Arg203His	Exon 3	Heterozygous	0.000008	rs587780357	129235	CM993816	PR	HNF1A_000137	Yes
P91, Female	HNF1A	Novel	c.713G>A	p.Arg238Lys	Exon 3	Heterozygous	NA	NA	NA	NA	Likely pathogenic, PS1, PM2, PP2, PP3	NA	NA
P78, Male	HNF1A	Novel	c.713 +2T>A	-	Intron 3	Heterozygous	NA	NA	NA	NA	Pathogenic, PVS1, PM2, PP1, PP2, PP3	NA	Yes
P82, Female	HNF1A	Known	c.779C>T	p.Thr260Met	Exon 4	Heterozygous	0.0000040	rs886039544	265436	CM971457	PR	HNF1A_000148	NA
P16, Female	HNF1A	Known	c.1522G > A	p.Glu508Lys	Exon 6	Heterozygous	0.00044	rs463353044	135665	CM082841	PR	HNF1A_000214	NA
P81, Male	HNF1A	Known	c.1768G>A	p.Val590Met	Exon 9	Heterozygous	0.0000042	rs1168108747	447484	NA	Uncertain significance, PM2, PP1, PP2, PP3	NA	Yes
P73, Male	HNF1A ABCC8	Known Known	c.160C>T c.1562G>A	p.Arg54* p.Arg521Gln	Exon 1 Exon 10	Heterozygous Heterozygous	0.0000042 0.000095	rs766956862 rs3681114790	805632 157683	CM032035 CM1212138	PR PR	HNF1A_000220 ABCC8_000172	Yes
P12, Male	ABCC8	Known	c.4369G>C	p.Ala1457Thr	Exon 36	Heterozygous	NA	rs72559717	NA	CM011260	PR	NA	Yes
P27, Female	HNF1B	Known	c.1006C>G	p.His336Asp	Exon 4	Heterozygous	0.0002	rs138986885	595653	CM067046	PR	HNF1B_000125	No

* RefSeq reference transcript: GCK (NM_000162.5), ABCC8 (NM_000352.3), HNF1B (NM_000458.2), and HNF1A (NM_000545.6). HGMD: Human Genome Mutation Database; LOVD database: Leiden Open Variation Database; NA: not available; PR: previously reported to be associated with a pathological phenotype (in the literature, in LOVD, ClinVar, or HGMD) and was not classified according to ACMG recommendations [21]. Variants identified for the first time are boldfaced.

To identify pathogenic variants at potential splice sites, we performed in silico testing, using dbscSNV (http://www.liulab.science/dbscsnv.html) for splice sites and regSNP-intron (https://regsnps-intron.ccbb.iupui.edu/) for both intronic and splice-altering SNVs. Nevertheless, these databases can be only a supplementary tool for the estimation of variant pathogenicity, in addition to the population and clinical data.

2.5. Verification Analysis

All selected SNVs were verified by Sanger direct automatic sequencing on an ABI 3500 DNA sequencer (Thermo Fisher Scientific, USA) by means of the BigDye Terminator v3.1 Cycle Sequencing Kit (Thermo Fisher Scientific, USA). Primer design for the selected SNVs was performed in the Primer-Blast software (https://www.ncbi.nlm.nih.gov/tools/primer-blast/).

At the second stage, segregation analysis was performed on the selected variants (novel and previously described) in the probands' family members available for the analysis.

2.6. MLPA Analysis

The third stage included an MLPA analysis of DNA samples from 50 randomly selected patients without detectable mutations in MODY-associated genes to search for major structural rearrangements (deletions and duplications). MLPA was performed using SALSA MLPA Probemix P241 MODY Mix 1 (MRC-Holland, Amsterdam, Netherlands), containing 52 specific MLPA probes for four genes: *HNF4A*, *GCK*, *HNF1A*, and *HNF1B* (https://www.mrcholland.com/product/P241/2528). The reaction was carried out in accordance with the manufacturer's recommendations. The resulting amplification products were detected by capillary electrophoresis on an ABI 3500 DNA sequencer (Thermo Fisher Scientific, USA). The data were processed in the Coffalyser.Net software.

3. Results

In 40 probands with a MODY phenotype, whole-exome analysis was performed; in 138 probands, we analyzed exons and adjacent splice sites of MODY-associated genes: *HNF4A, GCK, HNF1A, PDX1, HNF1B, NEUROD1, KLF11, CEL, PAX4, INS, BLK, KCNJ11, ABCC8*, and *APPL1*. In this work, we ignored common genetic variants and did not assess their possible effects on the phenotype. The results are presented in Table 2. We did not find any rare pathogenic variants in genes *HNF4A, PDX1, NEUROD1, KLF11, CEL, PAX4, INS, BLK, KCNJ11*, and *APPL1*. In 38 patients (37% males) out of the 178 subjects, mutations were identified in *HNF4A, GCK, HNF1A*, and *ABCC8* (one in a compound heterozygous state and 37 in a heterozygous state). The vast majority of them were carriers of rare variants of the *GCK* gene (26 probands; 68.4%), and nine probands (26.3%) had mutations in the *HNF1A* gene; one male (2.6%) carried a pathogenic variant in the *ABCC8* gene, and one female was a carrier of a rare variant in *HNF1B*. One male patient (73) was a compound heterozygote on two previously described mutations: Arg54* in *HNF1A* and Arg521Gln in *ABCC8*.

In total, we identified 36 rare variants in the studied genes: 12 of them (33.3%) are described for the first time, and the rest are present in databases (LOVD, HGMD, ClinVar, and/or gnomAD) or are previously reported in the literature. Among the identified variants, only three (all located in the *GCK* gene) were found twice in unrelated patients. Probands 3 and 77 both were found to carry Gly258Cys, probands 46 and 80 to carry undescribed Val181Asp, and probands 6 and 50 to carry Arg36Trp in the *GCK* gene. All the novel variants proved to be likely pathogenic or pathogenic according to the ACMG criteria [21]. For 28 families with identified relevant variants, a segregation analysis was performed. For most patients, segregation of the identified mutations with pathogenic phenotypes was found among their relatives.

An exception was the His336Asp mutation in *HNF1B* in a patient (P27) with gestational diabetes. The same mutation was found in her normoglycemic mother and her daughter.

In 50 patients without mutations in the studied genes, the MLPA analysis did not reveal any structural abnormalities in the genes HNF4A, GCK, HNF1A, and HNF1B.

4. Discussion

Genetic diagnosis is an important step in clinical practice, especially for family screening of individuals with borderline or moderate carbohydrate metabolic disorders. Clinical manifestations of MODY differ among patients and do not allow us to identify the type of diabetes unambiguously; therefore, it is important to employ timely genetic diagnostics for the optimal choice of a treatment. In the present study, we searched for mutations in MODY-associated genes by combining an examination of clinical criteria with NGS (the latter method has been effectively used as a first-line screening test for MODY-associated mutations). Next, the identified mutations were verified by Sanger sequencing followed by cascade genetic screening of available family members. In a Siberian population, we have previously reported some of the mutations: c.580 –1G>A in GCK [23], Ser6Arg in HNF1A [24], and Ala1457Thr in ABCC8 [25]. Among the studied patients (all from Western Siberia), the predominance of subtypes MODY2 (68.4%) and MODY3 (26.3%) was demonstrated here. We found eight novel genetic variants in GCK and four novel variants in HNF1A in this work (Figure 2, Table 2).

Routine or accidental blood glucose testing is the main route of hyperglycemia detection in GCK-MODY. The disease is characterized by an insignificant increase in the fasting glucose level (well controlled without medication) and low prevalence of micro- and macrovascular complications of diabetes [2]. Encoded by the GCK gene, glucokinase B (GlkB, hexokinase IV) is the first enzyme in the glycolytic pathway and phosphorylates glucose in pancreatic β-cells [26].

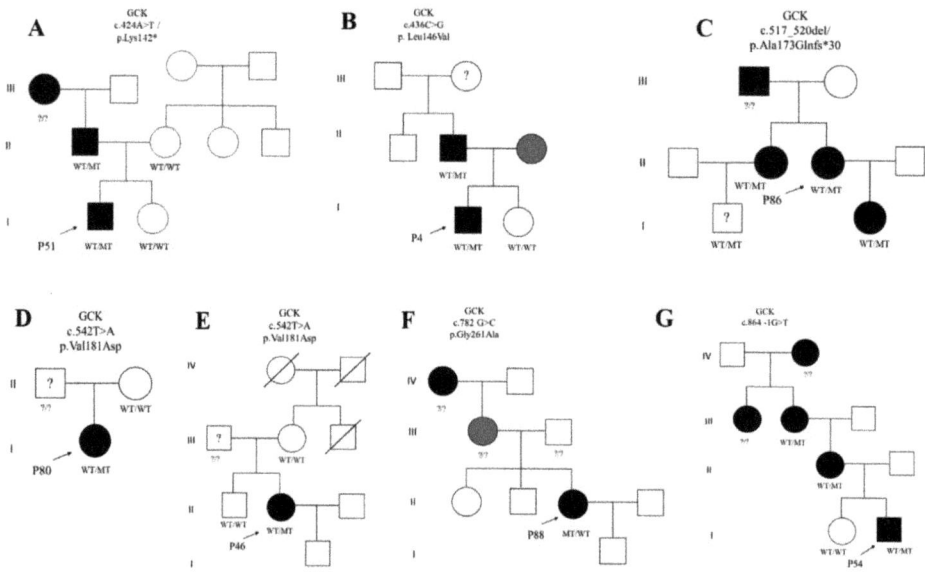

Figure 2. Cont.

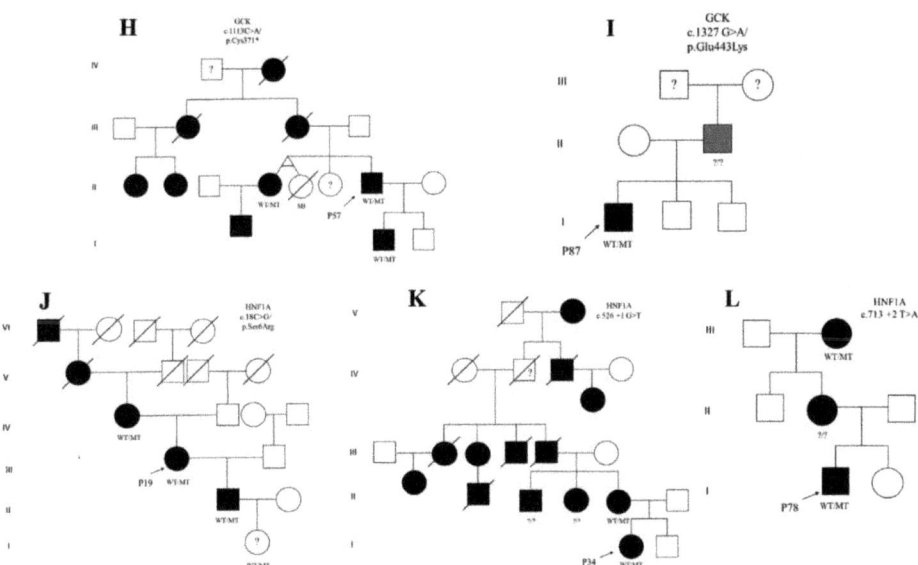

Figure 2. Screened MODY families (**A–L**) with novel identified variants in genes *GCK* and *HNF1A*. A grey filled symbol: a patient with prediabetes, MT: altered allele, SB: stillbirth, WT: wild type allele, ?/?: persons not genotyped, ?: a person with unknown health status. * RefSeq reference transcript: GCK (NM_000162.5), ABCC8 (NM_000352.3), HNF1B (NM_000458.2), and HNF1A (NM_000545.6).

The crystal structure of human glucokinase indicates that it has a large domain and small domain forming a deep cleft for glucose binding [27]. Amino acid residues 1–64 and 206–439 belong to the large domain, and residues 72–201 and 445–465 belong to the small domain; residues 65–71, 202–205, and 440–444 constitute three loops connecting the domains. Glucokinase is switched from an inactive to active conformation by ligand binding via a large rotation of the small domain [27,28]. Many mutations of this gene have been described (nonsense, missense, frameshift, and splice site mutations) in various populations [10]. Of note, all *GCK*-MODY patients have similar clinical phenotypes regardless of the mutation type [29].

p.Lys142* was found here in a 10-year-old boy (P51 in family A) with hyperglycemia. Lysine at codon 142 is adjacent to three basic amino acid residues (His-141, Lys-142, and Lys-143) that are phylogenetically conserved and form a positively charged surface. This basic patch in GlkB is believed to be a critical site for the binding of glucokinase-regulatory protein because substitutions at this site decrease this binding and nuclear entry of GlkB [30]. There are no reports on mutations in this codon in the literature.

The Leu146Val substitution is located in the small domain and was found in a 12-year-old male proband here (P4 in family B). Within codon 146, two other variants (Leu146Pro and Leu146Arg) have been described, both associated with MODY [10]. Research on enzyme kinetics has revealed that mutation Leu146Arg reduces enzymatic activity owing to decreased affinity for glucose [31].

A novel frameshift mutation, p.Ala173Glnfs*30, was identified here in family C with a MODY2 phenotype. Namely, this heterozygous deletion of four nucleotides in exon 5 was detected in a young woman 35 years of age (P86), in her son, and in her sibling. This AGGC deletion in codon 173 of the *GCK* gene changes the amino acid sequence and generates a premature stop codon at amino acid position 203. In our study, this variant segregated with the pathological phenotype in the proband and proband's daughter and sister. In view of the young age of the proband's nephew, monitoring of his carbohydrate metabolism parameters was recommended. Enzyme kinetics should be assessed to determine the functional basis of the disease.

In two unrelated female patients (P80 in family D and P46 in family E), a variant was found resulting in the replacement of valine in codon 181 with aspartic acid. In both families, the supposed carriers (fathers) of the Val181Ala variant were not available for the analysis; it turned out that healthy mothers of the probands and relatives of P46 are not carriers of this substitution. Val181Ala in a family of a MODY patient was described in Italy [32]. In the present study, a young patient (P88 in family F) with gestational diabetes mellitus and a family history of diabetes was found to have a previously undescribed missense substitution, Gly261Ala, in the *GCK* gene. Earlier, two substitution variants of this codon—Gly261Arg and Gly261Glu—were found in France [33,34], both associated with MODY.

Here, in a 2-year-old boy (P54 in family G) with hyperglycemia, the c.864 −1G>T substitution was identified in the acceptor site of *GCK* intron 7. This variant segregated with a pathological phenotype in the examined family members. Substitutions −1G>A and −1G>C at this position have been described in the United Kingdom and Czech Republic [35,36].

Several variants in codon Cys371 have been described [10]. We first identified a nonsense variant in this codon in patient P57 (family H). The substitution segregated with a pathological phenotype in other family members. Cys371 is a highly conserved amino acid residue located in the hydrophobic core of the protein [37], where it participates in disulfide bond formation [38].

It is known that L-arginine stimulates the production of glucose-6-phosphate and induces insulin secretion [39]. In a male patient (P87) in family I, the p.Glu443Lys variant was detected, which is involved in L-arginine binding and insulin secretion [39]. Glu443 is located in the α-13 helix of human GlkB [26]. During the domain reorganization between the active and inactive forms of the enzyme, helices α-13 and α-5 take part in the global conformational change [27].

Hepatocyte nuclear factor I homeobox A (HNF1A) is a transcription factor regulating the differentiation of pancreatic cells [40]. Mutations in the *HNF1A* gene are associated with MODY3, which is characterized by impaired insulin secretion, retention of sensitivity to sulfonylureas, and a decrease in the renal threshold for glucose. Cases of liver adenomatosis, renal dysplasia, and hypopituitarism in carriers of these mutations have been documented [41,42]. The clinical manifestations of MODY3 can vary within the same family and among unrelated mutation carriers. Moreover, carriers of *HNF1A* gene mutations may be normoglycemic, while their siblings can be hyperglycemic [43].

The Ser6Arg mutation of the *HNF1A* gene was found here in a family with diabetes mellitus in five generations [24] in proband P19 (family J). Another variant, c.526 +1 G>T in intron 2 of *HNF1A*, was detected in a 12-year-old patient (proband P34 in family K). She was found to have fasting hyperglycemia of 11.3 mmol/L and glycosuria of more than 55 mmol/L. In the proband's family, this variant segregated with a pathological phenotype and has not been described previously.

Proband P91 is a carrier of novel variant Arg238Lys. Two other substitutions at the same position, Arg238Met and Arg238Thr, have been previously described in the LOVD database as likely pathogenic (HNF1A_000306 and HNF1A_000417). One of them, Arg238Thr, is associated with MODY in the United Kingdom [44], and the other one, Arg238Met, is associated with hyperinsulinism diagnosed at birth (LOVD database). According to the proband, her ancestors had diabetes mellitus for three generations, but they were not available for analysis.

One of our young male patients (78 in family L) has substitution c.713 +2 T>A in intron 3 of the *HNF1A* gene. In an available relative of the proband, this mutation segregated with non-insulin-dependent diabetes mellitus and was found for the first time.

ATP-binding cassette superfamily transporter family C8 gene (*ABCC8*) encodes sulfonylurea receptor 1 (SUR1), which is a part of ATP-sensitive potassium channels on the islet β-cell membrane. Mutations in this gene can cause T2DM [45], a transient type of neonatal diabetes [46], neonatal diabetes [47], or MODY12 [6]. Previously, for the first time in Russia, we described the case of a patient with an *ABCC8* mutation [25]. In the current study, a 13-year-old male patient (73, family history is not shown) proved to be compound heterozygous on Arg521Gln of *ABCC8* and previously reported Arg54* of *HNF1A*. His mother, also with diabetes mellitus, has the same genotype. Elsewhere, the Arg521Gln substitution in the ABCC8 protein has been identified in a female with dominant hyperinsulinism [48] and in a case of a heterozygous carrier with diabetes [49]. In our case, neither the mother nor her son had any relevant complications.

A mutation in the *HNF1B* gene results in MODY5, which is characterized by reduced insulin secretion and usually a renal disease [50]. This gene plays the major part in the normal development of (and tissue-specific gene expression in) the kidneys, liver, pancreas, bile ducts, urogenital tract, lungs, thymus, and gut [50]. In patient P27 (family history is not shown), a diagnosis of gestational diabetes was made. Mutation His336Asp in *HNF1B* was detected in a proband and in her normoglycemic mother and daughter; no other *HNF1B*-associated clinical phenotypes, such as genital deformities or kidney involvement, were revealed in this proband [51]. The information on the pathogenicity of this variant is unclear. This mutation has been identified and categorized as pathogenic in two unrelated patients with severe renal anomalies, but healthy relatives of the patients are reported to be carriers of the mutation as well [52]. In another study, two out of three affected members from one family were carriers of this mutation, and it was found in one healthy individual [53]. In other studies, this variant was identified in a patient with suspected T1DM and absence of autoimmunity, but information about their parents was not available [54]. It is likely that the mutation does not have 100% penetrance and that other modulating pathological factors, including genetic ones, are required for disease manifestation.

In Russia, genetic screening of patients with MODY has been previously performed in the European part of Russia, and mutations in the *GCK* gene seem to be most prevalent among these MODY patients [55,56].

Direct sequencing of MODY genes is time-consuming and does not cover the entire spectrum of genes that can cause this type of diabetes. NGS techniques enable more efficient and cost-effective diagnosis of MODY subtypes [57]. High-tech sequencing also helps to determine the cause of a MODY phenotype if mutations in the genes known to be associated with MODY1–MODY14 are absent.

Limitations

This study has some limitations due to the unavailability of information about probands' family members (in some cases). This situation did not allow us to perform a segregation analysis of some rare potentially pathogenic variants identified in our patients (data not shown).

5. Conclusions

The spectrum of mutations in MODY genes was determined in a Western Siberian population by NGS. We believe that NGS techniques will lead to more effective and cost-efficient methods of MODY diagnosis. Apparently, mutations in the *GCK* gene are the predominant cause of MODY in Russia. We identified novel potentially causative mutations p.Lys142*, Leu146Val, Ala173Glnfs*30, Val181Asp, Gly261Ala, IVS7 c.864 −1G>T, Cys371*, and Glu443Lys in *GCK* and Ser6Arg, IVS 2 c.526 +1 G>T, IVS3 c.713 +2 T>A, and Arg238Lys in *HNF1A* (both are known MODY-associated genes). We did not find large rearrangements in MODY genes in a randomly selected cohort of 50 patients devoid of relevant point mutations.

Author Contributions: Conceptualization, M.I.V.; data curation, E.V.S., O.D.R., and A.K.O.; investigation, D.E.I.; methodology, D.E.I., E.S.V., and V.S.F.; project administration, M.I.V.; validation, S.V.M. and P.S.O.; writing—Original draft, D.E.I., E.V.S., E.S.V., and V.S.F.; writing—Review and editing, E.V.S. and S.V.M. All authors have read and agreed to the published version of the manuscript.

Funding: The collection of the samples and of clinical data and clinical examination were conducted as part of the main topic in state assignment No. AAAA-A17-117112850280-2, and NGS, Sanger sequencing, and bioinformatic analyses are financially supported as part of the publicly funded topic in state assignment No. AAAA-A19-119100990053-4.

Institutional Review Board Statement: The study protocol was approved by the Ethics Committee of the Institute of Internal and Preventive Medicine—Branch of the Institute of Cytology and Genetics, SB RAS, Novosibirsk, Russia, protocol number 7, 22 June 2008.

Informed Consent Statement: Informed consent was obtained from all subjects or his/her parent or legal guardian involved in the study.

Data Availability Statement: The data presented in this study are available on request from the corresponding author. The data are not publicly available due to privacy.

Acknowledgments: The authors thank the patients for the participation in this study.

Conflicts of Interest: The authors declare that they have no conflicts of interest related to the publication of this article.

References

1. Steele, A.M.; Shields, B.M.; Wensley, K.J.; Colclough, K.; Ellard, S.; Hattersley, A.T. Prevalence of vascular complications among patients with glucokinase mutations and prolonged, mild hyperglycemia. *JAMA* **2014**, *311*, 279–286. [CrossRef] [PubMed]
2. Murphy, R.; Ellard, S.; Hattersley, A.T. Clinical implication of a molecular genetic classification of monogenic β-cell diabetes. *Nat. Clin. Pract. Endocrinol. Metab.* **2008**, *4*, 200–213. [CrossRef]
3. Stanik, J.; Dusatkova, P.; Cinek, O.; Valentinova, L.; Huckova, M.; Skopkova, M.; Dusatkova, L.; Stanikova, D.; Pura, M.; Klimes, I.; et al. De novo mutations of GCK, HNF1A and HNF4A may be more frequent in MODY than previously assumed. *Diabetologia* **2014**, *57*, 480–484. [CrossRef] [PubMed]
4. Yorifuji, T.; Kurokawa, K.; Mamada, M.; Imai, T.; Kawai, M.; Nishi, Y.; Shishido, S.; Hasegawa, Y.; Nakahata, T. Neonatal diabetes mellitus and neonatal polycystic, dysplastic kidneys: Phenotypically discordant recurrence of a mutation in the hepatocyte nuclear factor-1beta gene due to germline mosaicism. *J. Clin. Endocrinol. Metab.* **2004**, *89*, 2905–2908. [CrossRef] [PubMed]
5. Shields, B.M.; McDonald, T.J.; Ellard, S.; Campbell, M.J.; Hyde, C.; Hattersley, A.T. The development and validation of a clinical prediction model to determine the probability of MODY in patients with young-onset diabetes. *Diabetologia* **2012**, *55*, 1265–1272. [CrossRef] [PubMed]
6. Firdous, P.; Nissar, K.; Ali, S.; Ganai, B.A.; Shabir, U.; Hassan, T.; Masoodi, S.R. Genetic Testing of Maturity-Onset Diabetes of the Young Current Status and Future Perspectives. *Front. Endocrinol.* **2018**, *9*, 253. [CrossRef]
7. Shields, B.M.; Hicks, S.; Shepherd, M.H.; Colclough, K.; Hattersley, A.T.; Ellard, S. Maturity-onset diabetes of the young (MODY): How many cases are we missing? *Diabetologia* **2010**, *53*, 2504–2508. [CrossRef]
8. Ellard, S.; Bellanné-Chantelot, C.; Hattersley, A.T. European Molecular Genetics Quality Network (EMQN) MODY group. Best practice guidelines for the molecular genetic diagnosis of maturity-onset diabetes of the young. *Diabetologia* **2008**, *51*, 546–553. [CrossRef]
9. Fajans, S.S.; Bell, G.I. MODY: History, genetics, pathophysiology, and clinical decision making. *Diabetes Care* **2011**, *34*, 1878–1884. [CrossRef]
10. Stenson, P.D.; Ball, E.V.; Mort, M.; Phillips, A.D.; Shiel, J.A.; Thomas, N.S.T.; Abeysinghe, S.; Krawczak, M.; Cooper, D.N. Human Gene Mutation Database (HGMD): 2003 update. *Hum. Mutat.* **2003**, *21*, 577–581. [CrossRef]
11. Dotto, R.P.; Mathez, A.L.G.; Franco, L.F.; de Sá, J.R.; Weinert, L.S.; Silveiro, S.P.; de Mello Almada Giuffrida, F.; da Silva, M.R.D.; Reis, A.F. Improving the identification of mody mutations by using MLPA technique in the molecular diagnostics routine. *Diabetol. Metab. Syndr.* **2015**, *11*, A246. [CrossRef]
12. Tatsi, E.B.; Kanaka-Gantenbein, C.; Scorilas, A.; Chrousos, G.P.; Sertedaki, A. Next generation sequencing targeted gene panel in Greek MODY patients increases diagnostic accuracy. *Pediatr. Diabetes* **2020**, *21*, 28–39. [CrossRef] [PubMed]
13. Stuppia, L.; Antonucci, I.; Palka, G.; Gatta, V. Use of the MLPA assay in the molecular diagnosis of gene copy number alterations in human genetic diseases. *Int. J. Mol. Sci.* **2012**, *13*, 3245–3276. [CrossRef] [PubMed]
14. American Diabetes Association. Standards of medical care in diabetes-2013. *Diabetes Care* **2013**, *36*, 11–66. [CrossRef] [PubMed]
15. Sambrook, J.; Russell, D.W. Purification of nucleic acids by extraction with phenol: Chloroform. *Cold Spring Harb. Protoc.* **2006**, *2006*, 4455. [CrossRef]
16. Li, H.; Durbin, R. Fast and accurate short read alignment with Burrows–Wheeler transform. *Bioinformatics* **2009**, *25*, 1754–1760. [CrossRef]
17. McKenna, A.; Hanna, M.; Banks, E.; Sivachenko, A.; Cibulskis, K.; Kernytsky, A.; Garimella, K.; Altshuler, D.; Gabriel, S.; Daly, M.; et al. The Genome Analysis Toolkit: A MapReduce framework for analyzing next-generation DNA sequencing data. *Genome Res.* **2010**, *20*, 1297–1303. [CrossRef]

18. Wang, K.; Li, M.; Hakonarson, H. ANNOVAR: Functional annotation of genetic variants from next-generation sequencing data. *Nucleic Acids Res* **2010**, *38*, e164. [CrossRef]
19. Karczewski, K.J.; Francioli, L.C.; Tiao, G.; Cummings, B.B.; Alföldi, J.; Wang, Q.; Collins, R.L.; Laricchia, K.M.; Ganna, A.; Birnbaum, D.P.; et al. The mutational constraint spectrum quantified from variation in 141,456 humans. *Nature* **2020**, *581*, 434–443. [CrossRef]
20. Landrum, M.J.; Lee, J.M.; Benson, M.; Brown, G.R.; Chao, C.; Chitipiralla, S.; Gu, B.; Hart, J.; Hoffman, D.; Jang, W.; et al. ClinVar: Improving access to variant interpretations and supporting evidence. *Nucleic Acids Res.* **2018**, *46*, D1062–D1067. [CrossRef]
21. Richards, S.; Aziz, N.; Bale, S.; Bick, D.; Das, S.; Gastier-Foster, J.; Grody, W.W.; Hegde, M.; Lyon, E.; Spector, E.; et al. Standards and guidelines for the interpretation of sequence variants: A joint consensus recommendation of the American College of Medical Genetics and Genomics and the Association for Molecular Pathology. *Genet. Med.* **2015**, *17*, 405–423. [CrossRef] [PubMed]
22. Wang, Z.; Diao, C.; Liu, Y.; Li, M.; Zheng, J.; Zhang, Q.; Yu, M.; Zhang, H.; Ping, F.; Li, M.; et al. Identification and functional analysis of *GCK* gene mutations in 12 Chinese families with hyperglycemia. *J. Diabetes Investig.* **2019**, *10*, 963–971. [CrossRef] [PubMed]
23. Ivanoshchuk, D.E.; Shakhtshneider, E.V.; Ovsyannikova, A.K.; Mikhailova, S.V.; Rymar, O.D.; Oblaukhova, V.I.; Yurchenko, A.A.; Voevoda, M.I. A rare splice site mutation in the gene encoding glucokinase/hexokinase 4 in a patient with MODY type 2. *Vavilov J. Genet. Breed.* **2020**, *24*, 299–305. [CrossRef]
24. Ovsyannikova, A.K.; Rymar, O.D.; Ivanoshchuk, D.E.; Mikhailova, S.V.; Shakhtshneider, E.V.; Orlov, P.S.; Malakhina, E.S.; Voevoda, M.I. A Case of Maturity Onset Diabetes of the Young (MODY3) in a Family with a Novel HNF1A Gene Mutation in Five Generations. *Diabetes Ther.* **2018**, *9*, 413–420. [CrossRef] [PubMed]
25. Ovsyannikova, A.K.; Rymar, O.D.; Shakhtshneider, E.V.; Klimontov, V.V.; Koroleva, E.A.; Myakina, N.E.; Voevoda, M.I. ABCC8-Related Maturity-Onset Diabetes of the Young (MODY12): Clinical Features and Treatment Perspective. *Diabetes Ther.* **2016**, *7*, 591–600. [CrossRef]
26. Pedelini, L.; Garcia-Gimeno, M.A.; Marina, A.; Gomez-Zumaquero, J.M.; Rodriguez-Bada, P.; López-Enriquez, S.; Soriguer, F.C.; Cuesta-Muñoz, A.L.; Sanz, P. Structure-function analysis of the alpha5 and the alpha13 helices of human glucokinase: Description of two novel activating mutations. *Protein Sci.* **2005**, *14*, 2080–2086. [CrossRef]
27. Kamata, K.; Mitsuya, M.; Nishimura, T.; Eiki, J.; Nagata, Y. Structural basis for allosteric regulation of the monomeric allosteric enzyme human glucokinase. *Structure* **2004**, *12*, 429–438. [CrossRef]
28. Capuano, M.; Garcia-Herrero, C.M.; Tinto, N.; Carluccio, C.; Capobianco, V.; Coto, I.; Cola, A.; Iafusco, D.; Franzese, A.; Zagari, A.; et al. Glucokinase (GCK) mutations and their characterization in MODY2 children of southern Italy. *PLoS ONE* **2012**, *7*, e38906. [CrossRef]
29. Stride, A.; Vaxillaire, M.; Tuomi, T.; Barbetti, F.; Njølstad, P.R.; Hansen, T.; Costa, A.; Conget, I.; Pedersen, O.; Søvik, O.; et al. The genetic abnormality in the beta cell determines the response to an oral glucose load. *Diabetologia* **2002**, *45*, 427–435. [CrossRef]
30. Fenner, D.; Odili, S.; Hong, H.K.; Kobayashi, Y.; Kohsaka, A.; Siepka, S.M.; Vitaterna, M.H.; Chen, P.; Zelent, B.; Grimsby, J.; et al. Generation of N-ethyl-N-nitrosourea (ENU) diabetes models in mice demonstrates genotype-specific action of glucokinase activators. *J. Biol. Chem.* **2011**, *286*, 39560–39572. [CrossRef]
31. Sagen, J.V.; Odili, S.; Bjørkhaug, L.; Zelent, D.; Buettger, C.; Kwagh, J.; Stanley, C.; Dahl-Jørgensen, K.; de Beaufort, C.; Bell, G.I. From clinicogenetic studies of maturity-onset diabetes of the young to unraveling complex mechanisms of glucokinase regulation. *Diabetes* **2006**, *55*, 1713–1722. [CrossRef] [PubMed]
32. Massa, O.; Meschi, F.; Cuesta-Munoz, A.; Caumo, A.; Cerutti, F.; Toni, S.; Cherubini, V.; Guazzarotti, L.; Sulli, N.; Matschinsky, F.M.; et al. High prevalence of glucokinase mutations in Italian children with MODY. Influence on glucose tolerance, first-phase insulin response, insulin sensitivity and BMI. *Diabetologia* **2001**, *44*, 898–905. [CrossRef] [PubMed]
33. Hager, J.; Blanché, H.; Sun, F.; Vaxillaire, N.V.; Poller, W.; Cohen, D.; Czernichow, P.; Velho, G.; Robert, J.J.; Cohen, N.; et al. Six mutations in the glucokinase gene identified in MODY by using a nonradioactive sensitive screening technique. *Diabetes* **1994**, *43*, 730–733. [CrossRef]
34. Stoffel, M.; Froguel, P.; Takeda, J.; Zouali, H.; Vionnet, N.; Nishi, S.; Weber, I.T.; Harrison, R.W.; Pilkis, S.J.; Lesage, S.; et al. Human glucokinase gene: Isolation, characterization, and identification of two missense mutations linked to early-onset non-insulin-dependent (type 2) diabetes mellitus. *Proc. Natl. Acad. Sci. USA* **1992**, *89*, 7698–7702. [CrossRef] [PubMed]
35. Ellard, S.; Beards, F.; Allen, L.; Shepherd, M.; Ballantyne, E.; Harvey, R.; Hattersley, A.T. A high prevalence of glucokinase mutations in gestational diabetic subjects selected by clinical criteria. *Diabetologia* **2000**, *43*, 250–253. [CrossRef] [PubMed]
36. Pruhova, S.; Dusatkova, P.; Sumnik, Z.; Kolouskova, S.; Pedersen, O.; Hansen, T.; Cinek, O.; Lebl, J. Glucokinase diabetes in 103 families from a country-based study in the Czech Republic: Geographically restricted distribution of two prevalent *GCK* mutations. *Pediatr. Diabetes* **2010**, *11*, 529–535. [CrossRef]
37. Aloi, C.; Salina, A.; Minuto, N.; Tallone, R.; Lugani, F.; Mascagni, A.; Mazza, O.; Cassanello, M.; Maghnie, M.; d'Annunzio, G. Glucokinase mutations in pediatric patients with impaired fasting glucose. *Acta Diabetol.* **2017**, *54*, 913–923. [CrossRef]
38. George, D.C.; Chakraborty, C.; Haneef, S.A.; Nagasundaram, N.; Chen, L.; Zhu, H. Evolution- and structure-based computational strategy reveals the impact of deleterious missense mutations on MODY 2 (maturity-onset diabetes of the young, type 2). *Theranostics* **2014**, *4*, 366–385. [CrossRef]

39. Cho, J.; Horikawa, Y.; Enya, M.; Takeda, J.; Imai, Y.; Imai, Y.; Handa, H.; Imai, T. L-Arginine prevents cereblon-mediated ubiquitination of glucokinase and stimulates glucose-6-phosphate production in pancreatic β-cells. *Commun. Biol.* **2020**, *3*, 497. [CrossRef]
40. Boj, S.F.; Parrizas, M.; Maestro, M.A.; Ferrer, J. A transcription factor regulatory circuit in differentiated pancreatic cells. *Proc. Natl. Acad. Sci. USA* **2001**, *98*, 14481–14486. [CrossRef]
41. Reznik, Y.; Dao, T.; Coutant, R.; Chiche, L.; Jeannot, E.; Clauin, S.; Rousselot, P.; Fabre, M.; Oberti, F.; Fatome, A.; et al. Hepatocyte nuclear factor-1 alpha gene inactivation: Cosegregation between liver adenomatosis and diabetes phenotypes in two maturity-onset diabetes of the young (MODY)3 families. *J. Clin. Endocrinol. Metab.* **2004**, *89*, 1476–1480. [CrossRef] [PubMed]
42. Simms, R.J.; Sayer, J.A.; Quinton, R.; Walker, M.; Ellard, S.; Goodship, T.H.J. Monogenic diabetes, renal dysplasia and hypopituitarism: A patient with a HNF1A mutation. *QJM Int. J. Med.* **2011**, *104*, 881–883. [CrossRef] [PubMed]
43. Fajans, S.S.; Bell, G.I. Phenotypic heterogeneity between different mutations of MODY subtypes and within MODY pedigrees. *Diabetologia* **2006**, *49*, 1106–1108. [CrossRef] [PubMed]
44. Colclough, K.; Bellanne-Chantelot, C.; Saint-Martin, C.; Flanagan, S.E.; Ellard, S. Mutations in the genes encoding the transcription factors hepatocyte nuclear factor 1 alpha and 4 alpha in maturity-onset diabetes of the young and hyperinsulinemic hypoglycaemia. *Hum. Mutat.* **2013**, *34*, 669–685. [CrossRef]
45. Zhou, X.; Chen, C.; Yin, D.; Zhao, F.; Bao, Z.; Zhao, Y.; Wang, X.; Li, W.; Wang, T.; Jin, Y.; et al. A Variation in the *ABCC8* Gene Is Associated with Type 2 Diabetes Mellitus and Repaglinide Efficacy in Chinese Type 2 Diabetes Mellitus Patients. *Intern. Med.* **2019**, *58*, 2341–2347. [CrossRef]
46. Vaxillaire, M.; Dechaume, A.; Busiah, K.; Cavé, H.; Pereira, S.; Scharfmann, R.; de Nanclares, G.P.; Castano, L.; Froguel, P.; Polak, M. SUR1-Neonatal Diabetes Study Group. New ABCC8 mutations in relapsing neonatal diabetes and clinical features. *Diabetes* **2007**, *56*, 1737–1741. [CrossRef]
47. Edghill, E.L.; Flanagan, S.E.; Ellard, S. Permanent neonatal diabetes due to activating mutations in ABCC8 and KCNJ11. *Rev. Endocr. Metab. Disord.* **2010**, *11*, 193–198. [CrossRef]
48. Calabria, A.C.; Li, C.; Gallagher, P.R.; Stanley, C.A.; De León, D.D. GLP-1 receptor antagonist exendin-(9–39) elevates fasting blood glucose levels in congenital hyperinsulinism owing to inactivating mutations in the ATP-sensitive K+ channel. *Diabetes* **2012**, *61*, 2585–2591. [CrossRef]
49. De Franco, E.; Saint-Martin, C.; Brusgaard, K.; Knight Johnson, A.E.; Aguilar-Bryan, L.; Bowman, P.; Arnoux, J.B.; Larsen, A.R.; Sanyoura, M.; Greeley, S.A.W.; et al. Update of variants identified in the pancreatic β-cell K_{ATP} channel genes *KCNJ11* and *ABCC8* in individuals with congenital hyperinsulinism and diabetes. *Hum. Mutat.* **2020**, *41*, 884–905. [CrossRef]
50. El-Khairi, R.; Vallier, L. The role of hepatocyte nuclear factor 1β in disease and development. *Diabetes Obes. Metab.* **2016**, *18*, 23–32. [CrossRef]
51. Klimontov, V.V.; Bulumbaeva, D.M.; Koroleva, E.A.; Ovsyannikova, A.K.; Rymar, O.D.; Ivanoshchuk, D.E.; Shakhtshneider, E.V. Maturity-onset diabetes of the young due to HNF1B mutation: A case report. In Proceedings of the Systems Biology and Biomedicine, SBioMed-2018\Systems Biology (BGRS\SB-2018), Novosibirsk, Russia, 20–25 August 2018; p. 64, ISBN 978-5-91291-040-1.
52. Weber, S.; Moriniere, V.; Knüppel, T.; Charbit, M.; Dusek, J.; Ghiggeri, G.M.; Jankauskiené, A.; Mir, S.; Montini, G.; Peco-Antic, A.; et al. Prevalence of mutations in renal developmental genes in children with renal hypodysplasia: Results of the ESCAPE study. *J. Am. Soc. Nephrol.* **2006**, *17*, 2864–2870. [CrossRef] [PubMed]
53. Karges, B.; Bergmann, C.; Scholl, K.; Heinze, E.; Rasche, F.M.; Zerres, K.; Debatin, K.M.; Wabitsch, M.; Karges, W. Digenic Inheritance of Hepatocyte Nuclear Factor-1α and -1β With Maturity-Onset Diabetes of the Young, Polycystic Thyroid, and Urogenital Malformations. *Diabetes Care* **2007**, *30*, 1613–1614. [CrossRef] [PubMed]
54. Urrutia, I.; Martínez, R.; Rica, I.; Martínez de LaPiscina, I.; García-Castaño, A.; Aguayo, A.; Calvo, B.; Castaño, L. Spanish Pediatric Diabetes Collaborative Group. Negative autoimmunity in a Spanish pediatric cohort suspected of type 1 diabetes, could it be monogenic diabetes? *PLoS ONE* **2019**, *14*, e0220634. [CrossRef]
55. Dedov, I.I.; Zubkova, N.A.; Arbatskaya, N.Y.; Akopova, A.G.; Tyul'pakov, A.N. MODY2: Clinical and molecular genetic characteristics of 13 cases of the disease. The first description of MODY in Russia. *Probl. Endokrinol.* **2009**, *55*, 3–7. [CrossRef] [PubMed]
56. Glotov, O.S.; Serebryakova, E.A.; Turkunova, M.E.; Efimova, O.A.; Glotov, A.S.; Barbitoff, Y.A.; Nasykhova, Y.A.; Predeus, A.V.; Polev, D.E.; Fedyakov, M.A.; et al. Whole-exome sequencing in Russian children with non-type 1 diabetes mellitus reveals a wide spectrum of genetic variants in MODY-related and unrelated genes. *Mol. Med. Rep.* **2019**, *20*, 4905–4914. [CrossRef]
57. GoodSmith, M.S.; Skandari, M.R.; Huang, E.S.; Naylor, R.N. The Impact of Biomarker Screening and Cascade Genetic Testing on the Cost-Effectiveness of MODY Genetic Testing. *Diabetes Care* **2019**, *42*, 2247–2255. [CrossRef]

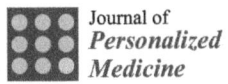

Journal of Personalized Medicine

Review
Gallstone Disease, Obesity and the Firmicutes/Bacteroidetes Ratio as a Possible Biomarker of Gut Dysbiosis

Irina N. Grigor'eva

Laboratory of Gastroenterology, Research Institute of Internal and Preventive Medicine-Branch of The Federal Research Center Institute of Cytology and Genetics of Siberian Branch of Russian Academy of Sciences, Novosibirsk 630089, Russia; niitpm.office@gmail.com; Tel.: +7-9137520702

Abstract: Obesity is a major risk factor for developing gallstone disease (GSD). Previous studies have shown that obesity is associated with an elevated *Firmicutes/Bacteroidetes* ratio in the gut microbiota. These findings suggest that the development of GSD may be related to gut dysbiosis. This review presents and summarizes the recent findings of studies on the gut microbiota in patients with GSD. Most of the studies on the gut microbiota in patients with GSD have shown a significant increase in the phyla *Firmicutes* (Lactobacillaceae family, genera *Clostridium, Ruminococcus, Veillonella, Blautia, Dorea, Anaerostipes*, and *Oscillospira*), *Actinobacteria* (*Bifidobacterium* genus), *Proteobacteria, Bacteroidetes* (genera *Bacteroides, Prevotella*, and *Fusobacterium*) and a significant decrease in the phyla *Bacteroidetes* (family *Muribaculaceae*, and genera *Bacteroides, Prevotella, Alistipes, Paludibacter, Barnesiella*), *Firmicutes* (genera *Faecalibacterium, Eubacterium, Lachnospira*, and *Roseburia*), *Actinobacteria* (*Bifidobacterium* genus), and *Proteobacteria* (*Desulfovibrio* genus). The influence of GSD on microbial diversity is not clear. Some studies report that GSD reduces microbial diversity in the bile, whereas others suggest the increase in microbial diversity in the bile of patients with GSD. The phyla *Proteobacteria* (especially family *Enterobacteriaceae*) and *Firmicutes* (*Enterococcus* genus) are most commonly detected in the bile of patients with GSD. On the other hand, the composition of bile microbiota in patients with GSD shows considerable inter-individual variability. The impact of GSD on the *Firmicutes/Bacteroidetes* ratio is unclear and reports are contradictory. For this reason, it should be stated that the results of reviewed studies do not allow for drawing unequivocal conclusions regarding the relationship between GSD and the *Firmicutes/Bacteroidetes* ratio in the microbiota.

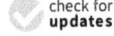

Keywords: Firmicutes; Bacteroidetes; gut microbiota; bile microbiota; gallstone patients

Citation: Grigor'eva, I.N. Gallstone Disease, Obesity and the Firmicutes/ Bacteroidetes Ratio as a Possible Biomarker of Gut Dysbiosis. *J. Pers. Med.* **2021**, *11*, 13. https://dx.doi.org/10.3390/jpm11010013

Received: 14 November 2020
Accepted: 22 December 2020
Published: 25 December 2020

Publisher's Note: MDPI stays neutral with regard to jurisdictional claims in published maps and institutional affiliations.

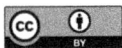

Copyright: © 2020 by the author. Licensee MDPI, Basel, Switzerland. This article is an open access article distributed under the terms and conditions of the Creative Commons Attribution (CC BY) license (https://creativecommons.org/licenses/by/4.0/).

1. Introduction

Obesity is defined as excessive fat accumulation that may impair health; obesity is a result of an imbalance between energy intake and expenditure [1,2]. Today obesity has become pandemic; about 1.9 billion people on the planet are overweight: overall, about 13% of the world's adult populations (11% of men and 15% of women) were obese in 2016 [3]. The World Health Organization (WHO) estimated that nearly 2.8 million deaths annually are a consequence of overweight and obesity-associated conditions [3], such as atherosclerosis, diabetes, gallstone disease (GSD), etc. [4–6].

GSD is a common benign gastrointestinal disease affecting 10–15% of adults around the world that greatly contributes to health care costs [7–10]. Risk factors of the GSD are age, female sex, obesity, insulin resistance, physical inactivity, genetic background, dietary factors (high carbohydrate, high-calorie intake), dyslipoproteinaemia, certain diseases (such as diabetes mellitus, nonalcoholic fatty liver disease (NAFLD), hypertension, and cardiovascular disease) and medications (hormone replacement therapy, fibrates, etc.), social and economic issues, fertility, and intestinal factors (with increased absorption of cholesterol, slow intestinal motility, and dysbiosis) [7–10]. Obesity is a major risk factor for developing GSD [9–12] because it is accompanied by increased synthesis and excretion of cholesterol into bile [13], wherein the amount of cholesterol produced is directly proportional to being overweight [11].Obesity is regarded as an inflammatory condition [14]. Inflammation may be the potential link between insulin resistance and gallstones [15]. Insulin resistance is considered a risk factor for GSD, as it may lead to excess biliary cholesterol production and saturation [16,17] and alone may be responsible for gallbladder dysmotility [18]. However, the absence of a relationship between body mass index (BMI) and GSD had been reported in several epidemiologic studies [7,8,19]. The possible pathogenesis for the close association between obesity and GSD iscomplex and not fully understood.

A significant relationship exists among food intake, energy balance and gut peptides that are secreted from gastrointestinal enteroendocrine cells, such as ghrelin, leptin, glucagon-like peptide-1, cholecystokinin (CCK), peptide tyrosine tyrosine (PYY), and serotonin [20]. Let's focus on two of them. Ghrelin, an orexigenic peptidyl hormone secreted from the stomach, was discovered in 1999 and is associated with feeding and energy balance [21]. Ghrelin increases appetite and energy expenditure and promotes the use of carbohydrates as a source of fuel at the same time as sparing fat [22]. The development of resistance to leptin andghrelin, hormones that are crucial for the neuroendocrine control of energy homeostasis, is a hallmark ofobesity [23]. The impact of acyl-ghrelin on glucose metabolism and lipid homeostasis may allow for novel preventative or early intervention therapeutic strategies to treat obesity-related type 2 diabetes and associated metabolic dysfunction [24]. There were no differences for total bile acids, insulin, ghrelin, and glucose-dependent insulinotropic polypeptide between patients with GSD and the control group without gallstones [25]. Mendez-Sanchez et al. (2006) found an inverse correlation of serum ghrelin levels and theprevalence of GSD in alogistic regression analysis (OR = 0.27, 95% CI 0.09–0.82, p = 0.02) [26]. Authors suggest that serum ghrelin concentrations are associated with a protective effect of GSD and this is related to a motilin-like effect of ghrelin on the gallbladder motility. However, themedian of serum ghrelin values did not show a difference between the patients and controls (660 vs. 682 ng/L) [26].

Leptin is associated with obesity: although it should reduce food intake and body weight, in obese patientsthe serum leptin levels are higher than in the lean individuals and do not manage reducing their food intake [27]. Insulin and leptin play an important role in the development of prediabetes and NAFLD, which is a risk factor for GSD. There could be the following pathogenic links: obesity promotes insulin resistance; high levels of insulin increase leptin levels; leptin cannot lead to decreased insulin levels and decreased appetite because of leptin resistance in the nervous system and the adipose tissue; and high levels of leptin promote hepatic steatosis which in turn increases insulin resistance [27]. Positive correlations between serum leptin and BMI, CCK, total cholesterol, and insulin were found in the gallstone group [28].

Gut microbiota can regulate levels of these gut peptides and thus regulate intestinal metabolism via the microbiota-gut-brain axis [20]. Serum ghrelin levels were negatively correlated with *Bifidobacterium*, *Lactobacillus* and *B. coccoides–Eubacterium rectale*, and positively correlated with *Bacteroides* and *Prevotella* [29]. Leptin was negatively correlated with *Clostridium*, *Bacteroides* and *Prevotella*, and positively correlated with *Bifidobacterium* and *Lactobacillus* [29].The results of the studies on the relationship between GSD, obesity, and incretin hormones remain controversial.

GSD and obesity have similar prevalence [10]. Most of the above risk factors are common to GSD and obesity. Despite the increasing number of scientific publications on the gut microbiota in obesity, there is a lack of studies that assess the gut microbiota in GSD. Research on this topic is limited and mainly focused on the study of certain genera and species of microorganisms, but not the *Firmicutes/Bacteroidetes* ratio. Many studies have shown that, in humans, obesity is associated with an increased *Firmicutes/Bacteroidetes* ratio in comparison with lean or "healthy obese" individuals [1,2,30–42]. This review presents and summarizes the recent findings of studies on the gut microbiota in patients with GSD regarding the *Firmicutes/Bacteroidetes* ratio, as a possible biomarker of obesity, given that obesity is a key risk factor for GSD.

The Gut Microbiome and Its Functions

Bacteria emerged 3.8 billion ago [43]. There are about 10 trillion human cells in the human body and about 100 trillion cells outside and inside our bodies being of microbial origin [44,45]. The gut microbiome is a dynamic assembly of microorganisms and the resultant products of their collective genetic and metabolic materials, containing from 2 to 20 million microbial genes by the human microbiome's predominantly in the gut [44]. The gut microbiome plays an array of biological functions ranging from controlling gut–immune system axis, providing several key metabolites and maintaining an optimal digestive system due to the presence of genes, which encode digestive enzymes that are not present in human cells but are associated with the metabolism and fermentation of many food compounds necessary for the host's nutrition [46]. A greater richness and diversity of bacterial species in the human intestine may be an indicator of health [45,47,48].

2. The Firmicutes/Bacteroidetes Ratio

2.1. Short Characteristics of the Firmicutes and the Bacteroidetes

As the dominant gut microbiota in healthy adult humans [4], intestinal bacteria include members of both the *Firmicutes* (range of quantitative data–20.5% up to 80% [49–53]) and the *Bacteroidetes* (from 13.85% up to 75.3% [20,49,51,52]). Major taxa of the *Firmicutes* to be included of more than 200 genera [53,54]. *Proteobacteria, Fusobacteria, Actinobacteria, Cyanobacteria*, and *Verrucomicrobia* phyla also are present as minor players [54].

Some *Bacteroides* spp. and *Prevotella* spp. have a variety of glycans and glycosidases that can utilize polysaccharides [53,55]. Other important functions of *Bacteroides* spp. include deconjugation of bile acids [56]. The gut microbiota, especially *Bacteroides intestinalis*, and to a certain extent *Bacteroides fragilis* and *E. coli*, also has the capacity to deconjugate and dehydrate the primary bile acids and convert them into the secondary bile acids in the human colon [57]. Bacteria belonging to the phylum *Bacteroidetes* have high functional redundancy, whereas the phylum *Firmicutes* was comprised of a large number of more functionally diverse core bacteria [53,54,58]. Commensal *Clostridial* clusters XIVa and IV plays an important role in the host and gut homeostasis from the metabolic point of view through the production of short-chain fatty acids, normalizes intestinal permeability, involved the brain–gut axis regulation, in the immune system development, etc. [59]. Many *Firmicutes'* abilities are related to the host's body weight: obesity-associated gut microbiota is enriched in *Clostridium leptum* [54], Roseburia intestinalis, Eubacterium ventriosum, *Eubacterium hallii* [60], *Lactobacillus reuteri* [42], *Blautia hydrogenotorophica, Coprococcus catus, Ruminococcus bromii, Ruminococcus obeum* [50]. However, other *Firmicutes* are abundant in non-obese individuals: *Clostridium cellulosi*, associated with the degradation of plant material [60,61], *Clostridium orbiscindens* (currently known as *Flavonifractor plautii*), capable of utilizing flavonoids [52], *Clostridium bolteae, Blautia wexlerae* [58], *Clostridium difficile*, the *Staphylococcus* genus [40], *Oscillospira guillermondii* [60], *Faecalibacterium (prausnitzii), Lactobacillus plantarum*, and *paracasei* [42]. Also, two *Bacteroides* species (*B. faecichinchillae* and *B. thetaiotaomicron*) [58] and *Akkermansia muciniphila*, and *Methanobrevibacter smithii* [42] were significantly more abundant in stool samples from non-obese compared with obese subjects. Such differences in the "behaviour" of bacteria cannot be explained only by their metabolic properties, because of the exact functions of bacteria are still unclear.

2.2. The Story of "Discovery" of the Firmicutes/Bacteroidetes Ratio

Increased efficiency of energy harvest, due to alterations in the gut microbiota has been implicated in obesity in mice [31,32,62] and humans [38]. Alterations affecting the dominant intestinal phyla the *Firmicutes* and the *Bacteroidetes* were first described by Ley et al. (2005) in obese animals [1]. In the analysis of the cecal microbiota (by the 16S rRNA gene sequences) of genetically obese ob/ob mice, lean ob/+ and wild-type +/+ siblings, ob/ob animals have a 50% reduction in the abundance of Bacteroidetes and a proportional increase in Firmicutes compared with lean mice [1]. The authors also pointed out that an increase of the *Firmicutes/Bacteroidetes* ratio may help promote adiposity in *ob/ob* mice.

The *Firmicutes/Bacteroidetes* ratio is also under debate as a possible biomarker of obesity and related dysfunctions [53,62–66]. A low *Firmicutes/Bacteroidetes* ratio was found to be associated with lean phenotypes, younger age, cardiovascular health, and a balanced immune system and is generally considered beneficial for health [67–69].

2.3. The Firmicutes/Bacteroidetes Ratio in Obesity: Pro

Ley et al. (2006) have shown that the microbiota in obese subjects shows an elevated proportion of the *Firmicutes* and a reduced population of the *Bacteroides*. Conversely, the relative proportion of the *Bacteroidetes* decreased in humans on a weight-loss program [30]. 16S rRNA gene sequencing revealed a lower proportion of *Bacteroidetes*, more *Actinobacteria* in obese versus lean individuals, but no significant difference in *Firmicutes* in 31 monozygotic twin pairs and 23 dizygotic twin pairs [33]. Armougom et al. [34] confirmed a reduction in the *Bacteroidetes* community in 20 obese patients compared with 20 normal-weight individuals ($p < 0.01$). Zuo et al. (2011) reported that obese people had fewer cultivable *Bacteroides* than their normal-weight counterparts [37]. In the gut in obese adolescents, the total microbiota was more abundant on the phylum *Firmicutes* (94.6%) as compared with *Bacteroidetes* (3.2%) [39]. In the systematic review (PubMed: 2005–2017) adecrease in the *Bacteroidetes* phylum and *Bacteroides/Prevotella* groups was related to high BMI and the *Firmicutes* phylum was positively correlated with weight gain in children between 0 and 13 years of age [40]. In an adult Ukrainian population, the *Firmicutes/Bacteroidetes* ratio was significantly associated with BMI (OR = 1.23, 95% CI 1.09–1.38) and this association continued to be significant after adjusting for confounders such as age, sex, smoking and physical activity (OR = 1.33, 95% CI 1.11–1.60) [41]. The recent systematic review confirmed that individuals with obesity have a greater the *Firmicutes/Bacteroidetes* ratio, more *Firmicutes, Fusobacteria, Proteobacteria, Mollicutes,* and less *Bacteroidetes* [42].

2.4. The Firmicutes/Bacteroidetes Ratio in Obesity: Contra

However, other human trials not only failed to confirm a high proportion of *Firmicutes* in obese patients [63,70–78] and, but reported even the opposite: about higher amounts of *Bacteroidetes*, and decreased amounts of *Clostridium* cluster XIVa in obese subjects as compared with lean donors [71]. Proportions of the genus *Bacteroides* were greater in overweight volunteers than lean and obese volunteers and the *Firmicutes/Bacteroidetes* ratio changed in favour of the *Bacteroidetes* in overweight and obese subjects [72]. Duncan et al. (2008) found that weight loss did not change the relative proportions of the *Bacteroides* spp, or the percentage of the *Firmicutes* present, in the human gut [73]. In another study, no significant differences in the *Firmicutes/Bacteroidetes* ratios were found between obese and normal-weight adults [74] or obese and normal-weight children [75]. Two meta-analyses have shown that the content of the *Firmicutes* and the *Bacteroidetes* and their ratio is not a consistent feature distinguishing lean from obese human microbiota generally [76,77].

Many authors have concluded that there is no simple taxonomic signature of obesity in the microbiota of the human gut and that significant technical and clinical differences exist between published studies [63] and that the phylum level difference of the gut microbiota between obese and lean individuals might not be universally true [78]. Likely explanations for these controversies are discussed below.

3. Role of the Microbiota in the Pathogenesis of Gallstone Disease

The pathogenesis of cholesterol GSD is multifactor, it is determined by five primary defects: genetic background and LITH genes, hepatic hypersecretion of biliary cholesterol, rapid precipitation of solid cholesterol crystals in bile, gallbladder dysmotility, and intestinal factors (with increased absorption of cholesterol, slow intestinal motility, and dysbiosis) [10].

In recent years, attention has been focused on the potential impact of the gut microbiota on the pathogenesis of pigment and cholesterol gallstones. It is proved that intestinal dysbiosis makes a significant contribution to the development of not only the GSD itself [5,6,79–82], but also to the development of numerous disorders that are risk factors for GSD, including obesity [31–42], type 2 diabetes [83], hypercholesterolemia [20,52], diet [84], NAFLD [85–88], cardiovascular diseases [68,89], physical inactivity [29,90,91], etc.

Gut microbiota affects the pathogenesis of GSD through several mechanisms. Some bacteria alter the composition of bile directly via β-glucuronidase, cholyl-glycyl hydrolase, phospholipase A1, or urease activities, or by biofilmformationthereby promoting calcium bilirubinate (pigment) stone generation [92,93]. Till now, it has not been clear whether bacterial pathogens of the biliary tree contribute to the stone formation or alternatively if the presence of gallstones promotes chronic colonization [15]. The activity of the gut microbiota could also be linked to the development of GSD by altering the concentration of serum lipids [94], and biliary lipids in bile and/or increasing the faecal excretion of bile salts [95]. Gut microbiota can modulate bile acid metabolism through the activity of bile salt hydrolases, which deconjugate bile acids, and the activity of 7α-dehydroxylase, which converts primary bile acids (cholic acid and chenodeoxycholic acid) to secondary bile acids (deoxycholic acid and lithocholic acid) [94].

Bile acids regulate metabolism via activation of specific nuclear receptors (e.g., farnesoid X receptor, pregnane X receptor, vitamin D receptor, and cell surface G protein-coupled receptors, such as the G protein-coupled bile acid receptor (TGR5 and Gpbar-1)) [96,97]. The effect of the farnesoid X receptor is antilithogenic:farnesoid X receptor activation in the intestine by bile acids induces fibroblast growth factor 15 expression, which suppresses the expression of cholesterol 7α-dehydroxylase in the liver [98]. Gallstone patients had significantly higher levels of 7α-dehydroxylating bacteria than individuals without gallstones [99]. The increase of 7α-dehydroxylation activity of the intestinal microflora promoted the deoxycholic acid excess in the bile acid pool [100], and the increase in the percentage of deoxycholic acid in bile and bile acid hydrophobicity leads to a decrease in the cholesterol microcrystal nucleation time and the formation of cholesterol gallstones [101].

4. The Firmicutes/BacteroidetesRatio and GSD

4.1. Gut Microbiota

4.1.1. Gut Microbiota in Mice and Cholelithiasis

Many reports are underlining the association of the gut microbiota with the pathogenesis of cholesterol cholelithogenesis in mice [15,102,103] and humans [5,6,80–82,93,100,104–119].

Alteration of indigenous gut microbiota by bacteria transferring has been shown to make germ-free mice more susceptible to the formation of cholesterol gallstones [102]. In a study of mice without and with cholesterol gallstones (induced by a lithogenic diet) using 16S rRNA gene sequencing, it was found that in the faeces of mice, the *Firmicutes/Bacteroidetes* ratio and the *Firmicutes* content decreased (from 59.71% under chow diet to 31.45% under lithogenic diet, $p < 0.01$), the richness and alpha diversity of the microbiota also significantly reduced [103]. Cholelithogenic enterohepatic *Helicobacter* spp. (phylum *Proteobacteria*) have been identified and their important role in the formation of cholesterol gallstones in mice and perhaps in humans has been shown [15].

4.1.2. Gut Microbiota in Humans and Gallstones

In the gallstone group included 30 patients, the diversity of intestinal bacteria and the abundances of certain phylogroups significantly decreased, especially *Firmicutes*, the *Firmicutes/Bacteroidetes* ratio was also significantly decreased compared with the control group included 30 healthy individuals [6]. 7α-dehydroxylating gut bacteria (the *Clostridium* genus) were significantly increased, whereas cholesterol-lowering bacteria (the *Eubacterium* genus) were significantly reduced. *Clostridium* was positively correlated with secondary bile acids. It can be assumed that an increase in *Clostridium* and a decrease in *Eubacterium* contribute to bile saturation with cholesterol in patients with gallstones [100]. In the gallstone group, *Ruminococcus gnavus* could be used as a biomarker, while in the control group–*Prevotella 9* and *Faecalibacterium* [6].

Keren et al. (2015) showed that intestinal microbial diversity, the abundances of the genus *Roseburia* and the species *Bacteroides uniformis* were decreased, and those of the family *Ruminococcaceae* and the genus *Oscillospira* were increased in patients with gallstones before cholecystectomy compared with the controls [5]. After cholecystectomy in the patients with gallstones, the abundance of the phylum *Bacteroidetes*, and also the family *Bacteroidaceae* and the genus *Bacteroides* showed a significant increase. Gallstone patients had higher overall concentrations of faecal bile acids [5]. *Roseburia* was significantly positively correlated with faecal cholesterol, but not with bile acids; *Oscillospira* correlated negatively with primary bile acids and faecal cholesterol concentration and positively–with the secondary bile lithocholic acid in the faeces. Thus, the authors suggest that *Oscillospira* may predispose individuals to cholesterol gallstones [5]. Cholecystectomy alters bile flow into the intestine and bidirectional interactions between bile acids and intestinal microbiota, thereby increasing bacterial degradation of bile acids into faecal secondary bile acids [104,105]. Deoxycholic acid can inhibit the growth of thececal microbiota in rats; moreover, members of the *Bacteroidetes* phylum (*Bacteroides vulgatus*, *Bacteroides sartorii*) are more sensitive to secondary bile acids exposure than members of the *Firmicutes* phylum (*Clostridium innocuum*, *Blautia coccoides*) [120]. Deoxycholic acid concentrations were negatively correlated with the *Bacteroidetes* phylum in patients with GSD [5]. Increasing levels of the cholic acid cause a dramatic shift toward the *Firmicutes* (from 54.1% before of administration of cholic acid up to 95% after [120]), particularly *Clostridium* cluster XIVa and increasing production of the harmful deoxycholic acid [104,121].

Wang W et al. (2018) identified ageing-associated faecal microbiota in a healthy population, which was lost in cholecystectomy patients [81]. Absent intestinal bacteria, such as *Bacteroides*, were also negatively related to secondary bile acids in cholecystectomy patients. The abundances of *Prevotella*, *Desulfovibrio*, *Barnesiella*, *Paludibacter*, and *Alistipes* all decreased, whereas those of *Bifidobacterium*, *Anaerostipes*, and *Dorea* all increased in the cholecystectomy patients [81].

In the frame of a case-control study, Yoon W et al. (2019) showed that *Blautia obeum* and *Veillonella parvula*, which have azoreductase activity, were more abundant in faecal samples in the 27 patients of the cholecystectomy group compared to the control group [82]. The abundance of family *Muribaculaceae* belonging to the phylum *Bacteroidetes* was decreased and that of the family *Lactobacillaceae* was increased in the cholecystectomy group. At the genus level, the abundance of *Ruminococcus* was greater in the cholecystectomy group [82].The actual number of taxa observed in a faecal sample was significantly lower in the cholecystectomy group. However, the difference in the diversity of the gut microbiota between the cholecystectomy and control groups was subtle [82].

Two years after cholecystectomy, eight patients with the symptomatic post-cholecystectomy syndrome, eight patients with the asymptomatic post-cholecystectomy syndrome, and eight healthy individuals were examined [106]. It was shown that *Firmicutes* and *Bacteroidetes* had similar abundance and contents among the three groups. The gut microbiome of the symptomatic post-cholecystectomy syndrome patients was dominated by *Proteobacteria* in faeces and contained little *Firmicutes* and *Bacteroidetes* [106].

Wu et al. (2013) studied the composition of bacterial communities of the gut, bile, and gallstones from 29 cholesterol gallstone patients and the gut of 38 healthy controls [107] by 16S rRNA gene sequencing method. They found a significant increment of the gut bacterial phylum *Proteobacteria* anddecrement of gut bacterial genera *Faecalibacterium*, *Lachnospira*, and *Roseburia*. When compared with gut, a significantly decreased level of the bacterial phylum *Bacteroidetes* in the biliary tract was found. The *Firmicutes*/*Bacteroidetes* ratio in faeces in patients with GSD did not differ in comparison with the control group [107].

Ren X et al. (2020) examined stool samples from 104 subjects (equally post-cholecystectomy patients and healthy controls) which were collected for 16S rRNA gene sequencing to analyze the bacterial profile [80]. It was shown noteworthy compositional and abundant alterations of bacterial microbiota in post-cholecystectomy patients, characterized as *Bacteroides ovatus*, *Prevotella copri*, and *Fusobacterium varium* remarkably increased;

Faecalibacterium prausnitzii, Roseburia faecis, and *Bifidobacterium adolescentis* significantly decreased. Machine learning-based analysis, that integrates gut microbiota and other anthropometric parameters, showed a pivotal role of *Megamonas funiformis* in discriminating post-cholecystectomy patients from healthy controls. Additionally, the duration after cholecystectomy notably affected bacterial composition in post-cholecystectomy patients [80].

Eventually, if we summarize the results of most studies of the microbiota in patients with GSD different authors found both a significant increment of gut bacterial phyla *Firmicutes* (*Lactobacillaceae* family, genera *Clostridium, Ruminococcus, Veillonella, Blautia, Dorea, Anaerostipes,* and *Oscillospira*), *Actinobacteria* (*Bifidobacterium* genus), *Proteobacteria, Bacteroidetes* (genera *Bacteroides, Prevotella,* and *Fusobacterium*) (Figure 1) and significant decrement of gut bacterial phyla *Bacteroidetes* (*Muribaculaceae* family, and *genera Bacteroides, Prevotella, Alistipes, Paludibacter, Barnesiella*), *Firmicutes* (genera *Faecalibacterium, Eubacterium, Lachnospira,* and *Roseburia*), *Actinobacteria* (*Bifidobacterium* genus), and *Proteobacteria* (*Desulfovibrio* genus) (Figure 2). In other words, in patients with GSD, an increase and decrease in almost all major intestinal bacterial phyla were detected. In one study the *Firmicutes/Bacteroidetes* ratio in faeces in patients with GSD was significantly decreased in comparison with the controls [6], in two studies–did not differ [106,107]. In addition to *Firmicutes* and *Bacteroidetes* as the main phyla, *Proteobacteria* and other phyla may contribute to the gut dysbiosis in patients with GSD.

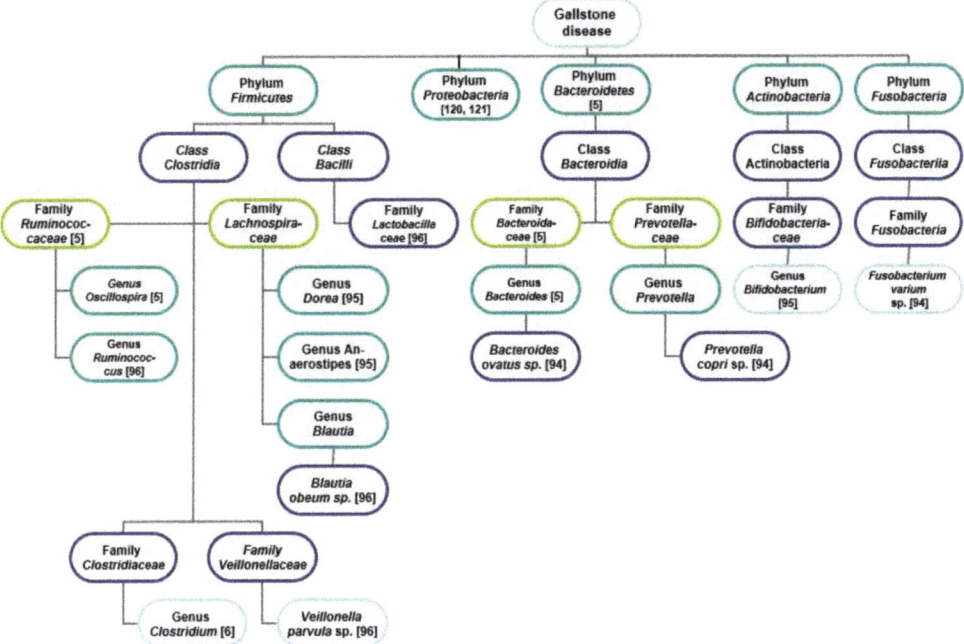

Figure 1. Characteristics of the gut microbiome of patients with GSD. A significant increase of the phyla *Firmicutes, Actinobacteria, Proteobacteria,* and *Bacteroidetes* is reflected. The number in square brackets indicates a reference in the list of references.

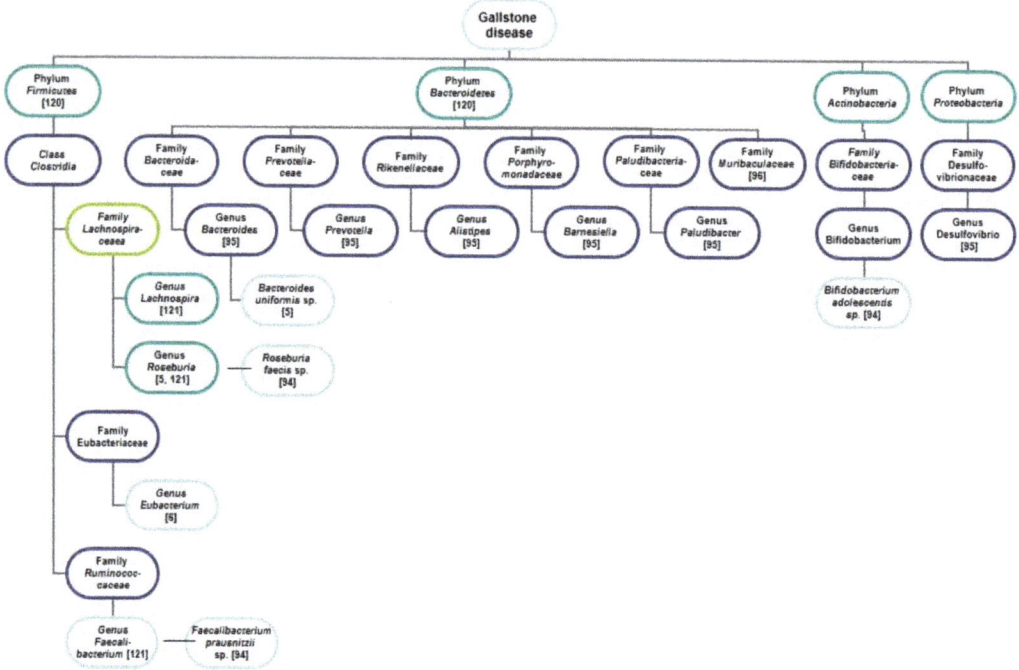

Figure 2. Characteristics of the gut microbiome of patients with GSD. A significant decrease of the phyla *Firmicutes*, *Actinobacteria*, *Proteobacteria*, and *Bacteroidetes* is reflected. The number in square brackets indicates a reference in the list of references.

Using metagenomic DNA sequencing, researchers have been able to categorize individuals as either high gene count (HGC) or low gene count (LGC) [44]. HGC individuals are generally considered to have a greater repertoire of microbial metabolic functions, a functionally more robust gut microbiome, and greater overall health, including a lower prevalence of obesity and metabolic disorders [48]. Examples of bacterial taxa that have been associated with human health and proper gastrointestinal function include *Bacteroides*, *Bifidobacterium*, *Clostridium* clusters XIVa and IVa (butyrate producers), *Eubacterium*, *Faecalibacterium*, *Lactobacillus*, and *Roseburia*. Bacterial species that might protect against weight gain and are enriched in HGC individuals include *Anaerotruncus colihominis*, *Butyrovibrio crossotus*, *Akkermansia* spp., and *Faecalibacterium* spp. [48]. The studies of the gut microbiota in patients with GSD included in our review demonstrated a reduction of bacterial taxa that have been associated with human health, i.e., genera *Bacteroides*, *Faecalibacterium*, *Roseburia*, *Eubacterium*, an increase in *Lactobacillaceae* family, and oppositely directed changes in *Bifidobacterium*.

4.1.3. Bile Microbiota in Humans and Gallstones

The presence of bacterial amplicons belonging to *Firmicutes*, *Bacteroidetes*, and *Actinobacteria*, and *Proteobacteria* phyla in the human intact gallbladder bile was proved by 16S rRNA gene sequencing [108,109]. Associations between alpha- and beta-diversity, a taxonomic profile of bile microbiota (*Bacteroidetes*, *Proteobacteria*, *Actinobacteria*, and *Firmicutes* phyla, analyzed with 16S rRNA gene sequencing), and taurocholic and taurochenodeoxycholic bile acid levels were evidenced in 37 Russian patients with GSD [110].

At the phylum level, *Bacteroidetes* was statistically more abundant in the bile of patients with GSD (24.00%) compared to the control (13.49%) [109]. Members of the families *Bacteroidaceae*, *Prevotellaceae*, *Porphyromonadaceae*, and *Veillonellaceae* were more frequently detected in patients with GSD. The genus *Dialister* and enterobacteria *Escherichia-Shigella* also showed a significantly higher representation in the bile in the patients with GSD [109]. The Shannon diversity index was statistically higher in the bile of the control group than that obtained in the patients with GSD [102].However, it was not taken into account that bile samples from the gallbladder of individuals from a control group were obtained from liver donors, and they were not only treated with antibiotics but also not fully examined to exclude hepatobiliary or other important pathology [109].

The *Proteobacteria, Firmicutes, Bacteroidetes,* and *Actinobacteria* phyla dominated the biliary microbiota in the persons, all of whom were diagnosed with GSD, at that biliary tract microbiota of participants with GSD showed substantial person-to-person variation [79]. Metagenomic sequencing of bile from gallstone patients showed that oral cavity/respiratory tract inhabitants were more prevalent than intestinal inhabitants [108]. At the same time, bile samples from gallstone patients had reduced microbial diversity compared to healthy faecal samples [108]. Among patients with the new onset of common bile duct stones, five dominant phyla were identified: *Proteobacteria* (60%), *Firmicutes* (27%), *Bacteroidetes* (4%), *Actinobacteria* (3%), and Unclassified_Bacteria (3%) in biliary microbiota [111]. At the genus level, the five genera with the highest relative abundances in patients with the new onset of common bile duct stones were *Escherichia/Shigella*, *Halomonas, Klebsiella, Streptococcus,* and *Enterococcus* [111].

In patients with cholangiolithiasis associated with sphincter of Oddi laxity, *Proteobacteria* and *Firmicutes* were the most widespread phylotypes, especially *Enterobacteriaceae*, in the bile, which was collected intraoperatively [112]. In the bile of the cholecystectomized gallstone patients *Escherichia coli, Salmonella* sp., and *Enterococcusgallinarum* were detected by using next-generation sequencing technology [113]. *Enterobacteriaceae* are frequently isolated from bile aspirates or gallbladder bile from GSD patients using cultural [114,115] and culture-independent techniques [116,117]. The biliary microbiota (investigated by using 16S rRNA amplicon sequencing) had a reduced diversity comparatively with the duodenal microbiota in gallstone patients [117]. Although the majority of identified bacteria were greatly diminished in bile samples, three *Enterobacteriaceae* genera (*Escherichia, Klebsiella*, and an Unclassified genus) and *Pyramidobacter* were abundant in bile [117].

In terms of bile microbial distribution, analyzed by the 16S rRNA encoding gene (V3-V4), patients with recurrent common bile duct stone had significantly higher *Proteobacteria*, while *Bacteroidetes* and *Actinobacteria* are significantly lower compared with the control group at the phylum level [117]. At the family level, *Enterobacteriaceae* was significantly abundant in the bile samples of the recurrence stone group compared with the control group. At the genus level, the recurrence stone group had significantly more *Escherichia*. The diversity of bile microbiome in patients with recurrent common bile duct stone is lower than that in the control non-cholelithiasis group [117].

During a cholecystectomy, mucosal DNA extraction and metagenomic sequencing were performed to evaluate changes in the microbiota between chronic calculous cholecystitis and gallbladder cancer patients [118]. At the phylum level, *Firmicutes, Bacteroidetes, Actinobacteria,* and *Proteobacteria* were found to be stable in both groups. The diversity of the biliary microbiota was significantly lower in the calculous cholecystitis group, compared with the gallbladder cancer group [118].

In four patients who underwent cholecystectomy for acute calculous cholecystitis metagenome analysis of bile, faeces, and saliva was performed [119]. In all the examined patients with acute calculous cholecystitis, *Escherichia coli* (*Enterobacteriaceae* family) was found in large quantities in the bile, in two of them-also in the faeces, in the third patient, *Bifidobacterium* prevailed in the faeces. This is not enough to conclude the relationship between the intestinal microbiota and acute calculous cholecystitis, since if bile samples were taken during surgery, then saliva and faeces were collected by patients during hospitalization (it is not clear before or after the cholecystectomy) [119].

During endoscopic retrograde cholangiopancreatography, a total of 44 bile samples of patients with GSD were collected. Bacterial infection in bile samples was detected in 54.5% of patients with GSD. *Escherichia coli* showed a significant association with gallstones [122].

Thus, bile samples from patients with GSD had reduced microbial diversity in some studies and increased microbial diversity in others compared to healthy faecal samples. Nevertheless, most authors recognize that patients with GSD have reduced bacterial diversity of intestinal and bile microbiota. The phyla *Proteobacteria* (especially family *Enterobacteriaceae*) and *Firmicutes* (*Enterococcus* genus) were more often detected in the bile of patients with GSD, and the phyla *Bacteroidetes* and *Synergistes* (*Pyramidobacter* genus) were less frequently detected.

Some reports described live bacteria and bacterial DNA as long-term constituents in different fat depots in obesity and diabetes mellitus type 2 [123,124]. In humans with the metabolic syndrome, altered microbiome composition together with a defective intestinal barrier has been suggested to facilitate translocation of microbes, thereby contributing to low-grade inflammation. A recent study demonstrated a bacterial signature in mesenteric adipose tissues without the obvious presence of blood: members of the *Enterobacteriaceae* family compartmentalize in the extra-intestinal tissues of people with diabetes mellitus type 2 independently of obesity [123]. The authors suggest that members of the *Enterobacteriaceae* family are key players in diet-induced dysmetabolism in the host. Unfortunately, the intriguing topic of possible translocation of living bacteria (perhaps even members of the *Enterobacteriaceae* family) from the gut to other body sites in patients with GSD remains undiscovered.

So, when analyzing available studies of intestinal and bile microbiota in animals and patients with GSD [5,6,15,79–82,92,93,100,102–119] there were no unidirectional changes in the *Firmicutes/Bacteroidetes* ratio. This situation with opposite results is typical not only for GSD. For comparison, we will briefly present the results of several studies reporting differences in phylum levels in patients with non-alcoholic fatty liver disease (usually associated with obesity): the phylum *Bacteroidetes*–increased [86], decreased [88,125], did not differ [87,126], the phylum *Firmicutes*–decreased [86,87], increased [126], and the *Firmicutes/Bacteroidetes* ratio decreased [88].

This variation in the relative abundance of the phylum of the gut corresponds to the analysis of seven studies in Finucane et al. (2014): *Bacteroidetes*–from 0% to 90%, *Firmicutes*–from 0 to 100% [63]. This also applies to GSD. For example, the highest abundance of *Firmicutes* phylum in the human gastrointestinal tract in one GSD patient was 93.30% and the lowest was 1.17% in another. A similar result was also seen in bile with a high of 55.10% and low of 0.08% [107]. In another study, the range of relative abundance of *Firmicutes* phylum was 0–92% in the bile of patients with GSD [79].

5. Some Reasons for the Lack of Unity in the Assessment of the *Firmicutes/Bacteroidetes* Ratio

Gut microbiota is changing with human development and is influenced by many confounding variables which could prevent the existence of a unique taxonomic signature as a standard feature for obesity and associated comorbidities such as GSD [64,83,89].

1. Gender, age, differences in host genetics [4]. There are differences in the gut microbiota between males and females, such as higher levels of **Bacteroides–Prevotella** group in males [127] and a higher proportion of *Firmicutes* in females [128]. However, Bezek et al. (2020) found the highest abundance of *Bacteroidetes* phylum in females [51]. The *Firmicutes/Bacteroidetes* ratio evolves during different life stages. For infants (up to 10 months), adults (25–45 years), and elderly individuals (70–90 years), these ratios were 0.4, 10.9, and 0.6, respectively [44].
2. Vaginal delivery or C-section, methods of milk feeding [129].
3. Changes in the gut microbiota under the influence of a variety of diets have been widely studied [30–32,35,36,38,47,52,62,72,73,84,91,129–131]. It was noted that the amount of stool energy in a proportion of ingested calories was positively correlated

with the abundance of the phylum *Bacteroidetes* and negatively–with the abundance of the phylum *Firmicutes* in the faeces [38]. As a rule, the "western diet" increases biliary secretion of bile acids and reshapes the gut microbiota in obesity by increasing the *Firmicutes* and decreasing the *Bacteroidetes* [35,62]. Several population-based studies have shown that populations given increased amounts of polyunsaturated fats have a significant risk of developing gallstones [9,12,132–134]. The MICOL study, however, showed no such association [135]. Gutiérrez-Díaz et al. (2018) support a link between diet, biliary microbiota, and GSD [84]. Comparing to health control in patients with GSD, dairy product intake was negatively associated with the proportions of *Bacteroidaceae* and *Bacteroides*, and several types of fibre, phenolics, and fatty acids were linked to the abundance of *Bacteroidaceae*, *Chitinophagaceae*, *Propionibacteraceae*, *Bacteroides*, and *Escherichia-Shigella* [84]. However, the timing of these changes is surprising. In response to dietary perturbations, the gut microbiota took from 24 h [130] to 3.5 days [36] to change detectably and reaches a new steady state. Repeated dietary shifts demonstrated that most changes to the gut microbiota are reversible [36]. Also, Carmody et al. (2015) suggest, that the effects of dietary intake overshadow any pre-existing differences between strains due to host genotype [36]. Add to this the inter-individual variability in the processing of dietary compounds by the human gastrointestinal tract [136] and the hope of finding patterns in the relationship "microbiota–host–diet" becomes quite vague.

4. The presence of pathological conditions (diabetes mellitus [83], cardiovascular disease [89], inflammatory bowel disease [64], etc.). For example, the sphincter of Oddi laxity is associated with cholangiolithiasis, probably due to enhanced reflux of intestinal contents that change the microenvironment [112]. Compared with patients with cholangiolithiasis with normal sphincter of Oddi, patients with sphincter of Oddi laxity possessed more varied microbiota [112].

5. Treatment (antibiotics [137], metformin [138], etc.). Metformin shifts gut microbiota composition through the enrichment of *Akkermansia muciniphila* as well as several SCFA-producing microbiotas (*Butyrivibrio*, *Bifidobacterium bifidum*, etc.) [138].

6. The influence of exercise training on the gut microbiome has also been examined [29,91,131] and it has been shown that exercise alone increased the *Firmicutes/Bacteroidetes* ratio, irrespective of diet [91].

7. Human microbiota differs according to the geographical location of the studies [113, 139–141]. It was found a positive correlation between *Firmicutes* and latitude and a negative correlation between *Bacteroidetes* and latitude [139]. In the frame of study of human gut microbiota community structures in urban and rural populations in Russia, two clusters were obtained: the first was driven by the genus *Prevotella*, and the second exhibited a high representation of *Bifidobacterium* and various genera of the phylum *Firmicutes*. The urban and rural metagenomes were distributed equally between the clusters: 53% of the first and 52% of the second cluster were urban [141].

8. Lifestyle. Sleep deprivation correlates with changes in the gut microbiome, with an increase of the *Firmicutes/Bacteroidetes* ratio, higher abundances of the families *Coriobacteriaceae* and *Erysipelotrichaceae*, and lower abundance of *Tenericutes* [51,142]. Stress, occupation, temporal dynamics and stability of the microbiome: diurnal oscillations in the relative abundance of almost 10% of all bacterial taxa were detected [143].

9. The extreme variability of the *Firmicutes/Bacteroidetes* ratio can be attributed to the different experimental designs (insufficient sample size [144]), microbiota fingerprinting, and genome analyses (choice of the primers for the 16S rRNA target region, DNA extraction technique [145], and sequencing platform) [50,146]. Besides, members of the *Bacteroidetes* and *Actinobacteria* were significantly more stable components of the microbiota than the population average, while the *Firmicutes* and *Proteobacteria* were significantly less stable [147]. The plasticity vs. stability dichotomy of the human microbiome was confirmed in a study by David et al. (2014): when analyzing microbiota samples over several months, only 5% of the gut species were defined as belonging to

a stable temporal core microbiome. Yet, each person still maintained a personalized microbiome [140].
10. There are also hard-to-determine factors, such as the Earth's geomagnetic field, weather, etc.

6. Conclusions

Meta-analysis has shown that the microbial changes associated with obesity may be minor shifts in the community that escape detection with significance tests [77]. It may be the case that the microbiome's effect on obesity is not mediated through its taxonomic composition but rather its function, since closely related taxa can have widely varying functions and distantly related taxa can have similar functions [63]. It is proved that variable combinations of species from different phyla could 'presumptively' fulfil overlapping and/or complementary functional roles required by the host, a scenario where minor bacterial taxa seem to be significant active contributors [39]. For example, the cocolonization of germ-free mice with *B. Thetaiotaomicron* and *E. rectale* constitutes a mutualism, in which both members show a clear benefit [148] and the efficiency of fermentation of dietary polysaccharides to short-chain fatty acids by *B. thetaiotaomicron* increases in the presence of *M. Smithii* [149].

Based on the analysis of the great number of contradictory results reported in the literature, it is currently difficult to associate specific microbial signatures or the *Firmicutes/Bacteroidetes* ratio with determining health status and more specifically to consider it as a hallmark of GSD and/or obesity. However, most authors believe that both obesity [33,34,40,48,64,130] and GSD [5,6,81,103,109,111,117–120] are associated with reduced microbial diversity.Therefore, it is important to look at the overall composition of the gut microbial population structure as an indicator of obesity and obesity-associated pathologies, such as GSD, rather than simply the *Firmicutes/Bacteroidetes* ratio [150]. However, in my opinion, it is possible to modify this ratio, e.g., to introduce a coefficient that characterizes BMI, to calculate the ratio not of the *Firmicutes* phylum, but only of the *Clostridia* class, and so on.

Further studies should focus on the possibility of modulating the intestinal microbiota to find out whether variations in the microbiota may be a target for lowering the risks and prevalence rates of GSD. Future studies to identify specific bacterial species or populations associated with the obesity or GSD phenotype will help optimize disease therapies through microbiome-informed patient stratification, through personalized treatment decisions. A better understanding of bacterial communities in both the gut and biliary tract of gallstone patients is crucial in developing strategies to promote personalized microbiome-based GSD prediction and treatment responsiveness.

Funding: This study was performed according to the framework of the budget theme of the State assignment no. AAAA-A17-117112850280-2 and with the financial support of the Biocodex MICROBIOTA Foundation, France.

Institutional Review Board Statement: Not applicable.

Informed Consent Statement: Not applicable.

Ethical Statement:: The author is accountable for all aspects of the work in ensuring that questions related to the accuracy or integrity of any part of the work are appropriately investigated and resolved.

Data Availability Statement: Not applicable.

Conflicts of Interest: The author declares no conflict of interest. The funders had no role in the design of the study; in the collection, analyses, or interpretation of data; in the writing of the manuscript, or in the decision to publish the results.

References

1. Ley, R.E.; Bäckhed, F.; Turnbaugh, P.; Lozupone, C.A.; Knight, R.D.; Gordon, J.I. Obesity alters gut microbial ecology. *Proc. Natl. Acad. Sci. USA* **2005**, *102*, 11070–11075. [CrossRef] [PubMed]

2. Mathur, R.; Barlow, G.M. Obesity and the microbiome. *Expert Rev. Gastroenterol. Hepatol.* **2015**, *9*, 1087–1099. [CrossRef]
3. WHO Overweight and Obesity. Available online: http://www.who.int/gho/ncd/risk_factors/overweight/en/ (accessed on 1 June 2019).
4. Woting, A.; Blaut, M. The Intestinal Microbiota in Metabolic Disease. *Nutrients* **2016**, *8*, 202. [CrossRef] [PubMed]
5. Keren, N.; Konikoff, F.M.; Paitan, Y.; Gabay, G.; Reshef, L.; Naftali, T.; Gophna, U. Interactions between the intestinal microbiota and bile acids in gallstones patients. *Environ. Microbiol. Rep.* **2015**, *7*, 874–880. [CrossRef] [PubMed]
6. Wang, Q.; Hao, C.; Yao, W.; Zhu, D.; Lu, H.; Li, L.; Ma, B.; Sun, B.; Xue, D.; Zhang, W. Intestinal flora imbalance affects bile acid metabolism and is associated with gallstone formation. *BMC Gastroenterol.* **2020**, *20*, 1–13. [CrossRef]
7. Salinas, G.; Velásquez, C.; Saavedra, L.; Ramírez, E.; Angulo, H.; Tamayo, J.C.; Orellana, A.; Huivin, Z.; Valdivia, C.; Rodríguez, W. Prevalence and Risk Factors for Gallstone Disease. *Surg. Laparosc. Endosc. Percutaneous Tech.* **2004**, *14*, 250–253. [CrossRef]
8. Chen, C.-H.; Huang, M.-H.; Yang, J.-C.; Nien, C.-K.; Etheredge, G.D.; Yang, C.-C.; Yeh, Y.-H.; Wu, H.-S.; Yueh, S.-K.; Chou, D.-A. Prevalence and risk factors of gallstone disease in an adult population of Taiwan: An epidemiological survey. *J. Gastroenterol. Hepatol.* **2006**, *21*, 1737–1743. [CrossRef]
9. Misciagna, G.; Centonze, S.; Leoci, C.; Guerra, V.; Cisternino, A.M.; Ceo, R.; Trevisan, M. Diet, physical activity, and gallstones—A population-based, case-control study in southern Italy. *Am. J. Clin. Nutr.* **1999**, *69*, 120–126. [CrossRef]
10. Di Ciaula, A.; Wang, D.Q.-H.; Portincasa, P. An update on the pathogenesis of cholesterol gallstone disease. *Curr. Opin. Gastroenterol.* **2018**, *34*, 71–80. [CrossRef]
11. Liu, T.; Wang, W.; Ji, Y.; Wang, Y.; Liu, X.; Cao, L.; Liu, S. Association between different combination of measures for obesity and new-onset gallstone disease. *PLoS ONE* **2018**, *13*, e0196457. [CrossRef]
12. Kiani, Q.; Farooqui, F.; Khan, M.S.; Khan, A.Z.; Tariq, M.N.; Akhtar, A. Association of Body Mass Index and Diet with Symptomatic Gall Stone Disease: A Case-Control Study. *Cureus* **2020**, *12*, e7188. [CrossRef] [PubMed]
13. Stahlberg, D.; Rudling, M.; Angelin, B.; Björkhem, I.; Forsell, P.; Nilsell, K.; Einarsson, K. Hepatic cholesterol metabolism in human obesity. *Hepatology* **1997**, *25*, 1447–1450. [CrossRef] [PubMed]
14. Wen, H.; Gris, D.; Lei, Y.; Jha, S.; Zhang, L.; Huang, M.T.-H.; Brickey, W.J.; Ting, J. Fatty acid-induced NLRP3-ASC inflammasome activation interferes with insulin signaling. *Nat. Immunol.* **2011**, *12*, 408–415. [CrossRef] [PubMed]
15. Maurer, K.J.; Carey, M.C.; Fox, J.G. Roles of Infection, Inflammation, and the Immune System in Cholesterol Gallstone Formation. *Gastroenterology* **2009**, *136*, 425–440. [CrossRef]
16. Biddinger, S.B.; Haas, J.T.; Yu, B.B.; Bezy, O.; Jing, E.; Zhang, W.; Unterman, T.G.; Carey, M.C.; Kahn, C.R. Hepatic insulin resistance directly promotes formation of cholesterol gallstones. *Nat. Med.* **2008**, *14*, 778–782. [CrossRef]
17. Paramsothy, P.; Knopp, R.H.; Kahn, S.E.; Retzlaff, B.M.; Fish, B.; Ma, L.; Ostlund, R.E., Jr. Plasma sterol evidence for decreased absorption and increased synthesis of cholesterol in insulin resistance and obesity. *Am. J. Clin. Nutr.* **2011**, *94*, 1182–1188. [CrossRef]
18. Nakeeb, A.; Comuzzie, A.G.; Al-Azzawi, H.; Sonnenberg, G.E.; Kissebah, A.H.; Pitt, H.A. Insulin Resistance Causes Human Gallbladder Dysmotility. *J. Gastrointest. Surg.* **2006**, *10*, 940–949. [CrossRef]
19. Dhamnetiya, D.; Goel, M.K.; Dhiman, B.; Pathania, O.P. Gallstone disease and its correlates among patients attending teaching hospital of North India. *J. Fam. Med. Prim. Care* **2019**, *8*, 189–193. [CrossRef]
20. Wang, S.-Z.; Yu, Y.; Adeli, K. Role of Gut Microbiota in Neuroendocrine Regulation of Carbohydrate and Lipid Metabolism via the Microbiota-Gut-Brain-Liver Axis. *Microorganisms* **2020**, *8*, 527. [CrossRef]
21. Ceranowicz, P.; Warzecha, Z.; Dembinski, A. Peptidyl hormones of endocrine cells origin in the gut—Their discovery and physiological relevance. *J. Physiol. Pharmacol.* **2015**, *66*, 11–27.
22. Abizaid, A. Stress and obesity: The ghrelin connection. *J. Neuroendocrinol.* **2019**, *31*, e12693. [CrossRef] [PubMed]
23. Cui, H.; López, M.; Rahmouni, H.C.K. The cellular and molecular bases of leptin and ghrelin resistance in obesity. *Nat. Rev. Endocrinol.* **2017**, *13*, 338–351. [CrossRef] [PubMed]
24. Churm, R.; Davies, J.; Stephens, J.W.; Prior, S.L. Ghrelin function in human obesity and type 2 diabetes: A concise review. *Obes. Rev.* **2017**, *18*, 140–148. [CrossRef] [PubMed]
25. Bugajska, J.; Gotfryd-Bugajska, K.; Szura, M.; Berska, J.; Pasternak, A.; Sztefko, K. Characteristics of amino acid profile and incretin hormones in patients with gallstone disease—A pilot study. *Pol. Arch. Intern. Med.* **2019**, *129*, 883–888. [CrossRef] [PubMed]
26. Mendez-Sanchez, N.; Ponciano-Rodriguez, G.; Bermejo-Martinez, L.; Villa, A.R.; Chavez-Tapia, N.C.; Zamora-Valdes, D.; Pichardo-Bahena, R.; Barredo-Prieto, B.; Uribe-Ramos, M.H.; Ramos, M.H.; et al. Low serum levels of ghrelin are associated with gallstone disease. *World J. Gastroenterol.* **2006**, *12*, 3096–3100. [CrossRef]
27. Bungau, S.; Behl, T.; Tit, D.M.; Banica, F.; Bratu, O.G.; Diaconu, C.C.; Nistor-Cseppento, C.D.; Bustea, C.; Aron, R.A.C.; Vesa, C.M. Interactions between leptin and insulin resistance in patients with prediabetes, with and without NAFLD. *Exp. Ther. Med.* **2020**, *20*, 1. [CrossRef]
28. Lei, Z.-M.; Ye, M.-X.; Fu, W.-G.; Chen, Y.; Fang, C.; Li, J. Levels of serum leptin, cholecystokinin, plasma lipid and lipoprotein differ between patients with gallstone or/and those with hepatolithiasis. *Hepatobiliary Pancreat. Dis. Int.* **2008**, *7*, 65–69.
29. Queipo-Ortuño, M.; Seoane, L.M.; Murri, M.; Pardo, M.; Gomez-Zumaquero, J.M.; Cardona, F.; Casanueva, F.; Tinahones, F.J. Gut Microbiota Composition in Male Rat Models under Different Nutritional Status and Physical Activity and Its Association with Serum Leptin and Ghrelin Levels. *PLoS ONE* **2013**, *8*, e65465. [CrossRef]

30. Ley, R.E.; Turnbaugh, P.J.; Klein, S.; Gordon, J.I. Human gut microbes associated with obesity. *Nature* **2006**, *444*, 1022–1023. [CrossRef]
31. Bäckhed, F.; Ding, H.; Wang, T.; Hooper, L.V.; Koh, G.Y.; Nagy, A.; Semenkovich, C.F.; Gordon, J.I. The gut microbiota as an environmental factor that regulates fat storage. *Proc. Natl. Acad. Sci. USA* **2004**, *101*, 15718–15723. [CrossRef]
32. Turnbaugh, P.J.; Ley, R.E.; Mahowald, M.A.; Magrini, V.; Mardis, E.R.; Gordon, J.I. An obesity-associated gut microbiome with increased capacity for energy harvest. *Nature* **2006**, *444*, 1027–1031. [CrossRef] [PubMed]
33. Turnbaugh, P.J.; Hamady, M.; Yatsunenko, T.; Cantarel, B.L.; Duncan, A.; Ley, R.E.; Sogin, M.L.; Jones, W.J.; Roe, B.A.; Affourtit, J.P.; et al. A core gut microbiome in obese and lean twins. *Nature* **2008**, *457*, 480–484. [CrossRef] [PubMed]
34. Armougom, F.; Henry, M.; Vialettes, B.; Raccah, D.; Raoult, D. Monitoring Bacterial Community of Human Gut Microbiota Reveals an Increase in Lactobacillus in Obese Patients and Methanogens in Anorexic Patients. *PLoS ONE* **2009**, *4*, e7125. [CrossRef] [PubMed]
35. Murphy, E.F.; Cotter, P.D.; Healy, S.; Marques, T.M.; O'Sullivan, O.; Fouhy, F.; Clarke, S.F.; O'Toole, P.W.; Quigley, E.M.; Stanton, C.; et al. Composition and energy harvesting capacity of the gut microbiota: Relationship to diet, obesity and time in mouse models. *Gut* **2010**, *59*, 1635–1642. [CrossRef] [PubMed]
36. Carmody, R.N.; Gerber, G.K.; Luevano, J.M.; Gatti, D.M.; Somes, L.; Svenson, K.L.; Turnbaugh, P. Diet Dominates Host Genotype in Shaping the Murine Gut Microbiota. *Cell Host Microbe* **2015**, *17*, 72–84. [CrossRef]
37. Zuo, H.-J. Gut bacteria alteration in obese people and its relationship with gene polymorphism. *World J. Gastroenterol.* **2011**, *17*, 1076–1081. [CrossRef]
38. Jumpertz, R.; Le, D.S.; Turnbaugh, P.J.; Trinidad, C.; Bogardus, C.; Gordon, J.I.; Krakoff, J. Energy-balance studies reveal associations between gut microbes, caloric load, and nutrient absorption in humans. *Am. J. Clin. Nutr.* **2011**, *94*, 58–65. [CrossRef]
39. Ferrer, M.; Ruiz, A.; Lanza, F.; Haange, S.-B.; Oberbach, A.; Till, H.; Bargiela, R.; Campoy, C.; Segura, M.T.; Richter, M.; et al. Microbiota from the distal guts of lean and obese adolescents exhibit partial functional redundancy besides clear differences in community structure. *Environ. Microbiol.* **2013**, *15*, 211–226. [CrossRef]
40. Indiani, C.M.D.S.P.; Rizzardi, K.F.; Castelo, P.M.; Ferraz, L.F.C.; Darrieux, M.; Parisotto, T.M. Childhood Obesity and Firmicutes/Bacteroidetes Ratio in the Gut Microbiota: A Systematic Review. *Child Obes.* **2018**, *14*, 501–509. [CrossRef]
41. Koliada, A.; Syzenko, G.; Moseiko, V.; Budovska, L.; Puchkov, K.; Perederiy, V.; Gavalko, Y.; Dorofeyev, A.; Romanenko, M.; Tkach, S.; et al. Association between body mass index and Firmicutes/Bacteroidetes ratio in an adult Ukrainian population. *BMC Microbiol.* **2017**, *17*, 120. [CrossRef]
42. Crovesy, L.; Masterson, D.; Rosado, E.L. Profile of the gut microbiota of adults with obesity: A systematic review. *Eur. J. Clin. Nutr.* **2020**, *74*, 1251–1262. [CrossRef] [PubMed]
43. Vandana, U.K. Linking gut microbiota with human diseases. *Bioinformation* **2020**, *16*, 196–208. [CrossRef] [PubMed]
44. Qin, J.; Li, R.; Raes, J.; Arumugam, M.; Burgdorf, K.S.; Manichanh, C.; Nielsen, T.; Pons, N.; Levenez, F.; Yamada, T.; et al. A human gut microbial gene catalogue established by metagenomic sequencing. *Nature* **2010**, *464*, 59–65. [CrossRef] [PubMed]
45. Gilbert, J.A.; Blaser, M.J.; Caporaso, J.G.; Jansson, J.K.; Lynch, S.V.; Knight, R. Current understanding of the human microbiome. *Nat. Med.* **2018**, *24*, 392–400. [CrossRef]
46. Cani, P.D. Human gut microbiome: Hopes, threats and promises. *Gut* **2018**, *67*, 1716–1725. [CrossRef] [PubMed]
47. Claesson, M.J.; Jeffery, I.B.; Conde, S.; Power, S.E.; O'Connor, E.M.; Cusack, S.; Harris, H.M.B.; Coakley, M.; Lakshminarayanan, B.; O'Sullivan, O.; et al. Gut microbiota composition correlates with diet and health in the elderly. *Nature* **2012**, *488*, 178–184. [CrossRef]
48. Le Chatelier, E.; Nielsen, T.; Qin, J.; Prifti, E.; Hildebrand, F.; Falony, G.; Almeida, M.; Arumugam, M.; Batto, J.-M.; Kennedy, S.; et al. Richness of human gut microbiome correlates with metabolic markers. *Nature* **2013**, *500*, 541–546. [CrossRef]
49. Arora, T.; Bäckhed, F. The gut microbiota and metabolic disease: Current understanding and future perspectives. *J. Intern. Med.* **2016**, *280*, 339–349. [CrossRef]
50. Abenavoli, L.; Scarpellini, E.; Colica, C.; Boccuto, L.; Salehi, B.; Sharifi-Rad, J.; Aiello, V.; Romano, B.; De Lorenzo, A.; Izzo, A.A.; et al. Gut Microbiota and Obesity: A Role for Probiotics. *Nutrients* **2019**, *11*, 2690. [CrossRef]
51. Bezek, K.; Petelin, A.; Pražnikar, J.; Nova, E.; Redondo-Useros, N.; Marcos, A.; Pražnikar, Z.J. Obesity Measures and Dietary Parameters as Predictors of Gut Microbiota Phyla in Healthy Individuals. *Nutrients* **2020**, *12*, 2695. [CrossRef]
52. Wu, M.; Yang, S.; Wang, S.; Cao, Y.; Zhao, R.; Li, X.; Xing, Y.; Liu, L.-T. Effect of Berberine on Atherosclerosis and Gut Microbiota Modulation and Their Correlation in High-Fat Diet-Fed ApoE−/− Mice. *Front. Pharmacol.* **2020**, *11*, 223. [CrossRef] [PubMed]
53. Rajilic-Stojanovic, M.; De Vos, W.M. The first 1000 cultured species of the human gastrointestinal microbiota. *FEMS Microbiol. Rev.* **2014**, *38*, 996–1047. [CrossRef] [PubMed]
54. Vos, P.; Garrity, G.; Jones, D.; Krieg, N.R.; Ludwig, W.; Rainey, F.A.; Schleifer, K.-H.; Whitman, W. (Eds.) *Bergey's Manual of Systematic Bacteriology: Volume 3: The Firmicutes*; Springer Science & Business Media: New York, NY, USA, 2010.
55. Morotomi, M.; Nagai, F.; Sakon, H.; Tanaka, R. *Paraprevotella clara* gen. nov., sp. nov. and *Paraprevotella xylaniphila* sp. nov., members of the family '*Prevotellaceae*' isolated from human faeces. *Int. J. Syst. Evol. Microbiol.* **2009**, *59*, 1895–1900. [CrossRef] [PubMed]
56. Narushima, S.; Itoh, K.; Miyamoto, Y.; Park, S.-H.; Nagata, K.; Kuruma, K.; Uchida, K. Deoxycholic acid formation in gnotobiotic mice associated with human intestinal bacteria. *Lipids* **2006**, *41*, 835–843. [CrossRef] [PubMed]

57. Fukiya, S.; Arata, M.; Kawashima, H.; Yoshida, D.; Kaneko, M.; Minamida, K.; Watanabe, J.; Ogura, Y.; Uchida, K.; Itoh, K.; et al. Conversion of cholic acid and chenodeoxycholic acid into their 7-oxo derivatives byBacteroides intestinalisAM-1 isolated from human feces. *FEMS Microbiol. Lett.* **2009**, *293*, 263–270. [CrossRef] [PubMed]
58. Kasai, C.; Sugimoto, K.; Moritani, I.; Tanaka, J.; Oya, Y.; Inoue, H.; Tameda, M.; Shiraki, K.; Ito, M.; Takei, Y.; et al. Comparison of the gut microbiota composition between obese and non-obese individuals in a Japanese population, as analyzed by terminal restriction fragment length polymorphism and next-generation sequencing. *BMC Gastroenterol.* **2015**, *15*, 1–10. [CrossRef]
59. Lopetuso, L.R.; Scaldaferri, F.; Petito, V.; Gasbarrini, A. Commensal clostridia: Leading players in the maintenance of gut homeostasis. *Gut Pathog.* **2013**, *5*, 1–23. [CrossRef]
60. Tims, S.; Derom, C.; Jonkers, D.; Vlietinck, R.; Saris, W.H.; Kleerebezem, M.; De Vos, W.M.; Zoetendal, E.G. Microbiota conservation and BMI signatures in adult monozygotic twins. *ISME J.* **2013**, *7*, 707–717. [CrossRef]
61. Yanling, H.; Youfang, D.; Yanquan, L. Two Cellulolytic Clostridium Species: *Clostridium cellulosi* sp. nov. and *Clostridium cellulofermentans* sp. nov. *Int. J. Syst. Bacteriol.* **1991**, *41*, 306–309. [CrossRef]
62. Turnbaugh, P.J.; Ridaura, V.K.; Faith, J.J.; Rey, F.E.; Knight, R.; Gordon, J.I. The Effect of Diet on the Human Gut Microbiome: A Metagenomic Analysis in Humanized Gnotobiotic Mice. *Sci. Transl. Med.* **2009**, *1*, 6ra14. [CrossRef]
63. Finucane, M.M.; Sharpton, T.J.; Laurent, T.J.; Pollard, K.S. A Taxonomic Signature of Obesity in the Microbiome? Getting to the Guts of the Matter. *PLoS ONE* **2014**, *9*, e84689. [CrossRef] [PubMed]
64. Magne, F.; Gotteland, M.; Gauthier, L.; Zazueta, A.; Pesoa, S.; Navarrete, P.; Balamurugan, R. The Firmicutes/Bacoidetes Ratio: A Relevant Marker of Gut Dysbiosis in Obese Patients? *Nutrients* **2020**, *12*, 1474. [CrossRef] [PubMed]
65. Mariat, D.; Firmesse, O.; Levenez, F.; Guimaraes, V.D.; Sokol, H.; Doré, J.; Corthier, G.; Furet, J.-P. The Firmicutes/Bacteroidetes ratio of the human microbiota changes with age. *BMC Microbiol.* **2009**, *9*, 123. [CrossRef] [PubMed]
66. Vaiserman, A.; Romanenko, M.; Piven, L.; Moseiko, V.; Lushchak, O.; Kryzhanovska, N.; Guryanov, V.; Koliada, A. Differences in the gut Firmicutes to Bacteroidetes ratio across age groups in healthy Ukrainian population. *BMC Microbiol.* **2020**, *20*, 1–8. [CrossRef] [PubMed]
67. Nicholson, J.K.; Holmes, E.; Kinross, J.; Burcelin, R.; Gibson, G.; Jia, W.; Pettersson, S. Host-Gut Microbiota Metabolic Interactions. *Science* **2012**, *336*, 1262–1267. [CrossRef]
68. Tang, W.W.H.; Kitai, T.; Hazen, S.L. Gut Microbiota in Cardiovascular Health and Disease. *Circ. Res.* **2017**, *120*, 1183–1196. [CrossRef]
69. Peter, J.; Fournier, C.; Keip, B.; Rittershaus, N.; Stephanou-Rieser, N.; Durdevic, M.; Dejaco, C.; Michalski, M.; Moser, G. Intestinal Microbiome in Irritable Bowel Syndrome before and after Gut-Directed Hypnotherapy. *Int. J. Mol. Sci.* **2018**, *19*, 3619. [CrossRef]
70. Fernandes, J.J.D.R.; Su, W.; Rahat-Rozenbloom, S.; Wolever, T.M.S.; Comelli, E.M. Adiposity, gut microbiota and faecal short chain fatty acids are linked in adult humans. *Nutr. Diabetes* **2014**, *4*, e121. [CrossRef]
71. Vrieze, A.; Van Nood, E.; Holleman, F.; Salojärvi, J.; Kootte, R.S.; Bartelsman, J.F.W.M.; Dallinga-Thie, G.M.; Ackermans, M.T.; Serlie, M.J.; Oozeer, R.; et al. Transfer of Intestinal Microbiota From Lean Donors Increases Insulin Sensitivity in Individuals With Metabolic Syndrome. *Gastroenterology* **2012**, *143*, 913–916. [CrossRef]
72. Schwiertz, A.; Taras, D.; Schaefer, K.; Beijer, S.; Bos, N.A.; Donus, C.; Hardt, P.D. Microbiota and SCFA in Lean and Overweight Healthy Subjects. *Obesity* **2010**, *18*, 190–195. [CrossRef]
73. Duncan, S.H.; E Lobley, G.; Holtrop, G.; Ince, J.; Johnstone, A.M.; Louis, P.; Flint, H.J. Human colonic microbiota associated with diet, obesity and weight loss. *Int. J. Obes.* **2008**, *32*, 1720–1724. [CrossRef] [PubMed]
74. Andoh, A.; Nishida, A.; Takahashi, K.; Inatomi, O.; Imaeda, H.; Bamba, S.; Kito, K.; Sugimoto, M.; Kobayashi, T. Comparison of the gut microbial community between obese and lean peoples using 16S gene sequencing in a Japanese population. *J. Clin. Biochem. Nutr.* **2016**, *59*, 65–70. [CrossRef] [PubMed]
75. Payne, A.N.; Chassard, C.; Zimmermann, M.B.; Muller, P.H.; Stinca, S.; Lacroix, C. The metabolic activity of gut microbiota in obese children is increased compared with normal-weight children and exhibits more exhaustive substrate utilization. *Nutr. Diabetes* **2011**, *1*, e12. [CrossRef] [PubMed]
76. Angelakis, E.; Armougom, F.; Million, M.; Raoult, D. The relationship between gut microbiota and weight gain in humans. *Future Microbiol.* **2012**, *7*, 91–109. [CrossRef] [PubMed]
77. Walters, W.A.; Xu, Z.; Knight, R. Meta-analyses of human gut microbes associated with obesity and IBD. *FEBS Lett.* **2014**, *588*, 4223–4233. [CrossRef] [PubMed]
78. Harris, K.; Kassis, A.; Major, G.; Chou, C.J. Is the Gut Microbiota a New Factor Contributing to Obesity and Its Metabolic Disorders? *J. Obes.* **2012**, *2012*, 1–14. [CrossRef]
79. Saltykova, I.V.; Petrov, V.A.; Logacheva, M.D.; Ivanova, P.G.; Merzlikin, N.V.; Sazonov, A.E.; Ogorodova, L.; Brindley, P.J. Biliary Microbiota, Gallstone Disease and Infection with Opisthorchis felineus. *PLoS Negl. Trop. Dis.* **2016**, *10*, e0004809. [CrossRef]
80. Ren, X.; Xu, J.; Zhang, Y.; Chen, G.; Zhang, Y.; Huang, Q.; Liu, Y. Bacterial Alterations in Post-Cholecystectomy Patients Are Associated With Colorectal Cancer. *Front. Oncol.* **2020**, *10*, 1418. [CrossRef]
81. Wang, W.; Wang, J.; Li, J.; Yan, P.; Jin, Y.; Zhang, R.; Yue, W.; Guo, Q.; Geng, J. Cholecystectomy Damages Aging-Associated Intestinal Microbiota Construction. *Front. Microbiol.* **2018**, *9*, 1402. [CrossRef]
82. Yoon, W.J.; Kim, H.-N.; Park, E.; Ryu, S.; Chang, Y.; Shin, H.; Kim, H.-L.; Yi, S.Y. The Impact of Cholecystectomy on the Gut Microbiota: A Case-Control Study. *J. Clin. Med.* **2019**, *8*, 79. [CrossRef]

83. Qin, J.; Li, Y.; Cai, Z.; Li, S.; Zhu, J.; Zhang, F.; Liang, S.; Zhang, W.; Guan, Y.; Shen, D.; et al. A metagenome-wide association study of gut microbiota in type 2 diabetes. *Nature* **2012**, *490*, 55–60. [CrossRef] [PubMed]
84. Gutiérrez-Díaz, I.; Molinero, N.; Cabrera, A.; Rodríguez, J.I.; Margolles, A.; Delgado, S.; González, S. Diet: Cause or Consequence of the Microbial Profile of Cholelithiasis Disease? *Nutrients* **2018**, *10*, 1307. [CrossRef] [PubMed]
85. Del Chierico, F.; Nobili, V.; Vernocchi, P.; Russo, A.; De Stefanis, C.; Gnani, D.; Furlanello, C.; Zandonà, A.; Paci, P.; Capuani, G.; et al. Gut microbiota profiling of pediatric nonalcoholic fatty liver disease and obese patients unveiled by an integrated meta-omics-based approach. *Hepatology* **2017**, *65*, 451–464. [CrossRef] [PubMed]
86. Zhu, L.; Baker, S.S.; Gill, C.; Liu, W.; Alkhouri, R.; Baker, R.D.; Gill, S.R. Characterization of gut microbiomes in nonalcoholic steatohepatitis (NASH) patients: A connection between endogenous alcohol and NASH. *Hepatology* **2013**, *57*, 601–609. [CrossRef]
87. Wong, V.W.-S.; Tse, C.-H.; Lam, T.T.-Y.; Wong, G.L.-H.; Chim, A.M.-L.; Chu, W.C.-W.; Yeung, D.K.-W.; Law, P.T.-W.; Kwan, H.-S.; Yu, J.; et al. Molecular Characterization of the Fecal Microbiota in Patients with Nonalcoholic Steatohepatitis—A Longitudinal Study. *PLoS ONE* **2013**, *8*, e62885. [CrossRef]
88. Da Silva, H.E.; Teterina, A.; Comelli, E.M.; Taibi, A.; Arendt, B.M.; Fischer, S.E.; Lou, W.; Allard, J.P. Nonalcoholic fatty liver disease is associated with dysbiosis independent of body mass index and insulin resistance. *Sci. Rep.* **2018**, *8*, 1–12. [CrossRef]
89. Cortés-Martín, A.; Iglesias-Aguirre, C.E.; Meoro, A.; Selma, M.V.; Espín, J.C. There is No Distinctive Gut Microbiota Signature in the Metabolic Syndrome: Contribution of Cardiovascular Disease Risk Factors and Associated Medication. *Microorganisms* **2020**, *8*, 416. [CrossRef]
90. Álvarez-Mercado, A.I.; Navarro-Oliveros, M.; Robles-Sánchez, C.; Plaza-Díaz, J.; Sáez-Lara, M.J.; Muñoz-Quezada, S.; Fontana, L.; Abadía-Molina, F. Microbial Population Changes and Their Relationship with Human Health and Disease. *Microorganisms* **2019**, *7*, 68. [CrossRef]
91. Evans, C.C.; LePard, K.J.; Kwak, J.W.; Stancukas, M.C.; Laskowski, S.; Dougherty, J.; Moulton, L.; Glawe, A.; Wang, Y.; Leone, V.; et al. Exercise Prevents Weight Gain and Alters the Gut Microbiota in a Mouse Model of High Fat Diet-Induced Obesity. *PLoS ONE* **2014**, *9*, e92193. [CrossRef]
92. Maki, T. Pathogenesis of calcium bilirubinate gallstone: Role of E. coli, beta-glucuronidase and coagulation by inorganic ions, polyelectrolytes and agitation. *Ann. Surg.* **2006**, *164*, 90–100. [CrossRef]
93. Stewart, L.; Smith, A.L.; Pellegrini, C.A.; Motson, R.W.; Way, L.W. Pigment Gallstones Form as a Composite of Bacterial Microcolonies and Pigment Solids. *Ann. Surg.* **1987**, *206*, 242–250. [CrossRef] [PubMed]
94. Ridlon, J.M.; Kang, D.-J.; Hylemon, P.B. Bile salt biotransformations by human intestinal bacteria. *J. Lipid Res.* **2005**, *47*, 241–259. [CrossRef] [PubMed]
95. Gérard, P. Metabolism of Cholesterol and Bile Acids by the Gut Microbiota. *Pathogens* **2013**, *3*, 14–24. [CrossRef] [PubMed]
96. Ridlon, J.M.; Harris, S.C.; Bhowmik, S.; Kang, D.-J.; Hylemon, P.B. Consequences of bile salt biotransformations by intestinal bacteria. *Gut Microbes* **2016**, *7*, 22–39. [CrossRef] [PubMed]
97. Long, S.L.; Gahan, C.G.M.; Joyce, S.A. Interactions between gut bacteria and bile in health and disease. *Mol. Asp. Med.* **2017**, *56*, 54–65. [CrossRef]
98. Li, F.; Jiang, C.; Krausz, K.W.; Li, Y.; Albert, I.; Hao, H.; Fabre, K.M.; Mitchell, J.B.; Patterson, A.D.; Gonzalez, F.J. Microbiome remodelling leads to inhibition of intestinal farnesoid X receptor signalling and decreased obesity. *Nat. Commun.* **2013**, *4*, 1–10. [CrossRef]
99. Wells, J.E.; Berr, F.; Thomas, L.A.; Dowling, R.; Hylemon, P.B. Isolation and characterization of cholic acid 7α-dehydroxylating fecal bacteria from cholesterol gallstone patients. *J. Hepatol.* **2000**, *32*, 4–10. [CrossRef]
100. Berr, F.; Kullak-Ublick, G.A.; Paumgartner, G.; Munzing, W.; Hylemon, P.B. 7 alpha-dehydroxylating bacteria enhance deoxycholic acid input and cholesterol saturation of bile in patients with gallstones. *Gastroenterology* **1996**, *111*, 1611–1620. [CrossRef]
101. Hussaini, S.H.; Pereira, S.P.; Murphy, G.M.; Dowling, R.H. Deoxycholic acid influences cholesterol solubilization and microcrystal nucleation time in gallbladder bile. *Hepatology* **1995**, *22*, 1735–1744.
102. Fremont-Rahl, J.J.; Ge, Z.; Umana, C.; Whary, M.T.; Taylor, N.S.; Muthupalani, S.; Carey, M.C.; Fox, J.G.; Maurer, K.J. An Analysis of the Role of the Indigenous Microbiota in Cholesterol Gallstone Pathogenesis. *PLoS ONE* **2013**, *8*, e70657. [CrossRef]
103. Wang, Q.; Jiao, L.; He, C.; Sun, H.; Cai, Q.; Han, T.; Hu, H. Alteration of gut microbiota in association with cholesterol gallstone formation in mice. *BMC Gastroenterol.* **2017**, *17*, 1–9. [CrossRef] [PubMed]
104. Grigor'eva, I.N.; Romanova, T.I. Gallstone Disease and Microbiome. *Microorganisms* **2020**, *8*, 835. [CrossRef] [PubMed]
105. Hepner, G.W.; Hofmann, A.F.; Malagelada, J.R.; Szczepanik, P.A.; Klein, P.D. Increased Bacterial Degradation of Bile Acids in Cholecystectomized Patients. *Gastroenterology* **1974**, *66*, 556–564. [CrossRef]
106. Kang, Z.; Lu, M.; Jiang, M.; Zhou, D.; Huang, H. Proteobacteria Acts as a Pathogenic Risk-Factor for Chronic Abdominal Pain and Diarrhea in Post-Cholecystectomy Syndrome Patients: A Gut Microbiome Metabolomics Study. *Med. Sci. Monit.* **2019**, *25*, 7312–7320. [CrossRef]
107. Wu, T.; Zhang, Z.; Liu, B.; Hou, D.; Liang, Y.; Zhang, J.; Shi, P. Gut microbiota dysbiosis and bacterial community assembly associated with cholesterol gallstones in large-scale study. *BMC Genom.* **2013**, *14*, 669. [CrossRef]
108. Shen, H.; Ye, F.; Xie, L.; Yang, J.; Li, Z.; Xu, P.; Meng, F.; Li, L.; Xiaochen, B.; Bo, X.; et al. Metagenomic sequencing of bile from gallstone patients to identify different microbial community patterns and novel biliary bacteria. *Sci. Rep.* **2015**, *5*, 17450. [CrossRef]

109. Molinero, N.; Ruiz, L.; Milani, C.; Gutiérrez-Díaz, I.; Sánchez, B.; Mangifesta, M.; Segura, J.; Cambero, I.; Campelo, A.B.; García-Bernardo, C.M.; et al. The human gallbladder microbiome is related to the physiological state and the biliary metabolic profile. *Microbiome* **2019**, *7*, 1–17. [CrossRef]
110. Petrov, V.A.; Fernández-Peralbo, M.A.; Derks, R.; Knyazeva, E.M.; Merzlikin, N.V.; Sazonov, A.E.; Mayboroda, O.A.; Saltykova, I.V. Biliary Microbiota and Bile Acid Composition in Cholelithiasis. *BioMed Res. Int.* **2020**, *2020*, 1–8. [CrossRef]
111. Chen, B.; Fu, S.W.; Lu, L.-G.; Zhao, H. A Preliminary Study of Biliary Microbiota in Patients with Bile Duct Stones or Distal Cholangiocarcinoma. *BioMed Res. Int.* **2019**, *2019*, 1–12. [CrossRef]
112. Liang, T.; Su, W.; Zhang, Q.; Li, G.; Gao, S.; Lou, J.; Zhang, Y.; Ma, T.; Bai, X. Roles of Sphincter of Oddi Laxity in Bile Duct Microenvironment in Patients with Cholangiolithiasis: From the Perspective of the Microbiome and Metabolome. *J. Am. Coll. Surg.* **2016**, *222*, 269–280. [CrossRef]
113. Tsuchiya, Y.; Loza, E.; Villa-Gomez, G.; Trujillo, C.C.; Baez, S.; Asai, T.; Ikoma, T.; Endoh, K.; Nakamura, K. Metagenomics of Microbial Communities in Gallbladder Bile from Patients with Gallbladder Cancer or Cholelithiasis. *Asian Pac. J. Cancer Prev.* **2018**, *19*, 961–967. [PubMed]
114. Capoor, M.R.; Nair, D.; Rajni; Khanna, G.; Krishna, S.V.; Chintamani, M.S.; Aggarwal, P. Microflora of bile aspirates in patients with acute cholecystitis with or without cholelithiasis: A tropical experience. *Braz. J. Infect. Dis.* **2008**, *12*, 222–225. [CrossRef] [PubMed]
115. Abeysuriya, V.; Deen, K.I.; Wijesuriya, T.; Salgado, S.S. Microbiology of gallbladder bile in uncomplicated symptomatic cholelithiasis. *Hepatobiliary Pancreat. Dis. Int.* **2008**, *7*, 633–637. [PubMed]
116. Liu, J.; Yan, Q.; Luo, F.; Shang, D.; Wu, D.; Zhang, H.; Shang, X.; Kang, X.; Abdo, M.; Liu, B.; et al. Acute cholecystitis associated with infection of Enterobacteriaceae from gut microbiota. *Clin. Microbiol. Infect.* **2015**, *21*, 851.e1–851.e9. [CrossRef]
117. Ye, F.; Shen, H.; Li, Z.; Meng, F.; Li, L.; Yang, J.; Chen, Y.; Bo, X.; Zhang, X.; Ni, M. Influence of the Biliary System on Biliary Bacteria Revealed by Bacterial Communities of the Human Biliary and Upper Digestive Tracts. *PLoS ONE* **2016**, *11*, e0150519. [CrossRef]
118. Song, X.; Wang, X.; Hu, Y.; Li, H.; Ren, T.; Li, Y.; Liu, L.; Li, L.; Li, X.; Wang, Z.; et al. A metagenomic study of biliary microbiome change along the cholecystitis-carcinoma sequence. *Clin. Transl. Med.* **2020**, *10*, 97. [CrossRef]
119. Kujiraoka, M.; Kuroda, M.; Asai, K.; Sekizuka, T.; Kato, K.; Watanabe, M.; Matsukiyo, H.; Saito, T.; Ishii, T.; Katada, N.; et al. Comprehensive Diagnosis of Bacterial Infection Associated with Acute Cholecystitis Using Metagenomic Approach. *Front. Microbiol.* **2017**, *8*, 685. [CrossRef]
120. Islam, K.S.; Fukiya, S.; Hagio, M.; Fujii, N.; Ishizuka, S.; Ooka, T.; Ogura, Y.; Hayashi, T.; Yokota, A. Bile Acid Is a Host Factor That Regulates the Composition of the Cecal Microbiota in Rats. *Gastroenterology* **2011**, *141*, 1773–1781. [CrossRef]
121. Ridlon, J.M.; Alves, J.M.P.; Hylemon, P.B.; Bajaj, J.S. Cirrhosis, bile acids and gut microbiota: Unraveling a complex relationship. *Gut Microbes* **2013**, *4*, 382–387. [CrossRef]
122. Tajeddin, E.; Sherafat, S.J.; Majidi, M.R.S.; Alebouyeh, M.; Alizadeh, A.H.M.; Zali, M.R. Association of diverse bacterial communities in human bile samples with biliary tract disorders: A survey using culture and polymerase chain reaction-denaturing gradient gel electrophoresis methods. *Eur. J. Clin. Microbiol. Infect. Dis.* **2016**, *35*, 1331–1339. [CrossRef]
123. Anhê, F.F.; Jensen, B.A.H.; Varin, T.V.; Servant, F.; Van Blerk, S.; Richard, D.; Marceau, S.; Surette, M.G.; Biertho, L.; Lelouvier, B.; et al. Type 2 diabetes influences bacterial tissue compartmentalisation in human obesity. *Nat. Metab.* **2020**, *2*, 233–242. [CrossRef] [PubMed]
124. Massier, L.; Chakaroun, R.; Tabei, S.; Crane, A.; Didt, K.D.; Fallmann, J.; Von Bergen, M.; Haange, S.-B.; Heyne, H.; Stumvoll, M.; et al. Adipose tissue derived bacteria are associated with inflammation in obesity and type 2 diabetes. *Gut* **2020**, *69*, 1796–1806. [CrossRef] [PubMed]
125. Mouzaki, M.; Comelli, E.M.; Arendt, B.M.; Bonengel, J.; Fung, S.K.; Fischer, S.E.; McGilvray, I.D.; Allard, J.P. Intestinal microbiota in patients with nonalcoholic fatty liver disease. *Hepatology* **2013**, *58*, 120–127. [CrossRef] [PubMed]
126. Raman, M.; Ahmed, I.; Gillevet, P.M.; Probert, C.S.; Ratcliffe, N.M.; Smith, S.; Greenwood, R.; Sikaroodi, M.; Lam, V.; Crotty, P.; et al. Fecal Microbiome and Volatile Organic Compound Metabolome in Obese Humans With Nonalcoholic Fatty Liver Disease. *Clin. Gastroenterol. Hepatol.* **2013**, *11*, 868–875.e3. [CrossRef] [PubMed]
127. Mueller, S.; Saunier, K.; Hanisch, C.; Norin, E.; Alm, L.; Midtvedt, T.; Cresci, A.; Silvi, S.; Orpianesi, C.; Verdenelli, M.C.; et al. Differences in Fecal Microbiota in Different European Study Populations in Relation to Age, Gender, and Country: A Cross-Sectional Study. *Appl. Environ. Microbiol.* **2006**, *72*, 1027–1033. [CrossRef] [PubMed]
128. Haro, C.; Rangel-Zúñiga, O.A.; Alcalá-Díaz, J.F.; Gómez-Delgado, F.; Pérez-Martínez, P.; Delgado-Lista, J.; Quintana-Navarro, G.M.; Landa, B.B.; Cortés, J.A.N.; Tena-Sempere, M.; et al. Intestinal Microbiota Is Influenced by Gender and Body Mass Index. *PLoS ONE* **2016**, *11*, e0154090. [CrossRef]
129. Rinninella, E.; Raoul, P.; Cintoni, M.; Franceschi, F.; Miggiano, G.A.D.; Gasbarrini, A.; Mele, M.C. What is the Healthy Gut Microbiota Composition? A Changing Ecosystem across Age, Environment, Diet, and Diseases. *Microorganisms* **2019**, *7*, 14. [CrossRef]
130. Wu, G.D.; Chen, J.; Hoffmann, C.; Bittinger, K.; Chen, Y.-Y.; Keilbaugh, S.A.; Bewtra, M.; Knights, D.; Walters, W.A.; Knight, R.; et al. Linking Long-Term Dietary Patterns with Gut Microbial Enterotypes. *Science* **2011**, *334*, 105–108. [CrossRef]
131. Clarke, S.F.; Murphy, E.F.; O'Sullivan, O.; Lucey, A.J.; Humphreys, M.; Hogan, A.; Hayes, P.; O'Reilly, M.; Jeffery, I.B.; Wood-Martin, R.; et al. Exercise and associated dietary extremes impact on gut microbial diversity. *Gut* **2014**, *63*, 1913–1920. [CrossRef]

132. Friedman, G.D.; Kannel, W.B.; Dawber, T.R. The epidemiology of gallbladder disease: Observations in the Framingham study. *J. Chronic Dis.* **2004**, *19*, 273–292. [CrossRef]
133. Wirth, J.; Song, M.; Fung, T.T.; Joshi, A.D.T.; Tabung, F.K.; Chan, A.T.; Weikert, C.; Leitzmann, M.; Willett, W.C.; Giovannucci, E.; et al. Diet-quality scores and the risk of symptomatic gallstone disease: A prospective cohort study of male US health professionals. *Int. J. Epidemiol.* **2018**, *47*, 1938–1946. [CrossRef] [PubMed]
134. Park, Y.; Kim, D.; Lee, J.S.; Na Kim, Y.; Jung, Y.K.; Lee, K.G.; Choi, D. Association between diet and gallstones of cholesterol and pigment among patients with cholecystectomy: A case-control study in Korea. *J. Health Popul. Nutr.* **2017**, *36*, 39. [CrossRef] [PubMed]
135. Attili, A.F.; Scafato, E.; Marchioli, R.; Marfisi, R.M.; Festi, D. The MICOL Group Diet and gallstones in Italy: The cross-sectional MICOL results. *Hepatology* **1998**, *27*, 1492–1498. [CrossRef] [PubMed]
136. Walther, B.; Lett, A.M.; Bordoni, A.; Tomás-Cobos, L.; Nieto, J.A.; Dupont, D.; Danesi, F.; Shahar, D.R.; Echaniz, A.; Re, R.; et al. GutSelf: Interindividual Variability in the Processing of Dietary Compounds by the Human Gastrointestinal Tract. *Mol. Nutr. Food Res.* **2019**, *63*, e1900677. [CrossRef] [PubMed]
137. Modi, S.R.; Collins, J.J.; Relman, D.A. Antibiotics and the gut microbiota. *J. Clin. Investig.* **2014**, *124*, 4212–4218. [CrossRef] [PubMed]
138. De La Cuesta-Zuluaga, J.; Mueller, N.T.; Corrales-Agudelo, V.; Velásquez-Mejía, E.P.; Carmona, J.A.; Abad, J.M.; Escobar, J.S. Metformin Is Associated With Higher Relative Abundance of Mucin-Degrading Akkermansia muciniphila and Several Short-Chain Fatty Acid-Producing Microbiota in the Gut. *Diabetes Care* **2017**, *40*, 54–62. [CrossRef]
139. Suzuki, T.A.; Worobey, M. Geographical variation of human gut microbial composition. *Biol. Lett.* **2014**, *10*, 20131037. [CrossRef]
140. David, L.A.; Materna, A.C.; Friedman, J.; Campos-Baptista, M.I.; Blackburn, M.C.; Perrotta, A.; Erdman, S.E.; Alm, E.J. Host lifestyle affects human microbiota on daily timescales. *Genome Biol.* **2014**, *15*. [CrossRef]
141. Tyakht, A.V.; Kostryukova, E.S.; Popenko, A.S.; Belenikin, M.S.; Pavlenko, A.V.; Larin, A.K.; Karpova, I.Y.; Selezneva, O.V.; Semashko, T.A.; Ospanova, E.A.; et al. Human gut microbiota community structures in urban and rural populations in Russia. *Nat. Commun.* **2013**, *4*, 2469. [CrossRef]
142. Benedict, C.; Vogel, H.; Jonas, W.; Woting, A.; Blaut, M.; Schuermann, A.; Cedernaes, J. Gut microbiota and glucometabolic alterations in response to recurrent partial sleep deprivation in normal-weight young individuals. *Mol. Metab.* **2016**, *5*, 1175–1186. [CrossRef]
143. Thaiss, C.A.; Zeevi, D.; Levy, M.; Zilberman-Schapira, G.; Suez, J.; Tengeler, A.C.; Abramson, L.; Katz, M.N.; Korem, T.; Zmora, N.; et al. Transkingdom Control of Microbiota Diurnal Oscillations Promotes Metabolic Homeostasis. *Cell* **2014**, *159*, 514–529. [CrossRef] [PubMed]
144. Sze, M.A.; Schloss, P.D. Looking for a Signal in the Noise: Revisiting Obesity and the Microbiome. *MBio* **2016**, *7*. [CrossRef] [PubMed]
145. Wesolowska-Andersen, A.; Bahl, M.I.; Carvalho, V.; Kristiansen, K.; Sicheritz-Pontén, T.; Gupta, R.; Licht, T.R. Choice of bacterial DNA extraction method from fecal material influences community structure as evaluated by metagenomic analysis. *Microbiome* **2014**, *2*, 19. [CrossRef] [PubMed]
146. Lozupone, C.A.; Stombaugh, J.; Gonzalez, A.; Ackermann, G.; Wendel, D.; Vázquez-Baeza, Y.; Jansson, J.K.; Gordon, J.I.; Knight, R. Meta-analyses of studies of the human microbiota. *Genome Res.* **2013**, *23*, 1704–1714. [CrossRef]
147. Faith, J.J.; Guruge, J.L.; Charbonneau, M.; Subramanian, S.; Seedorf, H.; Goodman, A.L.; Clemente, J.C.; Knight, R.; Heath, A.C.; Leibel, R.L.; et al. The Long-Term Stability of the Human Gut Microbiota. *Science* **2013**, *341*, 1237439. [CrossRef]
148. Mahowald, M.A.; Rey, F.E.; Seedorf, H.; Turnbaugh, P.J.; Fulton, R.S.; Wollam, A.; Shah, N.; Wang, C.; Magrini, V.; Wilson, R.K.; et al. Characterizing a model human gut microbiota composed of members of its two dominant bacterial phyla. *Proc. Natl. Acad. Sci. USA* **2009**, *106*, 5859–5864. [CrossRef]
149. Samuel, B.S.; Gordon, J.I. A humanized gnotobiotic mouse model of host-archaeal-bacterial mutualism. *Proc. Natl. Acad. Sci. USA* **2006**, *103*, 10011–10016. [CrossRef]
150. Jayasinghe, T.N.; Chiavaroli, V.; Holland, D.J.; Cutfield, W.S.; O'Sullivan, J.M. The New Era of Treatment for Obesity and Metabolic Disorders: Evidence and Expectations for Gut Microbiome Transplantation. *Front. Cell. Infect. Microbiol.* **2016**, *6*, 15. [CrossRef]

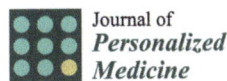

Article

Analysis of APPL1 Gene Polymorphisms in Patients with a Phenotype of Maturity Onset Diabetes of the Young

Dinara E. Ivanoshchuk [1,2,*], Elena V. Shakhtshneider [1,2], Oksana D. Rymar [2], Alla K. Ovsyannikova [2], Svetlana V. Mikhailova [1], Pavel S. Orlov [1,2], Yuliya I. Ragino [2] and Mikhail I. Voevoda [1]

1. Federal research center Institute of Cytology and Genetics, Siberian Branch of Russian Academy of Sciences (SB RAS), Prospekt Lavrentyeva 10, Novosibirsk 630090, Russia; 2117409@mail.ru or shakhtshneyderev@bionet.nsc.ru (E.V.S.); mikhail@bionet.nsc.ru (S.V.M.); orlovpavel86@gmail.com (P.S.O.); mvoevoda@ya.ru (M.I.V.)
2. Institute of Internal and Preventive Medicine—Branch of Institute of Cytology and Genetics, SB RAS, Bogatkova Str. 175/1, Novosibirsk 630004, Russia; orymar23@gmail.com (O.D.R.); aknikolaeva@bk.ru (A.K.O.); ragino@mail.ru (Y.I.R.)
* Correspondence: dinara2084@mail.ru or dinara@bionet.nsc.ru; Tel.: +7-(383)-363-4963; Fax: +7-(383)-333-1278

Received: 30 June 2020; Accepted: 22 August 2020; Published: 25 August 2020

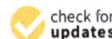

Abstract: The *APPL1* gene encodes a protein mediating the cross-talk between adiponectin and insulin signaling. Recently, it was found that *APPL1* mutations can cause maturity onset diabetes of the young, type 14. Here, an analysis of *APPL1* was performed in patients with a maturity-onset diabetes of the young (MODY) phenotype, and prevalence of these mutations was estimated in a Russian population, among type 2 diabetes mellitus (T2DM) and MODY patients. Whole-exome sequencing or targeted sequencing was performed on 151 probands with a MODY phenotype, with subsequent association analysis of one of identified variants, rs11544593, in a white population of Western Siberia (276 control subjects and 169 T2DM patients). Thirteen variants were found in *APPL1*, three of which (rs79282761, rs138485817, and rs11544593) are located in exons. There were no statistically significant differences in the frequencies of rs11544593 alleles and genotypes between T2DM patients and the general population. In the MODY group, AG rs11544593 genotype carriers were significantly more frequent (AG vs. AA + GG: odds ratio 1.83, confidence interval 1.15–2.90, $p = 0.011$) compared with the control group. An association of rs11544593 with blood glucose concentration was revealed in the MODY group. The genotyping data suggest that rs11544593 may contribute to carbohydrate metabolism disturbances.

Keywords: maturity onset diabetes of the young type 14; diabetes mellitus; APPL1; single-nucleotide variant; population

1. Introduction

Timely verification of a diabetes mellitus type is important because aside from diabetes mellitus types 1 and 2 and gestational diabetes, there are rarer types of this disease. Maturity onset diabetes of the young (MODY) is an inherited type of autosomal dominant diabetes mellitus with early onset and primarily involves a reduction in β-cell function without autoantibodies. MODY differs from the main diabetes types—type 1 diabetes mellitus (T1DM) and T2DM—in the clinical course, treatment strategies, and prognosis [1].

To date, 14 types of MODY (MODY1 through MODY14) have been identified, each associated with mutations in a specific gene: *HNF4A, GCK, HNF1A, PDX1, HNF1B, NEUROD1, KLF11, CEL, PAX4, INS, BLK, KCNJ11, ABCC8*, and *APPL1* [2–4]. Eleven percent to 30% of MODY cases are caused by impairment of functions of other genes [2,3].

The *APPL1* gene (adaptor protein, phosphotyrosine-interacting with the PH domain and leucine zipper 1) is located in chromosomal region 3p14.3 and contains 23 exons. APPL1 is a multifunctional adaptor protein that consists of 710 amino acid residues (aa) and is characterized by five key functional domains: an NH_2-terminal Bin/Amphiphysin/Rvs domain (BAR domain; aa 17–268, identified as a leucine zipper), a central pleckstrin homology domain (PH domain; aa 278–374), motif between PH and PTB domains (BPP domain, aa 375–499), a COOH-terminal phosphotyrosine-binding domain (PTB domain, aa 500–625), and a coiled-coil (CC domain, aa 625–710) [5,6]. All the domains of APPL1 can bind to lipids, and each domain has unique binding affinity [6].

In humans, high levels of *APPL1* expression have been found in the liver, adipose tissue, muscles, brain, and pancreas [6]. Chinese patients with newly diagnosed T2DM have elevated serum APPL1 levels [7].

APPL1 can interact with more than 50 different proteins regulating multiple signaling pathways depending on the cell type [8]. APPL1 binds to AKT2 (RAC-beta serine/threonine-protein kinase or AKT serine/threonine kinase 2), a key molecule in the insulin signaling pathway, thereby enhancing insulin-induced AKT2 activation and downstream signaling in the liver, skeletal muscle, adipocytes, and endothelium. In the liver, APPL1 potentiates the inhibitory effect of insulin on hepatic gluconeogenesis through activation of AKT protein kinases; APPL1 overexpression in the liver eliminates hyperglycemia in mice with diabetes. In skeletal muscle and adipocytes, APPL1 mediates insulin-stimulated glucose uptake by controlling the translocation of cytosolic glucose transporter 4 to the plasma membrane [5].

Additionally, APPL1 plays an important role in the regulation of insulin metabolism and insulin resistance, being an adaptor in the adiponectin signaling pathway. Adiponectin, a hormone secreted by white adipose tissue, has anti-inflammatory and antidiabetic effects, enhances insulin sensitivity, exerts various actions on fertility, and regulates the processes of sexual and general maturation, pregnancy, and lactation [9,10]. A decrease in adiponectin levels is associated with obesity and metabolic syndrome. The PTB domain of APPL1 directly interacts with the N-terminal intracellular region of adiponectin receptors: AdipoR1 and AdipoR2. In adiponectin signaling, APPL1 mediates fatty acid oxidation and glucose metabolism by activating AMPK (AMP-activated protein kinase) and p38 MAPK (P38 mitogen-activated protein kinases) [10]. It is reported that APPL1 protein isoforms APPL2 [11] and APPL1sv (which is encoded by a murine splice variant of *Appl1* mRNA [12]), apparently act as negative regulators of adiponectin signaling. In *Appl1* knockout mice, adipocyte differentiation is negatively affected, and lipolysis is enhanced in mature adipocytes; IN contrast, *APPL1* overexpression evidently does not influence these processes [13]. APPL1 mediates AMPK phosphorylation in response to adiponectin [14]. It affects the thermogenesis of brown adipocytes via an interaction with HDAC3 (Histone deacetylase 3); this phenomenon has promising implications for the treatment of obesity [15].

In a mouse model of T1DM, investigators have demonstrated a negative action of APPL1 on the regulation of inflammation and apoptosis in β-cells of the pancreas [16].

Furthermore, downregulation of *APPL1* expression by small interfering RNA reduces the synergistic effect of adiponectin on insulin-stimulated AKT phosphorylation. Hence, the APPL1-mediated cross-talk between insulin and adiponectin signaling pathways may be a critical mechanism underlying the insulin-sensitizing effect of adiponectin [6].

It has been shown that some variants of the gene have functional significance. An association of single-nucleotide polymorphisms rs3806622 and rs4640525 (of the *APPL1* gene) with a distribution of adipose tissue has been found among T2DM patients [17]. In that study, the G allele frequencies of rs3806622 and rs4640525 were significantly higher among the T2DM patients with greater waist circumference [17]. Additionally, rs4640525 is associated with increased risk of coronary heart disease in patients with T2DM [6,18] and the risk of nonalcoholic fatty liver disease in Chinese Han population [19].

Two rare mutations, rs869320673 (Leu552Ter) and rs796065047 (Asp94Asn), in the *APPL1* gene have been identified through whole-exome sequencing in two of 60 large families with high prevalence of diabetes not due to mutations in known MODY-associated genes (*HNF4A*, *GCK*, *HNF1A*, *PDX1*, *HNF1B*, and *NEUROD1*) [4]. The Leu552Ter mutation (rs869320673, introduction of a premature stop codon at aa position 552) causes a deletion of most of the PTB domain, thereby making APPL1 unable to bind to AKT and abrogates APPL1 protein expression in transfected HepG2 cells. In the above study, the substitution was found in all the 10 family members with diabetes or prediabetes. Most of the unaffected carriers of this substitution were younger than 38 years (the median age at diabetes diagnosis among the affected family members) [4]. Missense mutation Asp94Asn (rs796065047) was identified in three generations of a US family with MODY [4]. The mutation was found or inferred to be present in five of the seven family members with diabetes. The missense mutation affects the aspartic acid residue at position 94, which is located on the concave surface of the APPL1 BAR domain and is highly conserved among various species [20]. The Asp94Asn mutation significantly attenuates insulin-stimulated AKT2 and GSK3β phosphorylation. This mutation was not found in 1,639 unrelated individuals of European ancestry without diabetes mellitus and 2970 patients with T2DM [4].

The aims of our study were identification of potentially pathogenic variants in the *APPL1* gene in patients with early-onset diabetes mellitus corresponding to a MODY phenotype by whole-exome sequencing and estimation of their prevalence in a control Russian population and among patients with T2DM.

2. Materials and Methods

The study protocol was approved by the local Ethics Committee of the Institute of Internal and Preventive Medicine (a branch of the Institute of Cytology and Genetics, SB RAS, Novosibirsk, Russia), protocol number 7, 22.06.2008. Written informed consent to be examined and to participate in the study was obtained from each patient. For individuals younger than 18 years, the informed consent form was signed by a parent or legal guardian.

A group with a clinical diagnosis of MODY (MODY phenotype) consisted of 151 unrelated patients aged 8 to 35 years (26.1 ± 14.4 years (mean ± SD (standard deviation)); males: 47%). The inclusion criteria were as follows: a verified diagnosis of diabetes, a debut of the disease for probands at the age of 35 years and earlier, a family history of diabetes mellitus, the absence of obesity, the absence of antibodies against pancreas islet cells and glutamic acid decarboxylase, sufficient secretory function of β-cells, no need for insulin therapy, and the absence of ketoacidosis at the onset of the disease. The following exclusion criteria were applied: a history of tuberculosis or infection with the human immunodeficiency virus, an infectious disease caused by hepatitis B or C virus that requires antiviral treatment, and substance abuse or alcoholism for two years before the examination. The group with a MODY phenotype may have included patients with MODY, patients with T1DM and negative test results on antibodies, and patients with early-onset T2DM.

At first-time diagnosis of diabetes, most patients had no clinical symptoms of a carbohydrate metabolism disorder; hyperglycemia was diagnosed during routine examinations. In 33% of the females, diabetes manifested itself during pregnancy. In the patients with a MODY phenotype, glycated hemoglobin and C-peptide levels were close to normal. All the patients underwent continuous glucose monitoring for three days. The level of glycemia was 7.2 ± 2.7 mmol/L (mean ± SD); the minimum was 2.8 mmol/L, and maximum 12.8 mmol/L.

Blood samples were collected from the ulnar vein for biochemical analysis in the morning on an empty stomach. Lipid levels (cholesterol, triglycerides, and low-density and high-density lipoprotein cholesterols) and glucose concentration were determined on a biochemical analyzer KoneLab 300i (USA) with Thermo Fisher Scientific reagents (USA). Genomic DNA was isolated from venous-blood leukocytes by phenol–chloroform extraction [21]. Quality of the extracted DNA was assessed by means of a capillary electrophoresis system (Agilent 2100 Bioanalyzer; Agilent Technologies Inc., Santa Clara, CA, USA).

At the first stage, clinical exome sequencing was performed for 40 randomly selected patients from the MODY group. Clinical exome sequencing was carried out on an Illumina HiSeq 1500 instrument (Illumina, San Diego, CA, USA). The enrichment and library preparation were performed using the SureSelectXT Human All Exon v.5 + UTRs Kit. Whole-exome libraries were prepared with the AmpliSeq Exome Kit (Thermo Fisher Scientific). For other patients (111 unrelated probands), we performed targeted sequencing. In the target panel, we included coding parts and adjacent splicing sites of MODY-associated genes, e.g., APPL1. To prepare the libraries, oligodeoxynucleotide probes and the KAPA HyperPlus Kit (Roche, Switzerland) were employed. Quality of the analyzed DNA and of the prepared libraries was evaluated by means of a capillary electrophoresis system, Agilent 2100 Bioanalyzer (Agilent Technologies Inc., USA). Analysis of a fully prepared library was conducted on the Illumina MiSeq platform (Illumina, San Diego, CA, USA).

The sequence reads were mapped to the reference human genome (GRCh37) via the Burrow–Wheeler Alignment tool (BWA v.0.7.17) [22]. Polymerase chain reaction (PCR)-generated duplicates were removed in the Picard Tools (https://broadinstitute.github.io/picard/). A search for single-nucleotide variants (SNVs) was conducted using the Genome Analysis Toolkit v.3.3 package by the procedure for local remapping of short insertions/deletions and recalibration of read quality [23]. The depth of coverage was 34× to 53×. SNVs with genotype quality scores <20 and coverage depth <10× were filtered out and excluded from further analysis. In sequenced groups, we filtered sequence variants if they were present in 10 or more variant reads with a quality score ≥30. Annotation of the SNVs was performed in the ANNOVAR (ANNOtate VARiation) software [24] using gnomAD [25], ClinVar [26], and HGMD (The Human Gene Mutation Database) [27], and literature data were taken into account too. Possible functional and significant effects of SNVs were assessed by means of PolyPhen-2 v.2.2.5 [28], SIFT (The scale-invariant feature transform) [29], PROVEAN (Protein Variation Effect Analyzer) [30], LIST (Local Identity and Shared Taxa) [31], and MutationTaster [32]. Identified SNVs of the APPL1 gene were verified by Sanger sequencing.

At the second stage, segregation analysis was performed for two variants, rs138485817 and rs11544593, in probands' families.

At the third stage, minor allele frequency and prevalence of genotypes of rs11544593 was analyzed in a white population of West Siberia, among T2DM patients, and among patients with a MODY phenotype.

The control group consisted of 276 random residents of Novosibirsk aged 45 to 69 years (54.2 ± 0.4 years; males: 49%). The T2DM group consisted of 169 patients aged 45 to 69 years (59.0 ± 6.7 years; males: 45%) with glucose levels more than 11.1 mmol/L, according to the criteria of the American Diabetes Association. Both groups were randomly selected from the population of 9360 people interviewed within the framework of the HAPIEE (Health, Alcohol and Psychosocial factors in Eastern Europe) project (Wellcome Trust, Great Britain) "Determinants of cardiovascular diseases in Eastern Europe." An epidemiological survey of the population involved demographic and social data, smoking and alcohol abuse, a dietary survey, a history of chronic diseases, medication use, the Rose Angina Questionnaire, anthropometry, a threefold measurement of blood pressure, spirometry, ECG (Electrocardiogram) recording, and assessment of the blood glucose level, lipid profile, and other biochemical parameters [33]. Rs11544593 was genotyped by means of the TaqMan SNP assay (Biolink, Russia) and a StepOnePlus 7900HT Real-Time PCR System (Thermo Fisher Scientific, USA). Relative risk of MODY for a genotype or allele was calculated as an odds ratio (OR) via Fisher's exact test and Pearson's χ^2 test. Differences were considered statistically significant at $p < 0.05$. Verification of the Hardy–Weinberg equilibrium was carried out by the χ^2 method. Differences in means of the quantitative indicators between genotypes were calculated after adjustment for sex, age, and the body mass index (BMI) via the GLM (The generalized linear model) model of IBM SPSS Statistics 23.0.

3. Results and Discussion

Pathogenic sequence variants in MODY-associated genes were found in 37 probands out of the 151 persons examined by whole-exome sequencing or targeted sequencing of the panel of genomic loci. Discovered variants segregated with a pathological phenotype in the families of the probands. Among the 37 cases, 24 pathogenic variants were detected in the *GCK* gene, 11 variants in *HNF1A*, one variant in the *ABCC8* gene, and one in *HNF1b*.

In the *APPL1* gene, 13 SNVs were found. Rs79282761, rs11544593, and rs138485817 are located in the coding part of the gene (Table 1).

Table 1. The *APPL1* gene variants among the patients with a maturity-onset diabetes of the young phenotype in Russia, and the SNVs' (single nucleotide variants) minor allele frequency according to the gnomAD database.

Name of an SNV.	Location	Substitution (NM_012096.3)	Minor Allele Frequency (gnomAD)
rs113307246	5′UTR	c.-151=	0.005
rs79282761	Exon 1	Thr12Thr c.36G>C	C = 0.01
rs6789847	Intron 1	c.54+2907T>A	T = 0.07
rs200584055	Intron 12	c.1096-30del	delA = 0.03
rs62251992	Intron 17	c.1484-71A>G	G = 0.12
rs10510791	Intron 17	c.1658+38C>G	G = 0.46
rs1533272	Intron 18	c.1695+114T>A	C = 0.38
rs11544593	Exon 22	Glu700Gly c.2099A>G	G = 0.13
rs138485817	Exon 22	Ser673Cys c.2018 C>G	G = 0.0006
rs1046545	3′UTR	c.*1455=	T = 0.19
rs3204124	3′UTR	c.*1528=	G = 0.68
rs3087684	3′UTR	c.*2604=	C = 0.68
rs1913302	3′UTR	c.*3246=	A = 0.68

* Stop codon.

In one case, synonymous substitution rs79282761 (Thr12Thr) was found. Missense substitution rs11544593 (Glu700Gly) in exon 22 was detected in 49 patients; six of them carried a pathogenic mutation in the *GCK* gene, another one in the *HNF1A* gene, and 42 patients had no mutations in MODY1–13 genes. Rs138485817 (Ser673Cys) was found in one patient without mutations in other MODY-associated genes. In silico analysis of rs11544593 and rs138485817 predicted their potential damaging effect according to testing in PolyPhen-2 (score: 0.455 and 0.999), SIFT (score: 0.007 and 0.02), and LIST (score: 0.828 and 0.902), respectively. The PROVEAN software estimated these substitutions as neutral (score: −1.55 and −0.603). MutationTaster predicted rs11544593 to be neutral (score: 98) and rs138485817 to be disease causing (score: 112).

The Glu700Gly (rs11544593) substitution and Ser673Cys (rs138485817) are located in the C-C domain of APPL1; this domain is responsible for direct binding of this protein to insulin receptor β subunit (IRβ), TrkA receptor tyrosine kinase, and the GIPC1 protein [34]. Nevertheless, the identified variants did not segregate with the pathological phenotype in the families of the probands.

We assessed population prevalence and association with biochemical parameters for rs11544593 (as a more prevalent variant) in the control population, among T2DM patients, and among the patients with a MODY phenotype (Table 2).

The general-population group was in Hardy–Weinberg equilibrium for rs11544593: $\chi^2 = 3.05$. There were no significant differences in the prevalence rates of genotypes and alleles of the rs11544593 polymorphism between T2DM patients and the general-population group (Table 2).

Significantly lower prevalence of the A allele (OR = 1.57, 95% confidence interval (CI) 1.06–2.32, $p = 0.03$) was observed among the patients with a MODY phenotype (Table 2) compared with the general population. The frequency of the less common G allele of rs11544593 (in the *APPL1* gene) was 0.17 in group MODY and 0.13 in group T2DM. In the general-population group, G allele frequency was 0.12, in agreement with the gnomAD database (0.13). Thus, we found that in the Russian population, G allele frequency of rs11544593 is higher in the presence of a MODY phenotype, which is characterized by early onset of carbohydrate metabolism disorders (Table 2). In the MODY group, AG genotype carriers were significantly more frequent (AG vs. AA + GG: OR = 1.83, 95% CI 1.15–2.90, p = 0.011) and carriers of the AA genotype were less common (AA vs. AG + GG: OR = 0.57, 95% CI 0.36–0.89, p = 0.014) as compared with the general population (Table 2). For further investigation of the observed effect of heterozygous-variant carriage on the phenotype, a bigger sample size is needed.

Table 2. Frequencies of alleles and genotypes of rs11544593 in the general-population group (Western Siberia; control), in the type 2 diabetes mellitus group, and among patients with a maturity-onset diabetes of the young phenotype in Russia.

	MODY (n = 151)	T2DM (n = 169)	General Population (n = 276)	OR (An Odds Ratio), 95% CI (A Confidence Interval)	p
			Genotypes		
AA	67.55 (102)	76.33 (129)	78.62 (217)	1 vs. 3, 0.57 (0.36–0.89)	0.014
				2 vs. 3, 0.88 (0.56–1.38)	>0.05
AG	29.80 (45)	21.30 (36)	18.84 (52)	1 vs. 3, 1.83 (1.15–2.90)	0.011
				2 vs. 3, 1.17 (0.72–1.88)	>0.05
GG	2.65 (4)	2.37 (4)	2.54 (7)	1 vs. 3, 1.05 (0.30–3.63)	>0.05
				2 vs. 3, 0.93 (0.27–3.23)	>0.05
			Alleles		
A	82.3	86.98	88.04	1 vs. 3, 1.57 (1.06–2.32)	0.03
G	17.7	13.02	11.96	2 vs. 3, 0.91 (0.60–1.37)	>0.05

rs11544593 with the blood glucose level was revealed in the patients with a MODY phenotype. The highest average values of blood glucose levels were detected in the MODY patients with the GG genotype of rs11544593 (p = 0.004; Table 3). There was no association of rs11544593 with the blood glucose level among the patients with T2DM and in the control group.

Table 3. Mean blood glucose levels (mM/L).

rs11544593 Genotypes	MODY Phenotype Patients X (S_x)	T2DM Patients X (S_x)	General Population X (S_x)
AA	6.9 (0.2)	11.9 (0.4)	5.2 (0.1)
AG	6.0 (0.3)	12.2 (0.8)	5.8 (0.2)
GG	8.7 (0.8)	14.5 (2.)	5.4 (0.6)
Age (p)	0.000 *	0.508	0.508
Sex (p)	0.422	0.334	0.379
Genotype (p)	0.004 *	0.523	0.050

Continuous variables are presented as mean (X) ± standard error (S_x). * A statistically significant difference from the MODY group and general population.

We confirmed that mutations in the *APPL1* gene, depending on their location, may cause either autosomal dominant diabetes of the MODY14 type [4] or milder aberrations of blood glucose concentration.

There were no statistically significant associations of rs11544593 with sex, immunoreactive insulin, C-peptide, cholesterol, triglycerides, low-density and high-density lipoprotein cholesterols, triglyceride levels, BMI, atherogenicity index, waist circumference, and the waist/hip ratio.

Of note, there are some data on an association of rs11544593 with the BMI in a white American population consisting partly of individuals with T2DM [35]. We did not find an association of rs11544593 with either the BMI or T2DM. Apparently, this polymorphism can influence glucose and/or fatty acid metabolism, but its penetrance is incomplete. Although APPL1 is known to be an adaptor in multiple signaling pathways, phenotypic manifestations of its variants remain elusive. It is known that adiponectin has an antiatherosclerotic effect [36]. In atherosclerotic plaques of patients with T2DM, APPL1 is underexpressed relative to patients without diabetes [36]. In the latter study, in the group of patients with diabetes, subjects taking incretins showed higher APPL1 and adiponectin levels than did subjects who had never taken incretins [36]. This finding is interesting in terms of research into the association of *APPL1* variants with lipid metabolism disorders among patients with diabetes.

4. Conclusions

For the first time, a genetic analysis of the *APPL1* gene was performed on Russian patients with early-onset diabetes mellitus that phenotypically corresponds to MODY. Our whole-exome sequencing did not reveal novel or previously described rare pathogenic substitutions (Leu552Ter and Asp94Asn) in the *APPL1* gene that are associated with MODY14. The genotyping results and glucose level data obtained from the general-population group and patients with carbohydrate metabolism disorders suggest that rs11544593 (located in the *APPL1* gene) may contribute to earlier onset of carbohydrate metabolism disorders. Further research on rs11544593 in a larger study population and identification of polymorphisms of the genes encoding binding partners of APPL1 in signaling cascades hold promise for elucidation of the pathogenesis of diabetes phenotypes. The present study has some limitations. We examined only rs11544593 and traditional diabetes risk factors and thus could not rule out the influence of other factors, such as lifestyle factors and other genetic factors that may affect the results of observational studies. In some cases, MODY is caused by de novo mutations lacking a family history. In these situations, a clinician should focus on the specific clinical features of the patient's diabetes that are different from the typical course of T1DM and T2DM [37].

Author Contributions: Conceptualization, M.I.V.; Data curation, E.V.S., O.D.R., and A.K.O.; Investigation, D.E.I. and Y.I.R.; Methodology, D.E.I.; Project administration, M.I.V.; Validation, S.V.M. and P.S.O.; Writing—original draft, D.E.I., E.V.S., and P.S.O.; Writing—review and editing, E.V.S. and S.V.M. All authors have read and agreed to the published version of the manuscript.

Funding: Collection of the samples and clinical data, clinical examination, and high-throughput sequencing have been supported by the Russian Science Foundation (grant No. 14-15-00496-P). Sanger sequencing and bioinformatic analyses have been supported as part of the budget topic in state assignment No. AAAA-A19-119100990053-4.

Acknowledgments: The English language was corrected and certified by shevchuk-editing.com. The authors thank the patients for participation in this study.

Conflicts of Interest: The authors declare that they have no conflict of interest related to the publication of this article.

References

1. Murphy, R.; Ellard, S.; Hattersley, A.T. Clinical implication of a molecular genetic classification of monogenic β-cell diabetes. *Nat. Clin. Pract.* **2008**, *4*, 200–213. [CrossRef]
2. Bonnefond, A.; Philippe, J.; Durand, E.; Dechaume, A.; Huyvaert, M.; Montagne, L.; Marre, M.; Balkau, B.; Fajardy, I.; Vambergue, A.; et al. Whole-exome sequencing and high throughput genotyping identified KCNJ11 as the thirteenth MODY gene. *PLoS ONE* **2012**, *7*, e37423. [CrossRef]
3. Edghill, E.L.; Minton, J.A.; Groves, C.J.; Flanagan, S.E.; Patch, A.-M.; Rubio-Cabezas, O.; Shepherd, M.; Lenzen, S.; McCarthy, M.I.; Ellard, E.; et al. Sequencing of candidate genes selected by beta cell experts in monogenic diabetes of unknown aetiology. *J. Pancreas* **2010**, *11*, 14–17.
4. Prudente, S.; Jungtrakoon, P.; Marucci, A.; Ludovico, O.; Buranasupkajorn, P.; Mazza, T.; Hastings, T.; Milano, T.; Morini, E.; Mercuri, E.; et al. Loss-of-Function Mutations in APPL1 in Familial Diabetes Mellitus. *Am. J. Hum. Genet.* **2015**, *97*, 177–185. [CrossRef] [PubMed]

5. Cheng, K.K.; Lam, K.S.; Wu, D.; Wang, Y.; Sweeney, G.; Hoo, R.L.C.; Zhang, J.; Xu, A. APPL1 potentiates insulin secretion in pancreatic β cells by enhancing protein kinase Akt-dependent expression of SNARE proteins in mice. *Proc. Natl. Acad. Sci. USA* **2012**, *109*, 8919–8924. [CrossRef] [PubMed]
6. Liu, Z.; Xiao, T.; Peng, X.; Li, G.; Hu, F. APPLs: More than just adiponectin receptor binding proteins. *Cell Signal.* **2017**, *32*, 76–84. [CrossRef] [PubMed]
7. Wang, Y.; Zhang, M.; Yan, L.; Ding, S.; Xie, X. Serum APPL1 level is elevated in newly diagnosed cases of type 2 diabetes mellitus. *Nan Fang Yi Ke Da Xue Xue Bao* **2012**, *32*, 1373–1376.
8. Oughtred, R.; Stark, C.; Breitkreutz, B.J.; Rust, J.; Boucher, L.; Chang, C.; Kolas, N.; O'Donnell, L.; Leung, G.; McAdam, R.; et al. The BioGRID interaction database: 2019 update. *Nucleic Acids Res.* **2019**, *47*, D529–D541. [CrossRef]
9. Combs, T.P.; Marliss, E.B. Adiponectin signaling in the liver. *Rev. Endocr. Metab. Disord.* **2014**, *15*, 137–147. [CrossRef]
10. Dehghan, R.; Saidijam, M.; Mehdizadeh, M.; Shabab, N.; Yavangi, M.; Artimani, T. Evidence for decreased expression of APPL1 associated with reduced insulin and adiponectin receptors expression in PCOS patients. *J. Endocrinol. Investig.* **2016**, *39*, 1075–1082. [CrossRef]
11. Schmid, P.M.; Resch, M.; Schach, C.; Birner, C.; Riegger, G.A.; Luchner, A.; Endemann, D.H. Antidiabetic treatment restores adiponectin serum levels and APPL1 expression, but does not improve adiponectin-induced vasodilation and endothelial dysfunction in Zucker diabetic fatty rats. *Cardiovasc. Diabetol.* **2013**, *12*, 46. [CrossRef] [PubMed]
12. Galan-Davila, A.K.; Ryu, J.; Dong, K.; Xiao, Y.; Dai, Z.; Zhang, D.; Li, Z.; Dick, A.M.; Liu, K.D.; Kamat, A.; et al. Alternative splicing variant of the scaffold protein APPL1 suppresses hepatic adiponectin signaling and function. *J. Biol. Chem.* **2018**, *293*, 6064–6074. [CrossRef] [PubMed]
13. Wen, Z.; Tang, Z.; Li, M.; Zhang, Y.; Li, J.; Cao, Y.; Zhang, D.; Fu, Y.; Wang, C. APPL1 knockdown blocks adipogenic differentiation and promotes adipocyte lipolysis. *Mol. Cell Endocrinol.* **2020**, *506*, 110755. [CrossRef] [PubMed]
14. Pandey, G.K.; Vadivel, S.; Raghavan, S.; Mohan, V.; Balasubramanyam, M.; Gokulakrishnan, K. High molecular weight adiponectin reduces glucolipotoxicity-induced inflammation and improves lipid metabolism and insulin sensitivity via APPL1-AMPK-GLUT4 regulation in 3T3-L1 adipocytes. *Atherosclerosis* **2019**, *288*, 67–75. [CrossRef]
15. Fan, L.; Ye, H.; Wan, Y.; Qin, L.; Zhu, L.; Su, J.; Zhu, X.; Zhang, L.; Miao, Q.; Zhang, Q.; et al. Adaptor protein APPL1 coordinates HDAC3 to modulate brown adipose tissue thermogenesis in mice. *Metabolism* **2019**, *100*, 153955. [CrossRef]
16. Jiang, X.; Zhou, Y.; Wu, K.K.; Chen, Z.; Xu, A.; Cheng, K.K. APPL1 prevents pancreatic beta cell death and inflammation by dampening NFκB activation in a mouse model of type 1 diabetes. *Diabetologia* **2017**, *60*, 464–474. [CrossRef]
17. Fang, Q.C.; Jia, W.P.; Gao, F.; Zhang, R.; Hu, C.; Wang, C.-R.; Wang, C.; Ma, X.-M.; Lu, J.-X.; Xu, J.; et al. Association of variants in APPL1 gene with body fat and its distribution in Chinese patients with type 2 diabetic mellitus. *Zhonghua Yi Xue Za Zhi* **2008**, *88*, 369–373.
18. Ma, X.W.; Ding, S.; Ma, X.D.; Gu, N.; Guo, X.H. Genetic variability in adapter proteins with APPL1/2 is associated with the risk of coronary artery disease in type 2 diabetes mellitus in Chinese Han population. *Chin. Med. J.* **2011**, *124*, 3618–3621. [CrossRef]
19. Wang, B.; Wang, B.; Wang, Y.; Wen, B.; Liu, S.; Sang, L.; Chen, Y.; Zhang, D. Association of APPL1 Gene Polymorphism with Non-Alcoholic Fatty Liver Disease Susceptibility in a Chinese Han Population. *Clin. Lab.* **2015**, *61*, 1659–1666. [CrossRef]
20. Chial, H.J.; Wu, R.; Ustach, C.V.; McPhail, L.C.; Mobley, W.C.; Chen, Y.Q. Membrane targeting by APPL1 and APPL2: Dynamic scaffolds that oligomerize and bind phosphoinositides. *Traffic* **2008**, *9*, 215–229. [CrossRef]
21. Sambrook, J.; Russell, D.W. Purification of nucleic acids by extraction with phenol: Chloroform. *Cold Spring Harb. Protoc.* **2006**, *2006*, 4455. [CrossRef] [PubMed]
22. Li, H.; Durbin, R. Fast and accurate short read alignment with Burrows–Wheeler transform. *Bioinformatics* **2009**, *25*, 1754–1760. [CrossRef] [PubMed]
23. McKenna, A.; Hanna, M.; Banks, E.; Sivachenko, A.; Cibulskis, K.; Kernytsky, A.; Garimella, K.; Altshuler, D.; Gabriel, S.; Daly, M.; et al. The Genome Analysis Toolkit: A MapReduce framework for analyzing next-generation DNA sequencing data. *Genome Res.* **2010**, *20*, 1297–1303. [CrossRef] [PubMed]

24. Wang, K.; Li, M.; Hakonarson, H. ANNOVAR: Functional annotation of genetic variants from next-generation sequencing data. *Nucleic Acids Res.* **2010**, *38*, e164. [CrossRef]
25. Karczewski, K.J.; Francioli, L.C.; Tiao, G.; Cummings, B.B.; Alföldi, J.; Wang, Q.; Collins, R.L.; Laricchia, K.M.; Ganna, A.; Birnbaum, D.P.; et al. The mutational constraint spectrum quantified from variation in 141,456 humans. *Nature* **2020**, *581*, 434–443. [CrossRef]
26. Landrum, M.J.; Lee, J.M.; Benson, M.; Brown, G.R.; Chao, C.; Chitipiralla, S.; Gu, B.; Hart, J.; Hoffman, D.; Jang, W.; et al. ClinVar: Improving access to variant interpretations and supporting evidence. *Nucleic Acids Res.* **2018**, *46*, D1062–D1067. [CrossRef]
27. Stenson, P.D.; Ball, E.V.; Mort, M.; Phillips, A.D.; Shiel, J.A.; Thomas, N.S.T.; Abeysinghe, S.; Krawczak, M.; Cooper, D.N. Human Gene Mutation Database (HGMD): 2003 update. *Hum. Mutat.* **2003**, *21*, 577–581. [CrossRef]
28. Adzhubei, I.A.; Schmidt, S.; Peshkin, L.; Ramensky, V.E.; Gerasimova, A.; Bork, P.; Kondrashov, A.S.; Sunyaev, S.R. A method and server for predicting damaging missense mutations. *Nat. Methods* **2010**, *7*, 248–249. [CrossRef]
29. Sim, N.-L.; Kumar, P.; Hu, J.; Henikoff, S.; Schneider, G.; Ng, P.C. SIFT web server: Predicting effects of amino acid substitutions on proteins. *Nucleic Acids Res.* **2012**, *40*, W452–W457. [CrossRef]
30. Choi, Y.; Sims, G.E.; Murphy, S.; Miller, J.R.; Chan, A.P. Predicting the Functional Effect of Amino Acid Substitutions and Indels. *PLoS ONE* **2012**, *7*, e46688. [CrossRef]
31. Malhis, N.; Jones, S.J.M.; Gsponer, J. Improved measures for evolutionary conservation that exploit taxonomy distances. *Nat. Commun.* **2019**, *10*, 1556. [CrossRef] [PubMed]
32. Schwarz, J.M.; Cooper, D.N.; Schuelke, M.; Seelow, D. MutationTaster2: Mutation prediction for the deep-sequencing age. *Nat. Methods* **2014**, *11*, 361–362. [CrossRef] [PubMed]
33. Pajak, A.; Szafraniec, K.; Kubinova, R.; Malyutina, S.; Peasey, A.; Pikhart, H.; Nikitin, Y.; Marmot, M.; Bobak, M. Binge drinking and blood pressure: Cross-sectional results of the HAPIEE study. *PLoS ONE* **2013**, *8*, e65856. [CrossRef] [PubMed]
34. Deepa, S.S.; Dong, L.Q. APPL1: Role in adiponectin signaling and beyond. *Am. J. Physiol. Endocrinol. Metab.* **2009**, *296*, E22–E36. [CrossRef]
35. Cox, A.J.; Lambird, J.E.; An, S.S.; Register, T.C.; Langefeld, C.D.; Carr, J.J.; Freedman, B.I.; Bowden, D.W. Variants in adiponectin signaling pathway genes show little association with subclinical CVD in the diabetes heart study. *Obesity* **2013**, *21*, E456–E462. [CrossRef]
36. Barbieri, M.; Marfella, R.; Esposito, A.; Rizzo, M.R.; Angellotti, E.; Mauro, C.; Siniscalchi, M.; Chirico, F.; Caiazzo, P.; Furbatto, F.; et al. Incretin treatment and atherosclerotic plaque stability: Role of adiponectin/APPL1 signaling pathway. *J. Diabetes Complicat.* **2017**, *31*, 295–303. [CrossRef]
37. Özdemir, T.R.; Kırbıyık, Ö.; Dündar, B.N.; Abacı, A.; Kaya, Ö.Ö.; Çatlı, G.; Özyılmaz, B.; Acar, S.; Koç, A.; Güvenç, M.S.; et al. Targeted next generation sequencing in patients with maturity-onset diabetes of the young (MODY). *J. Pediatr. Endocrinol. Metab.* **2018**, *31*, 1295–1304. [CrossRef]

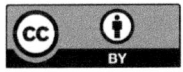

© 2020 by the authors. Licensee MDPI, Basel, Switzerland. This article is an open access article distributed under the terms and conditions of the Creative Commons Attribution (CC BY) license (http://creativecommons.org/licenses/by/4.0/).

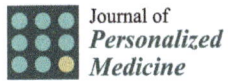

Article

The Blood Cytokine Profile of Young People with Early Ischemic Heart Disease Comorbid with Abdominal Obesity

Yulia I. Ragino, Veronika I. Oblaukhova *, Yana V. Polonskaya, Natalya A. Kuzminykh, Liliya V. Shcherbakova and Elena V. Kashtanova

Research Institute of Internal and Preventive Medicine—Branch of the Institute of Cytology and Genetics, Siberian Branch of Russian Academy of Sciences (IIPM–Branch of IC&G SB RAS), 175/1 B. Bogatkova Str., 630089 Novosibirsk, Russia; ragino@mail.ru (Y.I.R.); polonskayayv@bionet.nsc.ru (Y.V.P.); tina87@inbox.ru (N.A.K.); 9584792@mail.ru (L.V.S.); elekastanova@yandex.ru (E.V.K.)
* Correspondence: nikamedicine@mail.ru; Tel.: +7-923-149-08-84

Received: 22 June 2020; Accepted: 11 August 2020; Published: 13 August 2020

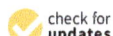

Abstract: Objective: The aim was to study the blood cytokine/chemokine profile of 25–44-year-old people with early ischemic heart disease (IHD) comorbid with abdominal obesity (AO). Methods: A cross-sectional medical examination of subjects in Novosibirsk, Russia, was conducted after random sampling of the above age group. A total of 1457 subjects, 804 females and 653 males, were analyzed. The epidemiological diagnosis of IHD was made in accordance with 17 validated and functional criteria, employing exercise ECG for confirmation. Simultaneous quantitative analyses of 41 cytokines/chemokines in blood serum were performed by a multiplex assay using the HCYTMAG-60K-PX41 panel (MILLIPLEX MAP) on a Luminex 20 MAGPIX flow cytometer, with additional ELISA testing. Results: Flt3 ligand, GM-CSF, and MCP-1 were significantly associated with the relative risk of early IHD. In the presence of AO, GM-CSF, MCP-1 and IL-4 also significantly correlated with the relative risk of early IHD. By univariate regression analysis, the relative risk of early IHD was associated with lowered blood concentrations of Flt3 ligand, whereas the relative risk of early IHD in the presence of AO was associated with lowered blood concentrations of GM-CSF. Employing multivariable regression analysis, only lower blood levels of Flt3 ligand were associated with a relative risk of early IHD, whereas the relative risk of early IHD in the presence of AO was limited to lower levels of IL-4. Conclusion: Findings related to Flt3 ligand, GM-CSF, and IL-4 are consistent with the international literature. Results from the present study are partly confirmative and partly hypothesis generating.

Keywords: early IHD; abdominal obesity; blood cytokines/chemokines complex; multiplex assay; Flt3 ligand; GM-CSF; MCP-1; IL-4

1. Introduction

Despite substantial progress in the diagnosis and treatment of ischemic heart disease (IHD), the prevalence of cardiovascular diseases (CVDs) among young people is steadily growing worldwide [1]. The main reason is the increasing prevalence of risk factors of CVDs. One of these risk factors is excess body weight, especially abdominal obesity (AO) [2,3].

The study of a wide range of biomolecules secreted by visceral adipocytes in AO and their effects is an important area in modern fundamental endocrinology. Much attention is given to the notion that AO causes a chronic, systemic, low-intensity, inflammatory process resulting from a combination of increased insulin resistance and higher production of inflammation mediators because of the expansion of the visceral/abdominaladipocyte pool [4,5]. Cytokines, which are endogenous, biologically active mediators of inflammation that are secreted by visceral adipocytes, regulate interactions between cells and between organ systems and determine cell survival, stimulation or suppression of cell growth, and cell differentiation and functional activity, as well as apoptotic processes. Cytokines ensure coordinated actions of immune, endocrine, and nervous systems under normal conditions and in response to pathological factors [6]. It is known that hypertrophied adipocytes, just likelymphocytes and macrophages, produce cytokines and participate in complement activation by launching a chain of inflammatory processes, with the inflammation becoming persistent and systemic. Many studies indicate that a cytokine imbalance is strongly linked with higher risks of cardiometabolic diseases and their complications [7–10].

Considering the influence of visceral obesity on human health in general, and on IHD in particular, our aim was to investigate the blood cytokine/chemokine profile of young people with early IHD comorbid with AO.

2. Materials and Methods

During 2014–2015, a cross-sectional populational medical examination was performed with random sampling of a young population in a typical borough of Novosibirsk, the capital of Western Siberia. The study protocol was authorized by a local ethical committee of IIPM—Branch of IC&G SB RAS (Minutes No. 9 dated 25 June 2013). To compile the study population, we employed a database of the Novosibirsk Territorial Fund of mandatory health insurance, from which 2500 people of both sexes at age 25–44 years were chosen by means of a random number generator. At our Screening Center, 1457 people underwent the medical examination: 804 females and 653 males. All participants gave informed consent to the medical examination and the use of personal data.

The screening was conducted by a team of physicians that had been trained in standardized epidemiological methods of screenings based on medical examination. The medicalexamination program involved the collection of social and demographic data, a socioeconomic questionnaire, questions about cigarettesmoking and alcoholdrinking habits, a nutritional survey, collection of a medication and chronicdisease history, the cardiological Rose questionnaire, three-time measurement of arterial blood pressure (BP), anthropometricdata collection, ECG recording with interpretation in accordance with the Minnesota Code (MC), spirometry, and assessment of other parameters.

The epidemiological diagnosis of IHD was made via validated epidemiological (using the Rose questionnaire) and functional (ECG recording with interpretation via the MC) criteria. The Rose questionnaire is widely used in epidemiological studies as a standardized method for assessing angina. Although it is a screening tool, rather than a diagnostic test, and was originally designed for use in men, it has been found to predict major coronary events in middle aged men and coronary heart disease mortality in both women and men. The diagnosis of "definite IHD" was made if the following criteria were present: a history of large-focal myocardial infarction (ECG with MC), ischemic changes on ECG without left ventricular hypertrophy (ECG with MC), tension angina pectoris (Rose questionnaire), and irregular rhythm and conductance (ECG with MC). Furthermore, the diagnosis of "definite IHD" was confirmed by conducting an ECG test with physical activity (stress test).

Based on diagnosed early IHD, 4 subgroups were formed from the study population (143 subjects total, Table 1):

(1) patients with IHD comorbid with AO, 24 subjects;
(2) patients with IHD without AO, 25 subjects;
(3) age- and sex-matched controls without IHD but with AO, 44 subjects;
(4) age- and sex-matched controls without IHD and without AO, 50 subjects.

Table 1. Clinical and anthropometric characteristics of the subgroups under study (median (lower; upper quartile)).

Parameters	Subjects without IHD		Subjects with IHD	
	without AO (n = 50)	with AO (n = 44)	without AO (n = 25)	with AO (n = 24)
Age, years	35.0 (31.0; 40.3)	37.0 (30.5; 42.0)	34.9 (30.7; 41.7)	40.8 (36.0; 45.3)
Systolic BP, mmHg	118.0 (108.0; 126.8)	118.2 (112.1; 130.0)	121.2 (108.3; 133.7)	124.0 (110.5; 148.7)
Diastolic BP, mmHg	77.5 (71.4; 83.4)	80.0 (71.6; 87.5)	79.5 (65.5; 85.7)	80.5 (72.0; 96.6)
Body mass index, kg/m^2	22.9 (20.8; 25.4)	28.9 (25.6; 33.1)	22.0 (18.9; 24.9)	28.5 (26.0; 34.0)
Heart rate, beats/min	73.5 (64.0; 79.0)	77.0 (68.5; 81.0)	69.5 (63.0; 83.1)	70.5 (65.5; 81.2)
Waist circumference, cm	74.9 (70.5; 76.2)	90.7 (84.0; 98.2)	67.6 (65.3; 78.9)	86.5 (82.8; 97.2)

Note: AO—abdominal obesity, BP—blood pressure.

Blood for biochemical analyses was collected from all subjects from the medial cubital vein in the morning after a ≥12 h fast on the day of the examination. Simultaneous quantitative analyses of cytokines/chemokines in blood serum were performed by a multiplex assay using the HCYTMAG-60K-PX41 panel (MILLIPLEX MAP) on a Luminex MAGPIX flow cytometer. This panel includes quantitation of the following 41 human cytokines/chemokines:

eotaxin (CCL11),
epidermal growth factor (EGF),
fibroblast growth factor 2 (FGF-2, also known as FGF-basic),
fractalkine (CX3CL1),
granulocyte colony-stimulating factor (G-CSF),
granulocyte-macrophage colony-stimulating factor (GM-CSF),
growth-regulated oncogene α (GROα),
interferonγ(IFNγ),
interferonα2 (IFNα2),
interferon γ–induced protein 10(IP-10, also known as CXCL10),
interleukin 1 receptor antagonist (IL-1Ra),
interleukin 1α (IL-1α),
interleukin 1β(IL-1β),
interleukin 10 (IL-10),
interleukin 12 (IL-12 (p40)),
interleukin 12 (IL-12 (p70)),
interleukin 13 (IL-13),
interleukin 15 (IL-15),
interleukin 17A (IL-17A, also known as CTLA8),
interleukin 2 (IL-2),
interleukin 3 (IL-3),
interleukin 4 (IL-4),
interleukin 5 (IL-5),
interleukin 6 (IL-6),
interleukin 7 (IL-7),
interleukin 8 (IL-8, also known as CXCL8),
interleukin 9 (IL-9),
ligand of Fms-like tyrosine kinase 3 (Flt3 ligand),
macrophage inflammatory protein1α (MIP-1α, also known as CCL3),
macrophage inflammatory protein1β (MIP-1β, also known as CCL4),
macrophage-derived chemokine (MDC, also known as CCL22),
monocyte chemoattractant protein 1(MCP-1, also known as CCL2),
monocyte chemoattractant protein 3 (MCP-3, also known as CCL7),

platelet-derived growth factor AA (PDGF-AA),
platelet-derived growth factor AB (PDGF-AB/BB),
regulated upon activation, normal T cell expressed and presumably secretedchemokine (RANTES, also known as CCL5),
soluble ligand of CD40 (sCD40L),
transforming growth factor α (TGFα),
tumor necrosis factor α (TNFα),
tumor necrosis factor β (TNFβ, also known as lymphotoxin-α (LTA)),
vascular endothelial growth factor A (VEGF-A).

In addition, some cytokines/chemokines were determined in blood serum by ELISA with the following test systems: Flt3 ligand (R&D), IL-7 (RayBiotech), GM-CSF, sCD40L, IL-2, IL-6, MCP-1, i.e., CCL2, MIP-1β, i.e., CCL4 and TNFα (Bender Medsystems) on ELISA analyzer MULTISCAN-II.

Statistical analysis of the data was performed using the SPSS software (version 17) for Windows, with assessment (for each variable) of the median, mean, confidence intervals (CIs), standard deviation, and lower and upper quartiles. Several methods of group comparison were utilized: Wilcoxon's test, one-way ANOVA with Dunnett's test for a multigroup comparison, the Mann–Whitney U test for a comparison of medians, odds ratio (OR) calculation in a logistical regression model, calculation of the OR via contingency tables, the t test, and χ^2 test. The 95% threshold of statistical significance was chosen.

3. Results

We uncovered differences in concentrations of some cytokines/chemokines between young people with early IHD and those without IHD (Table 2).

Table 2. Levels of the analyzed human cytokines/chemokines in IHD (median (lower; upper quartile)).

Analytes, pg/mL	Subjects without IHD (n = 94)	Subjects with IHD (n = 49)	p
EGF	46.93 [30.38; 77.36]	39.56 [24.12; 68.17]	0.247
FGF-2, i.e., FGF-basic	42.94 [32.02; 66.44]	43.12 [28.9; 53.15]	0.677
Eotaxin, i.e., CCL11	112.42 [79.64; 166.2]	102.85 [75.15; 149.87]	0.382
TGFα	4.44 [2.61; 6.49]	3.78 [2.13; 5.65]	0.119
G-CSF	25.62 [9.7; 41.13]	16.68 [7.61; 38.56]	0.278
Flt3 ligand	40.41 [27.76; 55.54]	28.19 [13.07; 41.99]	**0.003**
GM-CSF	8.36 [4.63; 13.73]	4.46 [2.16; 10.02]	**0.004**
Fractalkine, i.e., CX3CL1	31.49 [24.33; 58.85]	25.75 [22.21; 34.09]	0.159
IFNα2	13.2 [7.89; 23.63]	13.18 [7.97; 25.1]	0.897
IFNγ	9.84 [5.47; 14.98]	9.54 [5.92; 16.18]	0.745
GROα	1480.0 [855.35; 2169.0]	956.45 [580.18; 2019.12]	0.212
IL-10	5.28 [2.59; 7.41]	4.75 [1.31; 7.74]	0.564
MCP-3, i.e., CCL7	19.19 [13.13; 22.99]	20.32 [17.00; 26.8]	0.512
IL-12 (p40)	4.16 [2.55; 14.28]	6.23 [3.12; 15.45]	0.187
MDC, i.e., CCL22	717.04 [518.9; 1016.0]	635.85 [355.31; 998.56]	0.345
IL-12 (p70)	4.86 [1.37; 6.62]	5.12 [1.41; 6.22]	0.958
PDGF-AA	3306.0 [2026.0; 5050.0]	3125.9 [1615.15; 4263.45]	0.159
IL-13	9.13 [7.04; 13.54]	8.95 [6.35; 19.85]	0.687

Table 2. *Cont.*

Analytes, pg/mL	Subjects without IHD (n = 94)	Subjects with IHD (n = 49)	p
PDGF-AB/BB	17,351.25 [14,278.13; 22,158.08]	19,956.45 [13,125.12; 22,897.12]	0.715
IL-15	2.72 [1.5; 5.96]	2.87 [1.56; 5.49]	0.955
sCD40L	2230 [842.94; 4068]	1250.12 [185.56; 2974.64]	**0.046**
IL-17A, i.e., CTLA8	3.53 [1.49; 5.38]	2.45 [1.28; 6.11]	0.555
IL-1Ra	6.69 [4.09; 27.84]	6.24 [4.08; 36.88]	0.912
IL-1α	7.63 [5.24; 12.21]	9.56 [4.98; 26.87]	0.871
IL-9	4.14 [2.71; 5.42]	5.12 [2.11; 6.06]	0.412
IL-1β	1.57 [0.74; 2.23]	1.31 [0.59; 2.69]	0.649
IL-2	1.35 [0.64; 3.0]	1.68 [0.68; 2.97]	0.735
IL-3	1.63 [0.73; 2.12]	2.22	0.418
IL-4	71.95 [33.78; 115.43]	56.47 [41.11; 78.54]	0.247
IL-5	1.23 [0.67; 1.65]	1.38 [1.0; 2.68]	0.198
IL-6	2.27 [1.3; 3.6]	3.37 [1.36; 7.95]	0.157
IL-7	10.71 [6.18; 15.87]	7.64 [4.32; 12.85]	**0.029**
IL-8	9.75 [6.73; 13.93]	9.0 [5.11; 15.46]	0.512
IP-10, i.e., CXCL10	211.1 [163.16; 292.73]	165.48 [99.87; 269.45]	**0.035**
MCP-1, i.e., CCL2	516.9 [382.71; 672.92]	326.41 [164.11; 610.47]	**0.003**
MIP-1α, i.e., CCL3	6.79 [4.34; 10.1]	6.12 [4.61; 8.99]	0.748
MIP-1β, i.e., CCL4	29.98 [21.85; 38.91]	24.87 [16.54; 31.28]	**0.035**
RANTES, i.e., CCL5	2870.0 [1897.5; 4289.0]	2741.22 [1312.45; 3812.78]	0.299
TNFα	16.59 [11.99; 20.62]	12.95 [7.95; 18.55]	**0.035**
TNFβ, i.e., LTA	9.17 [7.73; 12.04]	9.87 [6.54; 15.87]	0.995
VEGF-A	97.0 [59.26; 138.69]	84.55 [51.56; 138.45]	0.745

In subjects with IHD, blood levels were lower for Flt3 ligand (1.4-fold), GM-CSF (1.9-fold), sCD40L (1.8-fold), IL-7 (1.4-fold), IP-10 (1.3-fold), MCP-1 (1.6-fold), MIP-1β (1.2-fold), and TNFα (1.3-fold) as compared with subjects without IHD.

Next, we carried out an identical analysis between groups of young people with or without AO (Table 3).

Table 3. Levels of the analyzed human cytokines/chemokines in IHD comorbid with AO and without AO (median (lower; upper quartile)).

Analytes, pg/mL	Subjects without AO (n = 75)			Subjects with AO (n = 68)		
	without IHD (n = 50)	with IHD (n = 25)	p	without IHD (n = 44)	with IHD (n = 24)	p
EGF	45.3 [29.5; 70.7]	42.3 [22.7; 72.5]	0.654	55.3 [32.2; 91.8]	39.5 [25.8; 67.9]	0.314
FGF-2, i.e., FGF-basic	42.1 [31.3; 63.1]	40.2 [28.1; 52.4]	0.658	45.5 [35.4; 76.3]	46.8 [35.4; 66.9]	0.755
Eotaxin, i.e., CCL11	114.3 [91.8; 165.7]	110.1 [71.5; 174.6]	0.611	98.5 [70; 179.1]	96.5 [75.68; 146.8]	0.689
TGFα	4.1 [2.8; 6.4]	4.32 [1.51; 5.87]	0.687	4.8 [2.47; 6.93]	3.12 [2.02; 4.69]	0.956
G-CSF	20.5 [10.0; 40.5]	18.0 [7.12; 33.56]	0.587	27.8 [9.7; 41.6]	16.8 [7.06; 47.88]	0.489
Flt3 ligand	40 [28.6; 54.9]	29.87 [14.03; 44.12]	0.021	40.9 [25.1; 58.8]	26.0 [12.9; 41.03]	0.048
GM-CSF	7.5 [4.1; 12.8]	4.98 [2.13; 13.13]	0.197	9.51 [5.64; 14.4]	4.06 [2.11; 9.41]	0.008
Fractalkine, i.e., CX3CL1	29.35 [24.3; 45.3]	25.9 [22.11; 32.97]	0.566	33.1 [23.3; 63.4]	26.8 [21.8; 49.8]	0.277
IFNα2	12.7 [7.4; 20.7]	10.13 [5.54; 22.79]	0.534	13.2 [7.89; 23.6]	17.9 [11.88; 27.03]	0.499
IFNγ	10.2 [4.9; 15.6]	8.98 [5.12; 16.56]	0.811	9.6 [6.2; 14.9]	10.21 [6.89; 19.34]	0.645
GROα	1297.5 [727; 1728.3]	1512.1 [567.3; 2239.78]	0.677	1738 [1034; 2624]	796.8 [511.23; 1389.45]	0.015
IL-10	6.4 [3.9; 8.7]	4.56 [1.31; 7.45]	0.278	3.67 [1.61; 5.92]	4.34 [1.01; 8.12]	0.512
MCP-3, i.e., CCL7	19.4 [16.3; 21.9]	21.51 [16.87; 95.46]	0.499	17.7 [12.3; 23.6]	19.5 [16.51; 23.56]	0.469
IL-12 (p40)	3.6 [2.2; 15.7]	9.78 [3.12; 54.84]	0.245	5.1 [3.07; 13.5]	5.47 [2.31; 15.87]	0.745
MDC, i.e., CCL22	672.4 [482.9; 921.1]	604.8 [214.8; 968.4]	0.498	819.7 [557.6; 1080]	647.87 [387.5; 1035.87]	0.389
IL-12 (p70)	5.5 [2.4; 6.8]	4.75 [1.07; 5.98]	0.389	3.15 [1.04; 5.9]	6.07 [1.14; 6.34]	0.359
PDGF-AA	3146 [2021.3; 5052]	2878.5 [1597; 4159.5]	0.311	3509 [2035; 5009.5]	3198.2 [1585; 4112.1]	0.325
IL-13	9.6 [7.0; 13.5]	8.48 [6.12; 44.51]	0.956	8.64 [7.08; 13.59]	8.85 [6.04; 11.88]	0.569
PDGF-AB/BB	16,303 [14,262; 20,616]	16,367 [13,232; 19,987]	0.745	18,111.4 [14,284.5; 22,804.3]	20,145 [12,366; 29,877]	0.355
IL-15	2.1 [1.2; 4.4]	2.54 [1.23; 4.25]	0.469	3.25 [1.97; 7.26]	3.16 [1.41; 6.31]	0.499
sCD40L	2176.5 [1047; 4057]	2123.7 [175.49; 3864.5]	0.379	2394 [421.5;4126]	1125.4 [197.3; 2705.6]	0.087

Table 3. Cont.

Analytes, pg/mL	Subjects without AO (n = 75)			Subjects with AO (n = 68)		
	without IHD (n = 50)	with IHD (n = 25)	p	without IHD (n = 44)	with IHD (n = 24)	p
IL-17A, i.e., CTLA8	3.5 [1.4; 5.3]	3.45 [1.23; 5.95]	0.867	3.09 [1.72; 6.3]	1.95 [1.01; 6.38]	0.345
IL-1Ra	5.4 [4.0; 33.2]	7.23 [4.03; 86.99]	0.697	8.12 [4.58; 27.7]	5.8 [3.99; 30.26]	0.678
IL-1α	8.1 [5.4; 13.7]	9.3 [5.15; 35.89]	0.311	7.15 [5.05; 11.24]	6.45 [4.01; 10.0]	0.789
IL-9	4.1 [2.7; 5.4]	4.24 [2.09; 8.45]	0.922	4.39 [3.53; 5.61]	4.26 [2.01; 5.12]	0.314
IL-1β	1.51 [0.76; 2.11]	1.45 [0.62; 1.76]	0.411	1.66 [0.62; 2.37]	2.03 [0.61; 2.55]	0.801
IL-2	1.65 [0.76; 3.11]	0.86 [0.61; 2.44]	0.071	0.93 [0.63; 2.76]	2.76 [1.65; 3.49]	**0.031**
IL-3	1.69 [0.98; 2.14]	1.71 [1.07; 2.19]	0.645	1.57 [0.55; 2.1]	1.51 [0.55; 2.11]	0.659
IL-4	52.3 [31.9; 125]	59.01 [50.88; 81.78]	0.899	80.3 [36.8; 110.2]	53.63 [38.64; 73.89]	0.089
IL-5	1.26 [0.6; 1.63]	1.31 [0.66; 2.41]	0.376	1.22 [0.78; 1.73]	1.29 [1.11; 1.89]	0.397
IL-6	2.02 [1.29; 3.12]	5.95 [1.87; 8.97]	**0.009**	2.6 [1.45; 4.03]	1.95 [1.02; 6.13]	0.613
IL-7	8.61 [6.02; 15.4]	6.47 [4.35; 11.55]	0.145	11.45 [6.18; 16.8]	8.67 [5.04; 14.23]	0.159
IL-8	9.65 [6.25; 12.9]	9.65 [4.03; 18.95]	0.957	9.75 [6.92; 15.14]	8.89 [5.56; 14.12]	0.379
IP-10, i.e., CXCL10	203.6 [167.88; 335]	177.1 [102.1; 247.56]	0.089	222.4 [141.6; 281.1]	160.12 [99.87; 270.44]	0.369
MCP-1, i.e., CCL2	474.8 [364.9; 646.1]	369.8 [239.5; 660.8]	0.229	593.8 [451.4; 717.3]	311.5 [173.0; 507.0]	**0.005**
MIP-1α, i.e., CCL3	6.97 [4.06; 9.96]	6.54 [4.31; 10.87]	0.961	6.53 [4.34; 1045]	6.12 [4.99; 8.45]	0.611
MIP-1β, i.e., CCL4	28 [21.4; 35.3]	25.46 [16.11; 30.1]	0.201	31.5 [22.5; 41.4]	26.31 [18.01; 36.31]	0.191
RANTES, i.e., CCL5	3021 [1905.8; 3949.5]	2887.2 [1312.4; 4569.2]	0.587	2795 [1735; 5134]	2749.5 [1365.4; 3645.45]	0.545
TNFα	15.9 [13.2; 20.6]	13.8 [7.45; 19.11]	0.197	17.4 [10.8; 20.9]	13.87 [8.01; 19.87]	0.159
TNFβ, i.e., LTA	8.7 [7.2; 12.6]	10.05 [6.45; 40.31]	0.397	9.46 [8.24; 11.67]	8.95 [6.62; 12.07]	0.405
VEGF-A	79.2 [54.7; 133.5]	86.45 [54.87; 202.45]	0.349	111.3 [65.1; 159.7]	72.45 [53.0; 109.48]	0.145

In subjects with IHD comorbid with AO, blood concentrations were lower for Flt3 ligand (1.5-fold), GM-CSF (2.3-fold), GROα (2.2-fold), and MCP-1 (1.9-fold), whereas IL-2 concentration in the blood was 3.0-fold higher relative to subjects with AO without IHD.

To confirm the obtained results for statistically significant differences in the values of cytokines/chemokines between the subgroups, we conducted an additional study of these cytokine/chemokines by ELISA (Table 4).

Table 4. Levels of the human cytokines/chemokines in IHD (median [lower; upper quartile]), ELISA data.

Analytes, pg/ml	Subjects without IHD (n = 39)	Subjects with IHD (n = 49)	p
Flt3 ligand	41.5 [26.5; 56.6]	26.5 [12.3; 40.6]	0.002
GM-CSF	9.5 [4.7; 15.8]	4.7 [2.1; 11.8]	0.004
sCD40L	2351.6 [854.6; 4178.9]	1348.7 [190.8; 3144.5]	0.049
IL-2	1.2 [0.4; 4.1]	1.9 [1.0; 3.7]	0.750
IL-6	3.4 [1.3; 5.1]	4.8 [1.5; 8.6]	0.255
IL-7	11.8 [6.0; 16.7]	8.0 [4.1; 13.5]	0.035
MCP-1, i.e., CCL2	550.7 [325.4; 670.6]	312.4 [125.8; 585.5]	0.005
MIP-1β, i.e., CCL4	31.4 [22.4; 40.7]	25.0 [15.5; 30.7]	0.045
TNFα	16.5 [10.7; 22.4]	13.1 [8.6; 17.8]	0.048

According to ELISA data, in subjects with IHD, blood levels were lower for Flt3 ligand (1.56-fold), GM-CSF (2.0-fold), sCD40L (1.7-fold), IL-7 (1.5-fold), MCP-1 (1.76-fold), MIP-1β (1.2-fold), and TNFα (1.26-fold) as compared with subjects without IHD. Thus, significant associations were shown between blood serum cytokine/chemokine measurements by multiplex analysis and ELISA.

The results of subsequent univariate and multivariate logistic regression analyses (with adjustment for age and sex) regarding possible correlations of cytokines/chemokines with the relative risk of early IHD in the whole study population are presented in Table 5.

Table 5. Results of regression analysis regarding correlations of cytokines/chemokines with IHD risk.

Factors	Univariate Analysis			Multivariate Analysis		
	Exp(B)[1]	95.0% CI	p	Exp(B)[1]	95.0% CI	p
Flt3 ligand	0.965	0.942–0.990	0.006	0.969	0.941–0.998	0.039
GM-CSF	0.904	0.832–0.982	0.017	0.972	0.896–1.06	0.499
sCD40L	0.999	0.998–1.001	0.075	1.001	0.999–1.003	0.726
IL-7	0.941	0.883–1.003	0.063	0.952	0.88–1.03	0.219
IP-10, i.e., CXCL10	0.999	0.995–1.002	0.378			
MCP-1, i.e., CCL2	0.998	0.996–0.999	0.007	0.999	0.997–1.001	0.403
MIP-1β, i.e., CCL4	0.969	0.939–1.000	0.051	0.997	0.961–1.034	0.871
TNFα	0.948	0.891–1.008	0.087			

[1] Exp(B): an odds ratio of a predictor.

The univariate regression analysis revealed that the relative risk of early IHD is significantly associated with lower blood levels of such cytokines/chemokines as Flt3 ligand (OR = 0.965, CI 0.942–0.990, p = 0.006), GM-CSF (OR = 0.904, CI 0.832–0.982, p = 0.017), and MCP-1 (OR = 0.998, CI 0.996–0.999, p = 0.007). Results of the multivariate logistic regression analysis showed that the relative risk of early IHD is significantly associated only with lowered blood concentration of Flt3 ligand (OR = 0.969, CI 0.941–0.998, p = 0.039).

Then, univariate and multivariate logistic regression analyses (with adjustment for age and sex) were performed to find possible associations between cytokines/chemokines and the relative risk of early IHD in the studied young people with AO (Table 6).

Table 6. Results of regression analysis regarding correlations of cytokines/chemokines with IHD risk in the presence of AO.

Factors	Univariate Analysis			Multivariate Analysis		
	Exp(B)[1]	95.0% CI	p	Exp(B)[1]	95.0% CI	p
Flt3 ligand	0.971	0.941–1.002	0.062	0.976	0.937–1.016	0.233
GM-CSF	**0.873**	**0.763–0.999**	**0.049**	0.967	0.847–1.104	0.620
GROα	0.999	0.998–1.001	0.097			
sCD40L	1.000	0.999–1.001	0.098			
IL-2	1.000	0.845–1.185	0.998			
IL-4	0.983	0.966–1.001	0.057	**0.979**	**0.958–0.999**	**0.049**
MCP-1, i.e., **CCL2**	**0.997**	**0.995–0.999**	**0.027**	0.998	0.995–1.001	0.275

[1] Exp(B): an odds ratio of a predictor.

According to the univariate regression analysis, the relative risk of early IHD among the subjects with AO is significantly associated with lower blood concentrations of such cytokines/chemokines as GM-CSF (OR = 0.873, CI 0.763–0.999, p = 0.049) and MCP-1 (OR = 0.997, CI 0.995–0.999, p = 0.027). Judging by the results of the multivariate logistic regression analysis, the relative risk of early IHD among subjects with AO is significantly associated only with a lower blood level of IL-4 (OR = 0.979, CI 0.958–0.999, p = 0.049).

Thus, we found that lowered blood concentrations of cytokines/chemokines such as Flt3 ligand, GM-CSF, and MCP-1 are significantly associated with the relative risk of early IHD in young people aged 25–44 years. In addition, in young people 25–44 years old with AO, lowered blood concentrations of cytokines/chemokines are significantly associated with the relative risk of early IHD comorbid with AO: GM-CSF, MCP-1, and IL-4.

4. Discussion

In the vast majority of cases, IHD, including early IHD, develops during coronary atherosclerosis, which is a chronic inflammatory process. Cytokines and chemokines are the main biomolecules mediating an inflammatory process. On the other hand, visceral/abdominal obesity is also a factor triggering the development of systemic inflammatory changes in the human body [4–6,10].

In biomedical research, the modern multiplex technology of biochemical assays allows us to evaluate blood concentrations of a large variety of cytokines and chemokines, including those with an unclear role in the pathogenesis of CVDs. Our results were hardly expected. For instance, not a single proinflammatory cytokine—among those known to be related to the pathogenesis of atherosclerosis—manifested a direct association with the risk of early IHD, including early IHD in the presence of AO. A possible reason is the small number of patients with IHD in our study, but we had to limit the study population to young subjects (aged 25–44 years).

Nonetheless, we detected significant inverse correlations of some cytokines/chemokines with the risk of early IHD. For example, we revealed that lowered blood concentrations of cytokines/chemokines such as Flt3 ligand, GM-CSF, and MCP-1 are significantly associated with the relative risk of early IHD in young people aged 25–44 years. Lowered blood concentrations of two of these cytokines/chemokines—GM-CSF and MCP-1—also significantly correlate with the relative risk of early IHD in the presence of AO. Additionally, a lowered blood level of IL-4 was found to be significantly associated with the relative risk of early IHD in the presence of AO.

Our findings related to Flt3 ligand, GM-CSF, and IL-4 are consistent with the international literature. For instance, Flt3 ligand (i.e., the ligand of Fms-like tyrosine kinase 3) is a cytokine stimulating the proliferation and differentiation of hematopoietic cells through activation of its receptor, Flt3. Besides this, it serves as the main growth factor of dendritic cells. It has been demonstrated that the number of dendritic cells is low in patients with IHD [11–13]. I. Van Brussel and coauthors [14] have reported that this phenomenon is linked with the downregulation of Flt3 ligand in patients with IHD. This observation is suggestive of a protective function of this ligand against IHD.

GM-CSF is a polypeptide cytokine belonging to the group of granulocyte-macrophage colony-stimulating factors. It stimulates the growth and differentiation of granulocytes, macrophages, and eosinophils. In response to inflammation mediators (IL-1, IL-6, and/or TNF-α), many types of cells start to express GM-CSF. It takes part in the pathogenesis of atherosclerosis. For example, there is evidence that mice deficient in GM-CSF are at a substantial risk of atherosclerosis [15]. In a murine experimental model of brain ischemia, GM-CSF reduces the volume of infarction-affected tissue in the brain and enhances the growth of collateral arteries [16]. GM-CSF can have a direct or indirect effect on CVDs by promoting neovascularization of an ischemic myocardium and by alleviating myocardial injury after an infarction [17]. Yiguan Xu and coauthors [18] have revealed that treatment with low doses of GM-CSF (5.0 g/kg) provides a benefit and reduces complications in patients with IHD and that GM-CSF administration at this dose can significantly improve myocardial perfusion and heart function in these patients. Nevertheless, owing to their small sample size, Yiguan Xu et al. stated that further research is needed and that this field holds promise. A study by M. Ditiatkovski and coworkers shows that, in apoE-deficient mice, the volume of atherosclerotic damage and macrophage accumulation increases if GM-CSF is downregulated, suggesting that, in vivo, GM-CSF protects from atherosclerosis [19]. The same authors demonstrated higher expression of adhesive moleculesin atherosclerotic lesions of GM-CSF-deficient mice, also indicating the anti-inflammatory role of GM-CSF in the development of such lesions.

IL-4 is acytokine inducing the differentiation of T helper cells into T helper 2 cells. IL-4 performs a multitude of biological functions, such as stimulation of activated proliferation of B and T cells and the differentiation of the former into plasma cells. This is a key regulator of adaptive (including humoral) immunity. IL-4 is considered an anti-inflammatory cytokine. In a study on a mouse model, Yu. Shintani and coauthors [20] demonstrated the effectiveness of long-acting IL-4 against acute myocardial infarctionin terms of improvements in both systolic and diastolic functions of ventricles.

Our data on the anti-inflammatory chemokine MCP-1 (i.e., CCL2) are hardly consistent with the results of other studies. For instance, it is known that MCP-1 is one of the factors linking obesity-induced inflammation and the development of atherosclerosis and acts by causing macrophage migration into the developing atherosclerotic plaque. Its blood concentration is increased in obese people, thereby recruiting monocytes from bone marrow to tissues via the blood stream [21,22]. MCP-1 can cause division of macrophagic cells in live-tissue implants, whereas MCP-1 deficiency in vivo diminishes the proliferation of adipose-tissue macrophages [23]. Although most of literature data support the involvement of MCP-1 in the pathologies related to obesity, there are some discrepancies. To give an example, K.E. Inouye and coworkers have reported the absence of changes in the number of macrophages in the adipose tissue of MCP-1-deficient mice during high-fat diet-induced obesity [24]. The same authors, however, found that these mice gained more weight and were glucose intolerant [24]. T.L. Cranford et al. have shown that MCP-1 deficiency can differently affect metabolic and inflammatory processes depending on genetic background [25]. A study by Y.W. Lee and colleagues [26] probably can also help to explain our findings about the inverse correlation of MCP-1with the risk of early IHD. These authors reported that IL-4 induces MCP-1 expression in a vascular endothelium, suggesting that this cytokine and this chemokine are unidirectionally linked. We also noted a "unidirectional link"betweenIL-4 and MCP-1, indicatingtheir significant inverse correlations (Table 5) with the relative risk of early IHD in 25–44-year-olds with AO.

In general, our findings related to Flt3 ligand, GM-CSF, and IL-4 are consistent with the international literature. Results from the present study are partly confirmative and partly hypothesis generating.

This study has its own strengths and limitations. The strength of the study is due to the research of a large complex of 41 cytokines/chemokines using a new biochemical technology (multiplex analysis) in young people with early IHD and abdominal obesity. The limitation of the study is the research of only one type of biological material in the examined persons - blood. The collection of other biological material (samples of organs and tissues) from the examined persons was not carried out.

5. Conclusions

We identified poorly studied biomolecules inversely correlating with early IHD, including early IHD comorbid with AO: Flt3 ligand, GM-CSF, MCP-1/CCL2, and IL-4. The results undoubtedly require further research on the development of IHD (especially early IHD) in the presence of AO. The use of multiplex biochemical express panels for this purpose should increase the effectiveness of the diagnosis, risk assessment, and prevention of these diseases, with major implications for the young employable population.

Author Contributions: Conceptualization, Y.I.R.; Data curation, Y.V.P., N.A.K. and E.V.K.; Formal analysis, L.V.S.; Investigation, Y.V.P., N.A.K. and E.V.K.; Methodology, Y.I.R. and E.V.K.; Writing—original draft, Y.I.R.; Writing—review and editing, V.I.O. All authors have read and agreed to the published version of the manuscript.

Funding: This work was done within the publicly funded topic in State Assignment No.AAAA-A17-117112850280-2 and with financial support from Russian Federation President grant for leading scientific schools No.НШ-2595.2020.7.

Conflicts of Interest: The authors declare no conflict of interest. The funders had no role in the design of the study; in the collection, analyses, or interpretation of data; in the writing of the manuscript, or in the decision to publish the results.

References

1. Roth, G.; Huffman, M.D.; Moran, A.E.; Feigin, V.; Mensah, G.A.; Naghavi, M.; Murray, C.J. Global and Regional Patterns in Cardiovascular Mortality from 1990 to 2013. *Circulation* **2015**, *132*, 1667–1678. [CrossRef] [PubMed]
2. Juonala, M.; Magnussen, C.G.; Berenson, G.S.; Venn, A.; Burns, T.L.; Sabin, M.A.; Srinivasan, S.R.; Daniels, S.R.; Davis, P.H.; Chen, W.; et al. Childhood Adiposity, Adult Adiposity, and Cardiovascular Risk Factors. *N. Engl. J. Med.* **2011**, *365*, 1876–1885. [CrossRef] [PubMed]
3. Bastien, M.; Poirier, P.; Lemieux, I.; Després, J.-P. Overview of Epidemiology and Contribution of Obesity to Cardiovascular Disease. *Prog. Cardiovasc. Dis.* **2014**, *56*, 369–381. [CrossRef] [PubMed]
4. Chait, A.; Hartigh, L.J.D. Adipose Tissue Distribution, Inflammation and Its Metabolic Consequences, Including Diabetes and Cardiovascular Disease. *Front. Cardiovasc. Med.* **2020**, *7*, 7–22. [CrossRef] [PubMed]
5. Kwaifa, I.K.; Bahari, H.; Yong, Y.K.; Noor, S.M. Endothelial Dysfunction in Obesity-Induced Inflammation: Molecular Mechanisms and Clinical Implications. *Biomolecules* **2020**, *10*, 291. [CrossRef] [PubMed]
6. Rea, I.M.; Gibson, D.S.; McGilligan, V.; McNerlan, S.E.; Alexander, H.D.; Ross, O.A. Age and Age-Related Diseases: Role of Inflammation Triggers and Cytokines. *Front. Immunol.* **2018**, *9*, 586. [CrossRef]
7. Ha, E.E.; Bauer, R.C. Emerging Roles for Adipose Tissue in Cardiovascular Disease. *Arter. Thromb. Vasc. Boil.* **2018**, *38*, e137–e144. [CrossRef]
8. Carbone, S.; Canada, J.M.; Billingsley, H.E.; Siddiqui, M.S.; Elagizi, A.; Lavie, C.J. Obesity paradox in cardiovascular disease: Where do we stand? *Vasc. Heal. Risk Manag.* **2019**, *15*, 89–100. [CrossRef]
9. Lavie, C.J.; Arena, R.; Alpert, M.A.; Milani, R.V.; Ventura, H.O. Management of cardiovascular diseases in patients with obesity. *Nat. Rev. Cardiol.* **2017**, *15*, 45–56. [CrossRef]
10. Lovren, F.; Teoh, H.; Verma, S. Obesity and Atherosclerosis: Mechanistic Insights. *Can. J. Cardiol.* **2015**, *31*, 177–183. [CrossRef]
11. Van Vre, E.A.; Hoymans, V.Y.; Bult, H.; Lenjou, M.; Van Bockstaele, D.R.; Vrints, C.J.; Bosmans, J.M. Decreased number of circulating plasmacytoid dendritic cells in patients with atherosclerotic coronary artery disease. *Coron. Artery Dis.* **2006**, *17*, 243–248. [CrossRef] [PubMed]
12. Van Vré, E.A.; Van Brussel, I.; De Beeck, K.O.; Hoymans, V.Y.; Vrints, C.J.; Bult, H.; Bosmans, J.M. Changes in blood dendritic cell counts in relation to type of coronary artery disease and brachial endothelial cell function. *Coron. Artery Dis.* **2010**, *21*, 87–96. [CrossRef] [PubMed]
13. Yilmaz, A.; Schaller, T.; Cicha, I.; Altendorf, R.; Stumpf, C.; Klinghammer, L.; Ludwig, J.; Daniel, W.G.; Garlichs, C.D. Predictive value of the decrease in circulating dendritic cell precursors in stable coronary artery disease. *Clin. Sci.* **2009**, *116*, 353–363. [CrossRef]

14. Van Brussel, I.; Van Vré, E.A.; De Meyer, G.; Vrints, C.J.; Bosmans, J.M.; Bult, H. Decreased numbers of peripheral blood dendritic cells in patients with coronary artery disease are associated with diminished plasma Flt3 ligand levels and impaired plasmacytoid dendritic cell function. *Clin. Sci.* **2011**, *120*, 415–426. [CrossRef] [PubMed]
15. Hamilton, J. Colony-stimulating factors in inflammation and autoimmunity. *Nat. Rev. Immunol.* **2008**, *8*, 533–544. [CrossRef]
16. Sugiyama, Y.; Yagita, Y.; Oyama, N.; Terasaki, Y.; Omura-Matsuoka, E.; Sasaki, T.; Kitagawa, K. Granulocyte Colony-Stimulating Factor Enhances Arteriogenesis and Ameliorates Cerebral Damage in a Mouse Model of Ischemic Stroke. *Stroke* **2011**, *42*, 770–775. [CrossRef]
17. Kovacic, J.C.; Muller, D.W.; Graham, R.M. Actions and therapeutic potential of G-CSF and GM-CSF in cardiovascular disease. *J. Mol. Cell. Cardiol.* **2007**, *42*, 19–33. [CrossRef]
18. Xu, Y.; Liu, Q.; Huang, D.; Zhang, D.; Bu, Y.; Yu, H.; Lei, Z.; Huang, X.; Xu, M. Effect of granulocyte-macrophage colony stimulating factor treatment on myocardial perfusion and heart function in patients with coronary artery disease. *Int. J. Clin. Exp. Med.* **2017**, *10*, 9407–9415.
19. Ditiatkovski, M.; Toh, B.-H.; Bobik, A. GM-CSF Deficiency Reduces Macrophage PPAR-γ Expression and Aggravates Atherosclerosis in ApoE-Deficient Mice. *Arter. Thromb. Vasc. Boil.* **2006**, *26*, 2337–2344. [CrossRef]
20. Shintani, Y.; Ito, T.; Fields, L.; Shiraishi, M.; Ichihara, Y.; Sato, N.; Podaru, M.; Kainuma, S.; Tanaka, H.; Suzuki, K. IL-4 as a Repurposed Biological Drug for Myocardial Infarction through Augmentation of Reparative Cardiac Macrophages: Proof-of-Concept Data in Mice. *Sci. Rep.* **2017**, *7*, 6877. [CrossRef]
21. Bremer, A.A.; Devaraj, S.; Afify, A.; Jialal, I. Adipose tissue dysregulation in patients with metabolic syndrome. *J. Clin. Endocrinol. Metab.* **2011**, *96*, E1782–E1788. [CrossRef] [PubMed]
22. Arner, E.; Mejhert, N.; Kulyté, A.; Balwierz, P.; Pachkov, M.; Cormont, M.; Lorente-Cebrián, S.; Ehrlund, A.; Laurencikiene, J.; Hedén, P.; et al. Adipose Tissue MicroRNAs as Regulators of CCL2 Production in Human Obesity. *Diabetes* **2012**, *61*, 1986–1993. [CrossRef] [PubMed]
23. Amano, S.U.; Cohen, J.L.; Vangala, P.; Tencerová, M.; Nicoloro, S.M.; Yawe, J.C.; Shen, Y.; Czech, M.P.; Aouadi, M. Local proliferation of macrophages contributes to obesity-associated adipose tissue inflammation. *Cell Metab.* **2013**, *19*, 162–171. [CrossRef]
24. Inouye, K.E.; Shi, H.; Howard, J.K.; Daly, C.H.; Lord, G.; Rollins, B.J.; Flier, J.S. Absence of CC Chemokine Ligand 2 Does Not Limit Obesity-Associated Infiltration of Macrophages Into Adipose Tissue. *Diabetes* **2007**, *56*, 2242–2250. [CrossRef] [PubMed]
25. Cranford, T.L.; Enos, R.T.; Velázquez, K.T.; McClellan, J.L.; Davis, J.M.; Singh, U.P.; Nagarkatti, M.; Nagarkatti, P.S.; Robinson, C.M.; Murphy, E.A. Role of MCP-1 on inflammatory processes and metabolic dysfunction following high-fat feedings in the FVB/N strain. *Int. J. Obes.* **2015**, *40*, 844–851. [CrossRef] [PubMed]
26. Lee, Y.W.; Lee, W.H.; Kim, P.H. Role of NADPH oxidase in interleukin-4-induced monocyte chemoattractant protein-1 expression in vascular endothelium. *Inflamm. Res.* **2010**, *59*, 755–765. [CrossRef]

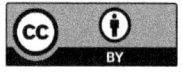

© 2020 by the authors. Licensee MDPI, Basel, Switzerland. This article is an open access article distributed under the terms and conditions of the Creative Commons Attribution (CC BY) license (http://creativecommons.org/licenses/by/4.0/).

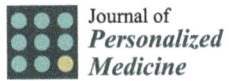

Article

The Risk of Osteoporotic Forearm Fractures in Postmenopausal Women in a Siberian Population Sample

Elena Mazurenko [1,2,*], Oksana Rymar [1], Liliya Shcherbakova [1], Ekaterina Mazdorova [1] and Sofia Malyutina [1]

1. Research Institute of Internal and Preventive Medicine–Branch of the Institute of Cytology and Genetics, Siberian Branch of Russian Academy of Sciences, 630089 Novosibirsk, Russia; orymar23@gmail.com (O.R.); 9584792@mail.ru (L.S.); mazdorova@mail.ru (E.M.); smalyutina@hotmail.com (S.M.)
2. Novosibirsk Research Institute of Traumatology and Orthopedics named after Ya. L. Tsivyan, 630112 Novosibirsk, Russia
* Correspondence: poltorackayaes@gmail.com; Tel.: +7-(952)-945-72-11

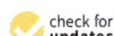

Received: 30 June 2020; Accepted: 30 July 2020; Published: 31 July 2020

Abstract: The reduction in bone and muscle mass increases in menopausal women and poses a threat to the loss of *self-dependence* in the elderly. The aim of the study was to assess the frequency of osteoporotic forearm fractures (OFF) in postmenopausal women and to study their association with risk factors for chronic non-communicable diseases (NCD). The study was based on the Russian arm of the Health, Alcohol and Psychosocial Factors In Eastern Europe (HAPIEE) project (Novosibirsk). In a subsample of postmenopausal women aged 55–84 years old (n = 2005), we assessed the history of OFF during the last 3 years and risk factors for fracture and common NCD/. Cross-sectional associations between OFF history and potential determinants were analyzed using multivariable-adjusted logistic regression. A history of OFF in the last 3 years was found in 3.9% women. In a multivariable-adjusted model, the risk of OFF was directly associated with smoking in the past (OR = 2.23; 95% Cl 1.10–4.55), total cholesterol level higher than 200 mg/dL (OR = 1.98; 95% Cl 1.19–3.29), and it was inversely associated with body mass index (OR = 0.91; 95% Cl 0.86–0.96). In studied population sample of postmenopausal women the cross-sectional determinants of osteoporotic forearm fractures were smoking in the past and high total cholesterol value; body mass index protectively related to the risk of osteoporotic fractures. These findings might have implications for fracture prevention in postmenopausal women.

Keywords: osteoporosis; fracture; menopause; population; chronic non-communicable diseases; risk factors

1. Introduction

The reduction in bone and muscle mass increases with age and poses a threat to the loss of *self-dependence* in the elderly and, specifically, during perimenopause. While the majority of women under the age of 50 years have normal bone mineral density (BMD), by the age of 80 years, 27% of them have osteopenia and 70% have osteoporotic BMD values when examining the thigh, lumbar spine or forearm [1]. According to the published data, the prevalence of osteoporotic forearm fractures (OFF) is the highest among fracture locations. At the age of about 50 years, Caucasian women have a lifetime risk of a wrist fracture about 16% [2]. Forearm fractures are clinically important outcomes from the perspective of morbidity, health care costs, and interruption of work [3]. In the Study of Osteoporotic Fractures, the elderly women with wrist fractures were almost 50% more likely to have a clinically important functional decline than those without fractures [4].

The risk of death within 5 years after an occurrence of OFF ranges from 12% among women aged 65 to 74 years to 43% for women aged 85 years and older [5]. Another study found that low BMD in the distal forearm, categorized as osteopenia and osteoporosis, was associated with increased mortality, and the association was only slightly attenuated by taking osteoporotic fractures into account [6]. This may suggest that low BMD is more powerful predictor of death than an increased risk of fracture [7].

For the Russian Federation, OFF is a serious problem, because most of these fractures occur during the cold season as a result of falling on the ice and this season might be from October to April. Referring the epidemiological study in 16 cities of Russia, the frequency of forearm fractures was 426/100,000 which exceeds the frequency of hip fracture by 3–7 times in men and 4–8 times in women, and it occurred significantly more in women [8,9]. Moreover, in such cities as Moscow, Tyumen, Khabarovsk and Yekaterinburg, women had a frequency of forearm fractures near 1200 per 100,000 and higher [10].

Forearm fractures may precede future secondary fractures. However, if a forearm fracture occurs in a patient with low BMD, this may result in even more severe fragility fractures such as femoral and vertebral fractures [11,12].

Dual-energy X-ray absorptiometry (DXA) screening is standard in the US (at the age of 65 years in women and age 70 in men, and in individuals over the age of 50 years who have suffered an adult fracture) [13], but, in the majority of other countries, population screening is not judged to be cost-effective and primary prevention is focused more on opportunistic case finding, triggered by the presence of clinical risk factors [14,15]. A recent randomized-controlled trial (the UK SCOOP) has investigated the effectiveness and cost-effectiveness of screening in older women in primary care for the prevention of fractures in seven centers where approximately 12,500 older women were randomized to either normal care or screening and subsequent treatment (based on the FRAX risk assessment tool). This study has demonstrated that this intervention leads to a 28% reduction in hip fracture risk [16]. As would be expected from this approach, the screening appeared to be the most effective in those at highest baseline fracture risk [17], and importantly, it was shown to be cost-effective [18,19]

Increased attention to OFF is important to identify women at increased risk for repeated future fractures and to apply preventive measures [20]. A high frequency of comorbidity of severe osteoporosis with NCD has been established [21]. Cardiovascular disease (CVD) is known to be associated with an increased risk of hip fractures [22]; similarly, it has been shown that low bone mass in women can be an independent predictor of CVD [23]. Diabetes mellitus (DM) is also a risk factor for hip fracture. Recent studies have shown that microstructural changes in bone tissue are more noticeable among people with diabetes with microvascular complications [24]. Commonly accepted risk factors for NCD probably contribute to the development of osteoporosis.

The aim of the study was to assess the frequency of osteoporotic forearm fractures in women aged over 55 years and to investigate the association between OFF and common risk factors for NCD.

2. Studied Population and Methods

2.1. Partisipants

The data came from the Russian arm of the Health, Alcohol, and Psychosocial Factors in Eastern Europe (HAPIEE) project. The random population sample (9360 men and women aged 45–69 years old) was examined in Novosibirsk (Russia) at baseline in 2003–2005 and re-examined twice. In 2015–2018, a sample of 3898 subjects was examined in the frame of the wave-3 (men, women aged 55–84 years). Current analysis was restricted to a random subset of women who gave answers to the question on history of fractures (n = 2005). Additionally, we excluded those with fractures that occurred more than 3 years ago who had no measurement of fasting blood glucose levels (FBG), and women in the reproductive period. The final sample for this analysis included 2005 women. The study was approved by the Ethics Committee of the Research Institute of Internal and Preventive Medicine NIITPM (Protocol, dated 12/26/2014).

2.2. Study Questionnaire

The program of examination of the HAPIEE project is published elsewhere [25] (http://www.ucl.ac.uk/easteurope/hapiee-cohort.htm). The data on fractures of the forearm in the last 3 years, the history of DM2, the duration of menopause in women, smoking and alcohol intake habits, physical functioning and other risk factors for CVD and NCD, and socio-demographic data were collected using the structured questionnaire.

The osteoporotic forearm fracture was defined as the history of fracture within the last 3 years which occurred when the subject fell from his own growth or spontaneously.

The smoking questionnaire included information about current smoking one or more cigarettes per day and smoking history in the past. A person was considered as a current smoker if he or she smokes at least one cigarette per day. Alcohol consumption was estimated using the Graduated Frequency Questionnaire (GFR). Physical activity was assessed using the Physical Functioning scale (PF10, subscale from SF-36). The value of PF10 scale distribution <75‰ was considered as low.

2.3. Anthropometry and Blood Pressure Measurement

Anthropometric measurements were performed including height, weight, waist and hip circumference. The height was measured standing, without outerwear and shoes, on a standard height meter with an accuracy of 0.5 cm. Body weight was determined without outerwear and shoes, on standard lever scales that underwent metrological control (with measurement accuracy 0.1 kg).

Waist hip ratio (WHR) and body mass index (BMI) was calculated by a common formula:

$$\text{BMI (kg/m}^2\text{)} = \text{body weight (kg)/height}^2 \text{ (m}^2\text{)} \tag{1}$$

$$\text{WHR (units)} = \text{waist circumference/hip circumference} \tag{2}$$

Blood pressure (BP) measurement was performed three times on the right hand in a sitting position after five minutes of rest at intervals of 2 min between measurements. The average value of three blood pressure measurements was used in the current analysis.

2.4. Biochemical Measurements

Blood sampling was performed after 8 h fasting. After centrifugation, the serum was stored in a low-temperature chamber (−70 °C). A biochemical blood test was performed at the Clinical Biochemistry Laboratory of NIITPM, standardized for Federal quality control at regular basis. The concentration of total cholesterol, high-density lipoprotein cholesterol (HDL-C), triglycerides (TG) and glucose in blood serum was carried out by the enzymatic method using commercial standard Biocon kits (Germany) on a KoneLab autoanalyzer (USA). The concentration of low-density lipoprotein cholesterol (LDL-C) was calculated by Fridewald formula. The conversion of serum glucose to plasma glucose (GP) was done by formula

$$\text{GP (mmol/L)} = -0.137 + 1.047 \times \text{serum glucose (mmol/L) (EASD, 2005)}. \tag{3}$$

Diabetes mellitus, type 2 (DM2) was established by epidemiological criteria with FBG ≥7.0 mmol/L (WHO, 2003) and/or normoglycemia in patients with a medical history of established DM2.

2.5. Statistical Analysis

Statistical analysis was performed using the SPSS software package (v.13.0). The statistical significance of differences in average values was evaluated by Student's criterion (t) for normally distributed characters. To determine the statistical significance of differences in qualitative characteristics, the Pearson method (χ^2) was used. Comparison of two independent groups by quantitative characteristics with an abnormal distribution was made using the nonparametric Mann–Whitney criterion. The measures are presented as relative values (n, %), and average values (M ± SD), where M is the arithmetic mean value and SD is the standard deviation. Differences were considered statistically significant at *p*-value < 0.05. To assess the relationship between OFF in the last three years and common risk factors, the logistic regression method was used in age- and multivariable-adjusted models.

3. Results

3.1. Comparative Characteristics of the Studied Groups

In studied population sample of 2005 postmenopausal women the incidence of OFF comprised 3.9% (n = 71). The frequency of OFF in the last 3 years did not differ in women with DM2—3.0% and without DM2—4.3% (*p* = 0.218)

The subjects examined were split into two groups: those with a history of OFF and those without a history of OFF; comparative characteristics are presented in Table A1. Women with OFF had lower weight (*p* = 0.003), BMI (*p* = 0.001), waist circumference (*p* = 0.001), hip circumference (*p* = 0.013), WHR (*p* = 0.001), compared to those without OFF. The groups did not differ by age, BP values, lipid values, physical functioning, smoking, frequency of DM2 and education level.

3.2. The Relationship Between NCD Risk Factors and OFF by Logistic Regression Analysis

Logistic regression analysis was used to assess the association between the history of OFF in the last 3 years and common risk factors for NCD. Regression was performed in age-adjusted Model 1 and in multivariable–adjusted Model 2 and Model 3. The history of OFF in the last 3 years was used as a dependent variable. The tested factors were used as independent variables and include age (continuous measure; per 1 year), presence of DM2 (categorized as yes/no), smoking (categorized as never smoking/smoking in the past/present smoking), BMI (continuous measure; per 1 kg/m^2), duration of menopause (categorized as ≥10 years/<10 years), physical performance (categorized in 2 categories having low pf10 < 75‰ and preserved pf10 value ≥ 75‰), total cholesterol value (categorized as total cholesterol ≥ 200 mg/dL and < 200 mg/dL) Model 2 was controlled for the following covariates: age, DM2, BMI, smoking, menopause, physical performance. Model 3 was controlled for the following covariates: age, DM2, smoking, physical performance, total cholesterol value.

The results of logistic regression are presented on Figure A1. In age-adjusted analysis, the risk of OFF in postmenopausal women was positively associated with history of past smoking (OR = 2.29; 95% Cl 1.13–4.65), total cholesterol ≥ 200 mg/dL (OR = 2.03; 95% Cl 1.25–3.41), and negatively associated with BMI (OR = 0.92; 95% Cl 0.87–0.97). In multivariable-adjusted analysis, these relationship remained significant and the risk of OFF was positively associated with history of past smoking (OR = 2.23; 95% Cl 1.10–4.55), elevated total cholesterol value ≥ 200 mg/dL (OR=1.98; 95% Cl 1.19–3.29), and negatively associated with BMI (OR = 0.91; 95% Cl 0.86–0.96) regardless of other factors (Figure A1).

4. Discussion

In a studied population sample of postmenopausal women aged 55–80 years old, we revealed that substantial frequency of osteoporotic forearm fractures occurred during the last 3 years— 3.9% OFF. In our cross-sectional analysis, the risk of OFF was associated with several risk factors of NCD, specifically, it was directly associated with past smoking, elevated total cholesterol and it was inversely related to BMI value independent of other factors.

The prevalence of OFF in the world is high and continues to increase. In the southern part of the Skane region (Sweden), the incidence of OFF is 278 cases per 100,000 persons. From 1999 to 2010, the total annual number of OFF in women increased from 1779 to 2323 [26]. Abrahamsen et al. [27], in a recent large-scale study in Denmark, showed that the incidence in women (530 per 100,000 persons) was slightly higher than in the Jerrhag D study [26].

We found the frequency of OFF occurred during the last 3 years among postmenopausal women in Novosibirsk of 3.9%. The results of our study confirm the high incidence of OFF in the Russian population. In the city of Pervouralsk (Russia), 586 OFF were registered over a two-year period, which amounted to an average of 540.7/100,000 persons, moreover, women experienced fractures five times more often than men (787.9/100,000 and 171.1/100,000 in women and men, respectively, $p < 0.00001$) [28]. According to study of Zavodsky B.V. et al. conducted in the period 2008–2014 in the Volgograd region, fractures of the radial bones dominated among all fractures both among those with osteoporosis and with normal bone mineral density ($p < 0.0001$) [29]. In the city of Ulan-Ude, the medical documentation of trauma centers was studied for the period of 2009–2011 and it was revealed that women most often underwent OFF—in 44.4% of cases among all fractures [30]. When calculating the rate per 100,000 persons of the corresponding nationality, it turned out that the Buryats suffered from complications of osteoporosis two times more often than Russians: 648.8 cases per 100,000 of inhabitants of the Mongoloid race and 323.6 cases per 100,000 of inhabitants of Slavic origin. However, women, regardless of nationality, most often suffered from the fractures of the distal forearm [30]. These published data [29,30] repeatedly focus on the fact that the BMD of the wrist might be underestimated in common medical practice. In our earlier study, we found that the BMD in the distal third of the wrist was 0.4–0.6 SD lower than in the lumbar spine and femoral neck sites [31]. Perhaps this parameter has the greatest sensitivity in predicting the risk of fractures.

The frequency of OFF over 3 years in women with DM2 aged 55–84 years in our study was 3.0%. Similar data were obtained by Yalochkina et al., 2016, among 214 individuals with DM2 (44–88 years old); 5.1% of patients had OFF [32].

The investigations of association between osteoporotic fractures and risk factors for NCD are actively carried out in international and Russian studies. According to the multivariate analysis in our study, the odds of forearm fractures among postmenopausal women independently increased in those with past smoking by 2.23 times, in those with elevated level of total cholesterol higher than 200 mg/dL by two times, and the chance of a fracture was inversely related to BMI value.

Tobacco is the most common risk factor for osteoporosis. In a meta-analysis of 48 studies [33], bone density in smoking women decreased by about 2% for every 10 years, with a difference of 6% at the age of 80 years. In another meta-analysis [34], Kanis JA et al., 2005, showed that smoking is associated with an increased risk of any fracture compared to non-smokers both in men and women. Smoking in the past was associated with a significantly increased risk of fracture compared to non-smokers, but the risk was lower than that of current smokers. In addition, those who quit smoking had a lower risk of fracture than those who continued to smoke, but higher than those who had never smoked [34].

In our study, the risk of fractures increased in those women who smoked in the past, but we did not find an association between OFF and present smoking. We studied a population sample of postmenopausal women and the frequency of smoking in elderly women is quite rare in Russia. Therefore, it is possible the association between current smoking and OFF was not identified due to small numbers of smokers in our sample. The study limitation is that we have no data available on the duration and intensity of smoking. It might be that those who quit smoking had higher duration and intensity of smoking and/or had greater health problems as a result of which they quit smoking, compared to those who continue to smoke.

In general, possible mechanism by which smoking can increase bone loss is age at smoking initiation and its effect on body weight. Some studies have shown that initiation of smoking at age 13 affected bone accrual and was associated with low mean BMD at age 17 [35,36]. Thus, BMD deficiency at a young age led to a more rapid decrease in BMD in those over 50. By middle age, smokers weigh an average of 7–8 pounds less than nonsmokers [37]. Another study found quitting smoking significantly associated with increased body weight, fat, muscles, and functional mass that affected BMD [38].

Smoking cessation is significantly associated with increased body weight, fat, which ambiguously affects BMD and these mechanisms require further study.

The results of assessment of correlation between osteoporotic fractures and total cholesterol and BMD are contradictory. The effect of total cholesterol and its metabolites on osteoblastic activity was shown in vivo and in vitro [39]. Luegmayr E., et al., have shown that elevated plasma total cholesterol levels may decrease BMD and increase the incidence of fractures. In in vitro study, total cholesterol prolonged the survival of osteoclast-like cells that contribute to osteoporosis [40]. In addition, it was shown that a high level of total cholesterol was associated with a low level of 25 (OH) D, which was necessary for calcium absorption. [41,42]. In recent meta-analysis of Y.-Y. Chen et al., 2018, has shown that serum levels of total cholesterol are higher in women with postmenopausal osteoporosis than in the group with normal bone density. These data are consistent with the results in our study [43].

In our study, in unadjusted analysis, BMI in women with fractures was significantly lower than in those without fractures. However, after controlling for covariates, the risk of fractures was inversely related to BMI. Obesity is traditionally perceived as a protective effect on bone. This might be explained by an increase in the mechanical load on the skeleton and the ability of adipocytes to convert androgens to 17β-estradiol, which increases BMD [44].

The OFF is the most common type of fracture, and even a slight increase in the number of fracture cases significantly affects the need for health resources, especially among people of working age, when patients are to be "on sick leave" for 5–12 weeks or more depending on their profession. The NORA study has demonstrated that OFF at the age of ≥45 years increases the future risk of fracture of the proximal femur by 1.9 times [45]. These facts allow discussion about the "osteoporotic cascade" of fractures, when the next, and sometimes a series of new fractures occur after one fracture. Bone Health Alliance National Working Group experts note that OFF are characterized as osteoporotic fractures if there is concomitant osteopenia or osteoporosis by measuring BMD (T-score less than −1.0 SD) at the level of the lumbar spine or femur [46]. This allows us to suggest a shift of a paradigm shift from hip fractures to wrist fractures, and given the data from our study in Novosibirsk population, we could suppose the rationale for modification of criteria for osteoporosis diagnosis for the National Expert Working Group (USA).

However, current Russian recommendations on osteoporosis, 2017 [9] and the recommendations of the National Osteoporosis Foundation of the United States, 2014 [13], do not consider wrist fractures (in patients without preliminary hip/vertebral fractures or with BMD in the range of osteoporosis values) as an indication for pharmacotherapy [9,13].

Thus, there is currently no consensus among specialized bone research societies regarding whether low-energy wrist fractures should be considered as a criterion for diagnosing osteoporosis. Therefore, the identification and monitoring of these patients as a high-risk group for fractures is one of the important tasks of public health.

5. Conclusions

In the studied Siberian population sample of postmenopausal women aged 55–80 years old, the frequency of osteoporotic forearm fractures during the last 3 years was 3.9%. The cross-sectional determinants of OFF were smoking in the past and high total cholesterol value; body mass index value was inversely related to the risk osteoporotic fractures. The identification of mutual risk factors suggests deeper relationships between NCD and osteoporotic fracture development. The obtained data might have implications for fracture prevention in postmenopausal women.

Author Contributions: E.M. (Elena Mazurenko)—data receiving, material processing and analysis writing the text of the manuscript; O.R.—scientific coordination of current study, analysis, editing the text of the manuscript; L.S.— database managment, statistical analysis; E.M. (Ekaterina Mazdorova)—data receiving, critical comments to the text; S.M.—leading the HAPIEE project in Russia and ageing study coordination of population survey, analysis, editing the text of the manuscript. All authors made a significant contribution to the research and preparation of the article, read and approved the final version before publication. All authors have read and agreed to the published version of the manuscript.

Funding: This study was supported by the Russian Scientific Foundation (20-15-00371) and the Russian Academy of Science, State target (AAAA-A17-117112850280-2); the HAPIEE study was funded by the Welcome Trust (WT064947, WT081081), the US National Institute of Aging (1RO1AG23522).

Acknowledgments: The authors acknowledge Eu. Verevkin for the database constructing, J. Ragino for the organization of biochemical research and M.Bobak, H. Pikhart, A. Peasey, M. Holmes, D. Stefler, J. Hubacek for valuable advices in paper planning and discussion.

Conflicts of Interest: The authors declare no conflict of interest.

Appendix A

Table A1. Characterizatics in groups of postmenopausalwomen aged 55-80 yesars with a history of OFF over the past 3 years and without a history of OFF.

Characteristics	OFF + n = 79	OFF − n = 1926	p
Age, years	68.8 ± 6.3	69.2 ± 6.8	0.611
Height, cm	157.7 ± 7.1	157.2 ± 6.1	0.453
Weight, kg	70.9 ± 13.2	75.9 ± 14.7	0.003
BMI, kg/m^2	28.5 ± 4.7	30.7 ± 5.7	0.001
Waist circumference, cm	89.7 ± 11.9	95.2 ± 12.4	0.001
Hip circumference, cm	105.9 ± 10.3	109.1 ± 10.7	0.013
Waist circumference/Hip circumference	0.85 ± 0.6	0.87 ± 0.7	0.001
SBP, mmHg	143.4 ± 20.9	144.9 ± 21.6	0.528
DBP, mmHg	83.4 ± 10.1	82.3 ± 10.8	0.362
FBG, mmol/l	6.3 ± 5.1	6.3 ± 1.8	0.937
Total cholesterol, mg/dL	225.9 ± 37.1	219.1 ± 46.7	0.201
TG, mg/dL	133.5 ± 103.1	136.8 ± 84.1	0.739
HDL-C, mg/dL	53.2 ± 14.1	53.0 ± 14.9	0.918
PF10, n/%			
>75‰	24/30.4%	732/38%	0.171
≤75‰	55/69.6%	1194/62%	0.171
Education (n/%)			
Univer education	28/35.4%	580/30.1%	0.313
Secondary education	48/60.8%	1214/63.0%	0.682
Primary education	3/3.8%	132/6.9%	0.288
DM2 (n/%)	13/16.5%	423/22.0%	0.245
Smoking, n (%)			
Smoking present n (%)	3/3.9%	90/4.6%	0.717
Smoking in the past n (%)	8/10.3%	107/5.6%	0.087
Non smoking	67/85.9%	1727/89.8%	0.168
Postmenopause duration, years	19.5 ± 7.9	19.7 ± 8.4	0.834

The values are presented as M±SD or n/%

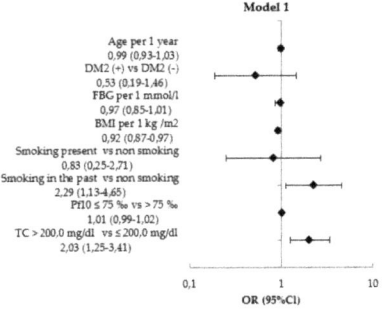

Figure A1. *Cont.*

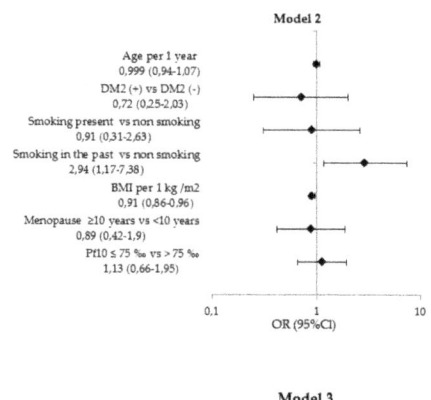

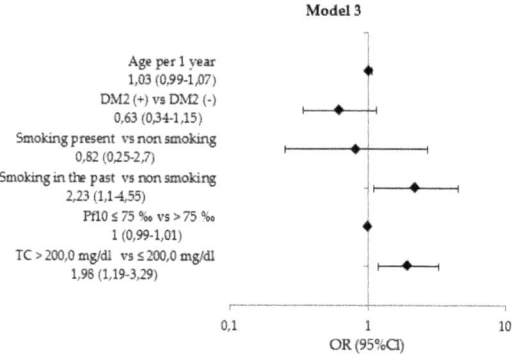

Figure A1. The results of a logistic regression analysis of the relationship OFF over the past 3 years and studied risk factors. Model 1—age-adjusted. Model 2 adjusted for age, DM2, BMI, smoking, duration of menopause, physical performance. Model 3 adjusted for age, DM2, smoking, physical performance, total cholesterol.

References

1. Dawson-Hughes, B.; Tosteson, A.N.A.; Melton, L.J., 3rd; Baim, S.; Favus, M.J.; Khosla, S.; Lindsay, R.L. Implications of absolute fracture risk assessment for osteoporosis practice guidelines in the USA. *Osteoporos. Int.* **2008**, *19*, 449–458. [CrossRef] [PubMed]
2. Litwic, A.; Lekarz, W.D.; Dennison, E. Distal radius fracture: Cinderella of the osteoporotic fractures. *Orthopedic. Muscul. Syst.* **2014**, *3*, 162. [CrossRef]
3. Yu, W.; Ying, Q.; Guan, W.; Lin, Q.; Zhang, Z.; Chen, J.; Engelke, K.; Hsieh, E. Impact of reference point selection on DXA-based measurement of forearm bone mineral density. *Arch. Osteoporos.* **2019**, *14*, 107. [CrossRef] [PubMed]
4. Edwards, B.J.; Song, J.; Dunlop, D.D.; Fink, H.A.; Cauley, J.A. Functional decline after incident wrist fractures-study of osteoporotic fractures: Prospective cohort study. *BMJ* **2010**, *341*, c3324. [CrossRef] [PubMed]
5. Curtis, J.R.; Beukelman, T.; Onofrei, A.; Cassell, S.; Greenberg, J.D.; Kavanaugh, A.; Reed, G.; Strand, V.; Kremer, J.M. Elevated liver enzyme tests among patients with rheumatoid arthritis or psoriatic arthritis treated with methotrexate and/or leflunomide. *Ann. Rheum. Dis.* **2010**, *69*, 43–47. [CrossRef] [PubMed]
6. Hauger, A.V.; Bergland, A.; Holvik, K.; Ståhle, A.; Emaus, N.; Strand, B.H. Osteoporosis and osteopenia in the distal forearm predict all-cause mortality independent of grip strength: 22-year follow-up in the population-based Tromsø Study. *Osteoporos. Int.* **2018**, *29*, 2447–2456. [CrossRef] [PubMed]
7. Hauger, A.V.; Bergland, A.; Holvik, K.; Emaus, N.; Strand, B.H. Can bone mineral density loss in the non-weight bearing distal forearm predict mortality? *Bone* **2020**, *136*, 115347. [CrossRef] [PubMed]

8. Mikhailov, E.E.; Benevolenskaya, L.I.; Anikin, S.G. The frequency of fractures of the proximal femur and distal forearm among the urban population of Russia. *Osteoporos. Osteopathy* **1999**, *3*, 2–6.
9. Mel'nichenko, G.A.; Belaya, Z.E.; Rozhinskaya, L.Y.; Toroptsova, N.V.; Alekseeva, L.I.; Biryukova, E.V.; Grebennikova, T.A.; Dzeranova, L.K.; Dreval, A.V.; Zagorodniy, N.V.; et al. Russian clinical guidelines on the diagnostics, treatment, and prevention of osteoporosis. *Probl. Endocrinol.* **2017**, *63*, 392–426. [CrossRef]
10. International Osteoporosis Foundation. *The Eastern European & Central Asian Regional Audit: Epidemiology, Costs & Burden of Osteoporosis in 2010*; International Osteoporosis Foundation: Washington, DC, USA, 2011; pp. 1–68.
11. Bozkurt, H.H.; Atik, O.Ş.; Tokgöz, M.A. Can distal radius or vertebra fractures due to low-energy trauma be a harbinger of a hip fracture? *Jt. Dis. Relat. Surg.* **2018**, *29*, 100–103. [CrossRef]
12. Kanda, T.; Endo, N.; Kondo, N. Low Bone Mineral Density of the Forearm and Femur among Postmenopausal Women with Metaphyseal Comminuted Fracture of the Distal Radius. *Tohoku. J. Exp. Med.* **2019**, *249*, 147–154. [CrossRef] [PubMed]
13. Cosman, F.; de Beur, S.J.; LeBoff, M.S.; Lewiecki, E.M.; Tanner, B.; Randall, S.; Lindsay, R. Clinician's Guide to Prevention and Treatment of Osteoporosis. *Osteoporos. Int.* **2014**, *25*, 2359–2381. [CrossRef] [PubMed]
14. Kanis, J.A.; McCloskey, E.V.; Johansson, H.; Cooper, C.; Rizzoli, R.; Reginster, J.Y. European guidance for the diagnosis and management of osteoporosis in postmenopausal women. *Osteoporos. Int.* **2013**, *24*, 23–57. [CrossRef] [PubMed]
15. Compston, J.; Cooper, A.; Cooper, C.; Gittoes, N.; Gregson, C.; Harvey, N.; Hope, S.; Kanis, J.A.; McCloskey, E.V.; Poole, K.E.; et al. UK clinical guideline for the prevention and treatment of osteoporosis. *Arch. Osteoporos.* **2017**, *12*, 43. [CrossRef] [PubMed]
16. Shepstone, L.; Lenaghan, E.; Cooper, C.; Clarke, S.; Fong-Soe-Khioe, R.; Fordham, R.; Gittoes, N.; Harvey, I.; Harvey, N.; Heawood, A.; et al. Screening in the community to reduce fractures in older women (SCOOP): A randomised controlled trial. *Lancet* **2018**, *391*, 741–747. [CrossRef]
17. Condurache, C.I.; Chiu, S.; Chotiyarnwong, P.; Johansson, H.; Shepstone, L.; Lenaghan, E.; Cooper, C.; Clarke, S.; Khioe, R.F.S.; Fordham, R.; et al. Screening for high hip fracture risk does not impact on falls risk: A post hoc analysis from the SCOOP study. *Osteoporos. Int.* **2020**, *31*, 457–464. [CrossRef]
18. Turner, D.A.; Khioe, R.F.S.; Shepstone, L.; Lenaghan, E.; Cooper, C.; Gittoes, N.; Harvey, N.C.; Holland, R.; Howe, A.; McCloskey, E.; et al. The cost-effectiveness of screening in the community to reduce osteoporotic fractures in older women in the UK: Economic evaluation of the SCOOP study. *J. Bone Miner. Res.* **2018**, *33*, 845–851. [CrossRef]
19. Liu, J.; Curtis, E.M.; Cooper, C.; Harvey, N.C. State of the art in osteoporosis risk assessment and treatment. *J. Endocrinol. Investig.* **2019**, *42*, 1149–1164. [CrossRef]
20. Crandall, C.J.; Hovey, K.M.; Cauley, J.A.; Andrews, C.A.; Curtis, J.R.; Wactawski-Wende, J.; Wright, N.C.; Li, W.; LeBoff, M.S. Wrist Fracture and Risk of Subsequent Fracture: Findings from the Women's Health Initiative Study. *J. Bone Miner. Res.* **2015**, *30*, 2086–2095. [CrossRef]
21. Thayer, S.W.; Stolshek, B.S.; Gomez Rey, G.; Seare, J.G. Impact of osteoporosis on high-cost chronic diseases. *Value Health* **2014**, *17*, 43–50. [CrossRef]
22. Sennerby, U.; Melhus, H.; Gedeborg, R.; Byberg, L.; Garmo, H.; Ahlbom, A.; Pedersen, N.L.; Michaëlsson, K. Cardiovascular diseases and risk of hip fracture. *JAMA* **2009**, *302*, 1666–1673. [CrossRef] [PubMed]
23. Marcovitz, P.A.; Tran, H.H.; Franklin, B.A.; O'Neill, W.W.; Yerkey, M.; Boura, J.; Kleerekoper, M.; Dickinson, C.Z. Usefulness of bone mineral density to predict significant coronary artery disease. *Am. J. Cardiol.* **2005**, *96*, 1059–1063. [CrossRef] [PubMed]
24. Shanbhogue, V.V.; Hansen, S.; Frost, M.; Jørgensen, N.R.; Hermann, A.P.; Henriksen, J.E.; Brixen, K. Compromised cortical bone compartment in type 2 diabetes mellitus patients with microvascular disease. *Eur. J. Endocrinol.* **2016**, *174*, 115–124. [CrossRef] [PubMed]
25. Peasey, A.; Bobak, M.; Kubinova, R.; Malyutina, S.; Pajak, A.; Tamosiunas, A.; Pikhart, H.; Nicholson, A.; Marmot, M. Determinants of cardiovascular disease and other non-communicable diseases in Central and Eastern Europe: Rationale and design of the HAPIEE study. *BMC Public Health* **2006**, *6*, 255. [CrossRef] [PubMed]
26. Jerrhag, D.; Englund, M.; Karlsson, M.K.; Rosengren, B.E. Epidemiology and time trends of distal forearm fractures in adults—A study of 11.2 million person-years in Sweden. *BMC Musculoskelet. Disord.* **2017**, *18*, 240. [CrossRef] [PubMed]

27. Abrahamsen, B.; Jorgensen, N.R.; Schwarz, P. Epidemiology of forearm fractures in adults in Denmark: National age- and gender-specific incidence rates, ratio of forearm to hip fractures, and extent of surgical fracture repair in inpatients and outpatients. *Osteoporos. Int.* **2015**, *26*, 67–76. [CrossRef]
28. Gladkova, E.N.; Khodyrev, V.N.; Lesnyak, O.M.; Chodyrev, V.N. Analysis of epidemiology of osteoporotic fracturesusing data from primary care physicians. *Osteoporos. Bone Dis.* **2011**, *14*, 14–18. [CrossRef]
29. Zavodovsky, B.V.; Seewordova, L.E.; Polyakova, Y.V.; Simacova, E.S.; Kravtsov, V.I.; Fofanova, N.A. Leading risk factors of osteoporosis among education workers in Volgograd region. *Med. Tr. Prom. Ekol.* **2017**, *7*, 52–55.
30. Batudayeva, T.I. Rasprostranennost' osteoporoticheskikh perelomov sredi zhiteley respubliki Buryatiya 40 let i starshe. *Osteoporos. Bone Dis.* **2016**, *19*, 12. [CrossRef]
31. Mazurenko, E.S.; Malutina, S.K.; Shcherbakova, L.V.; Hrapova, Y.V.; Isaeva, M.P.; Rymar, O.D. 10-year risk of fractures (FRAX) in people with diabetes type 2 in the elderly. *Ther. Arch.* **2019**, *91*, 76–81. [CrossRef]
32. Yalochkina, T.O.; Belaya, J.E.E.; Rozhinskaya, L.Y.; Antsiferov, M.B.; Dzeranova, L.K.; Melnichenko, G.A.E. Bone fractures in patients with type 2 diabetes mellitus: Prevalence and risk factors. *Diabetes Mellit.* **2016**, *19*, 359–365. [CrossRef]
33. Law, M.R.; Hackshaw, A.K. A meta-analysis of cigarette smoking, bone mineral density and risk of hip fracture: Recognition of a major effect. *BMJ* **1997**, *315*, 841–846. [CrossRef] [PubMed]
34. Kanis, J.A.; Johnell, O.; Odén, A.; Johansson, H.; De Laet, C.; Eisman, J.A.; Fujiwara, S.; Kroger, H.; McCloskey, E.V.; Mellstrom, D.; et al. Smoking and fracture risk: A meta-analysis. *Osteoporos. Int.* **2005**, *16*, 155–162. [CrossRef] [PubMed]
35. Emaus, N.; Wilsgaard, T.; Ahmed, L.A. Impacts of body mass index, physical activity, and smoking on femoral bone loss: The tromso study. *J. Bone Miner. Res.* **2014**, *29*, 2080–2089. [CrossRef] [PubMed]
36. Lucas, R.; Fraga, S.; Ramos, E.; Barros, H. Early Initiation of Smoking and Alcohol Drinking as a Predictor of Lower Forearm Bone Mineral Density in Late Adolescence: A Cohort Study in Girls. *PLoS ONE* **2012**, *7*, e46940. [CrossRef] [PubMed]
37. Javed, F.; Al-Kheraif, A.A.; Salazar-Lazo, K.; Yanez-Fontenla, V.; Aldosary, K.M.; Alshehri, M.; Malmstrom, H.; Romanos, G.E. Periodontal inflammatory conditions among smokers and never-smokers with and without type 2 diabetes mellitus. *J. Periodontol.* **2015**, *86*, 839–846. [CrossRef] [PubMed]
38. Kleppinger, A.; Litt, M.D.; Kenny, M.D.; Litt, A.M.; Oncken, C.A. Effects of smoking cessation on body composition in postmenopausal women. *J. Women's Health* **2010**, *19*, 1651–1657. [CrossRef]
39. Parhami, F.; Garfinkel, A.; Demer, L.L. Role of lipids in osteoporosis. *Arterioscler. Thromb. Vasc. Biol.* **2000**, *20*, 2346–2348. [CrossRef]
40. Luegmayr, E.; Glantschnig, H.; Wesolowski, G.A.; Gentile, M.A.; Fisher, J.E.; Rodan, G.A.; Reszka, A.A. Osteoclast formation, survival and morphology are highly dependent on exogenous cholesterol/lipoproteins. *Cell Death Differ.* **2004**, *11*, S108–S118. [CrossRef]
41. Chung, J.Y.; Kang, H.T.; Lee, D.C.; Lee, H.R.; Lee, Y.J. Body composition and its association with cardiometabolic risk factors in the elderly: A focus on sarcopenic obesity. *Arch. Gerontol. Geriatr.* **2013**, *56*, 270–278. [CrossRef]
42. Ponda, M.P.; Dowd, K.; Finkielstein, D.; Holt, P.R.; Breslow, J.L. The short-term effects of vitamin D repletion on cholesterol: A randomized, placebo-controlled trial. *Arterioscler. Thromb. Vasc. Biol.* **2012**, *32*, 2510–2515. [CrossRef] [PubMed]
43. Chen, Y.Y.; Wang, W.W.; Yang, L.; Chen, W.W.; Zhang, H.X. Association between lipid profiles and osteoporosis in postmenopausal women: A meta-analysis. *Eur. Rev. Med. Pharmacol. Sci.* **2018**, *22*, 1–9. [CrossRef] [PubMed]
44. Muka, T.; Trajanoska, K.; Kiefte-de Jong, J.C.; Oei, L.; Uitterlinden, A.G.; Hofman, A.; Dehghan, A.; Zillikens, M.C.; Franco, O.H.; Rivadeneira, F. The Association between Metabolic Syndrome, Bone Mineral Density, Hip Bone Geometry and Fracture Risk: The Rotterdam Study. *PLoS ONE* **2015**, *10*, e0129116. [CrossRef] [PubMed]

45. Barrett-Connor, E.; Sajjan, S.G.; Siris, E.S.; Miller, P.D.; Chen, Y.T.; Markson, L.E. Wrist fracture as a predictor of future fractures in younger versus older postmenopausal women: Results from the National Osteoporosis Risk Assessment (NORA). *Osteoporos. Int.* **2008**, *19*, 607–613. [CrossRef] [PubMed]
46. Siris, E.S.; Adler, R.; Bilezikian, J.; Bolognese, M.; Dawson-Hughes, B.; Favus, M.J.; Harris, S.T.; De Beur, S.J.; Khosla, S.; Lane, N.E.; et al. The clinical diagnosis of osteoporosis: A position statement from the National Bone Health Alliance Working Group. *Osteoporos. Int.* **2014**, *25*, 1439–1443. [CrossRef] [PubMed]

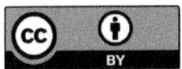

© 2020 by the authors. Licensee MDPI, Basel, Switzerland. This article is an open access article distributed under the terms and conditions of the Creative Commons Attribution (CC BY) license (http://creativecommons.org/licenses/by/4.0/).

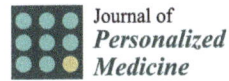

Article

Correlations between Iron Metabolism Parameters, Inflammatory Markers and Lipid Profile Indicators in Patients with Type 1 and Type 2 Diabetes Mellitus

Nadezhda N. Musina [1,*], Tatiana V. Saprina [1], Tatiana S. Prokhorenko [1,2], Alexander Kanev [1] and Anastasia P. Zima [1]

1. Siberian State Medical University, 634050 Tomsk, Russia; trck.tomsk@mail.ru or tanja.v.saprina@mail.ru (T.V.S.); mmikld.ssmu@gmail.com (T.S.P.); alexkanev92@gmail.com (A.K.); zima2302@gmail.com (A.P.Z.)
2. Tomsk Regional Blood Center, 634034 Tomsk, Russia
* Correspondence: nadiezhda-musina@mail.ru; Tel.: +7-961-891-16-55

Received: 25 June 2020; Accepted: 23 July 2020; Published: 25 July 2020

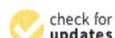

Abstract: This study aims to establish relationships between inflammatory status, ferrokinetics and lipid metabolism in patients with diabetes mellitus. Subclinical inflammation was assessed by levels of high-sensitive C-reactive protein, tumor necrosis factor-α and erythrocyte sedimentation rate. Iron metabolism parameters included complete blood count, serum iron, transferrin and ferritin. Metabolic status assessment included lipid profile, glycated hemoglobin and microalbuminuria measurement. As a result of the study it was possible to establish both general (universal) and diabetes mellitus (DM) type-dependent relationships between the parameters of lipid profile and metabolic control in DM. High-density lipoprotein cholesterol (HDL-C) levels negatively correlated with microalbuminuria ($r = -0.293$; $p < 0.05$ for type 1 diabetes and $r = -0.272$; $p < 0.05$ for type 2 diabetes). Ferritin concentration positively correlated with triglyceride level ($r = 0.346$; $p < 0.05$ for type 1 diabetes and $r = 0.244$; $p < 0.05$ for type 2 diabetes). In type 1 diabetes, a negative correlation was discovered between estimated glomerular filtration rate (eGFR) and LDL-C ($r = -0.480$; $p < 0.05$), very low-density-lipoprotein cholesterol (VLDL-C) ($r = -0.490$; $p < 0.05$) and triglycerides ($r = -0.553$; $p < 0.05$), and a positive one between C-reactive protein concentration and triglyceride level ($r = 0.567$; $p < 0.05$). Discovered relationships between lipid profile indices, inflammatory status and microalbuminuria confirmed mutual influence of hyperlipidemia, inflammation and nephropathy in diabetes patients. Obtained results justify the strategy of early hypolipidemic therapy in patients with diabetes mellitus to prevent the development and progression of microvascular complications.

Keywords: diabetes mellitus; anemia of chronic disease; iron deficiency anemia; hyperlipidemia; inflammation; C-reactive protein; tumor necrosis factor-α; erythrocyte sedimentation rate

1. Introduction

It is now well-established that diabetes mellitus (DM) is associated with a proinflammatory immune status and is accompanied by an increase in the level of circulating inflammatory markers. Indeed, type 1 DM is directly caused by an autoimmune response against pancreatic beta-cells [1–3], while chronic subclinical inflammation evidenced in type 2 DM is usually attributed to the proinflammatory activity of adipose tissue [4–7]. Evidence exists, however, that the level of cytokines in diabetes patients remains high even after weight loss [8]. This fact outlines the important, yet not the exclusive, role that excessive adipose tissue plays in the inflammatory process in type 2 DM. For example, hyperglycemia itself can induce the expression of proinflammatory molecules by β-cells and lead to the activation of fibroblast growth factors and inflammatory markers [9,10]. There are enough data confirming the contribution of low-intensity systemic inflammation to the development and progression of the atherosclerotic disease in individuals with or without impaired carbohydrate metabolism [11–13]. Therefore, insulin resistance, dysglycemia, atherosclerosis and chronic inflammation can be considered as links of the same pathogenetic process. It is worth mentioning that the existing studies were mainly focused on the state of lipid metabolism and inflammatory status, as well as their mutual influence, in separate cohorts of patients with either type 1 or type 2 DM. That did not allow for the comparative assessment of the contribution of diabetes-specific metabolic disorders to the development of both systemic inflammation and the disorders of lipid metabolism and ferrokinetics.

The role of chronic low-grade inflammation in the development of anemic syndrome has been acknowledged. The process involves the promotion of myelopoiesis at the expense of erythropoiesis induced by the cytokines, suppression of erythroid-committed precursor proliferation and macrophage activation for erythrophagocytosis by tumor necrosis factor α (TNF-α) and decrease in iron delivery to plasma from macrophages, which is governed by interleukin 6 (IL-6) through its effects on hepcidin production [14]. At present, studying the features of iron metabolism in individuals with impaired carbohydrate metabolism seems to be rather relevant [15–17]. However, quite a few studies to date have investigated the relationship between lipid metabolism and other metabolic parameters, inflammatory status and ferrokinetics in patients with type 1 and type 2 DM in comparative aspects. Therefore, the aim of the present study was to establish the relationship between inflammatory markers, ferrokinetics parameters and lipid metabolism in patients with type 1 and 2 DM.

2. Materials and Methods

2.1. Study Design

Study design—an observational single-center, one-stage, cross-sectional controlled study. Patients with type 1 and type 2 DM were included in the study during planned hospitalization in the endocrinology clinics of Siberian State Medical University after evaluating the inclusion and exclusion criteria. Diabetes mellitus was diagnosed anamnestically. Patients were stratified into main groups 1 and 2 according to the type of DM. After inclusion in the study, patients underwent a block of all laboratory tests indicated below in the text. The control group included healthy volunteers. Before inclusion in the study, in order to exclude disorders of carbohydrate metabolism, a standard glucose tolerance test with 75 g of glucose was performed for healthy controls. All healthy volunteers of the control group underwent the same laboratory tests as patients with type 1 and type 2 DM.

2.2. Inclusion and Exclusion Criteria

Inclusion criteria for the diabetes groups. Patients with an established diagnosis of type 1 or type 2 DM and a disease history of 1 to 30 years, aged 18 to 70 years, with glycated hemoglobin level between 6.5% and 10.5% and estimated glomerular filtration rate (eGFR) > 15 mL/min/1.73 m^2 as assessed by the CKD-EPI creatinine equation (chronic kidney disease stages 1–4), were included in the study.

Inclusion criteria for the control group. Patients aged 18 to 70 years, with body mass index (BMI) from 18.5 to 29.9 kg/m^2. and the absence of carbohydrate metabolism disorders as assessed by glycated hemoglobin concentration and 75 g oral glucose tolerance test, were included in the study.

Exclusion criteria: infectious diseases in the acute stage, specific infectious diseases such as: HIV/AIDS; viral hepatitis with any degree of activity; liver cirrhosis of viral or autoimmune etiology; tuberculosis; malignancy; chronic obstructive pulmonary disease or bronchial asthma; active smoking at the time of inclusion in the study; blood transfusion within 1 month prior to the inclusion in the study or at the moment; iron supplements intake; pre or postoperative period; acute renal, hepatic or heart failure; eGFR below 15 mL/min/1.73 m^2; presence of proteinuria; decompensation of DM manifest in the form of ketoacidosis/hyperosmolar hyperglycemic state; refusal of the patient to participate in the study, refusal to sign the informed consent form.

2.3. Methods

The study was conducted on the basis of the endocrinology clinics of Siberian State Medical University, Tomsk. A total of 146 people who underwent planned hospitalizations were enrolled over the span of two years (2017–2019), 48 of which had a diagnosis of type 1 DM (group 1), while 81 had type 2 DM (group 2). The control group consisted of 17 healthy volunteers.

Ten milliliter samples of venous plasma and serum were collected from the cubital vein in the morning after a fasting period using vacutainer tubes. All patients underwent comprehensive anthropometric evaluation. To assess the state of carbohydrate metabolism and its level of compensation, evaluation of glycated hemoglobin concentration was performed using a D10 analyzer (BIO-RAD, Hercules, CA, USA). Serum creatinine concentration was evaluated, with the subsequent calculation of eGFR using the CKD-EPI equation. Quantitative assessment of microalbuminuria (MA) (mg/L) was performed using an Abbott Architect c4000 analyzer (USA). Main hematological parameters (red blood cell count (RBC), reticulocyte count, hemoglobin concentration and hematocrit level) were evaluated using an XN1000 analyzer (Sysmex, Kobe, Japan). Iron metabolism indices (serum iron (μmol/L), transferrin (mg/dL) and ferritin (ng/mL) concentrations) were assessed using an ARCHITECT i2000SR analyzer (Abbott, Abbott Park, IL, USA). Lipid profile values (total cholesterol (TC), high-density lipoprotein cholesterol (HDL-C), low-density lipoprotein cholesterol (LDL-C), very low-density-lipoprotein cholesterol (VLDL-C), and triglyceride (TG) concentrations (mmol/L)) were estimated using an ARCHITECT i2000SR analyzer (Abbott, USA). Atherogenic coefficient was calculated according to the formula TC-HDL cholesterol/HDL cholesterol (TC-HDL-c)/HDL-c). Among the evaluated inflammatory markers were erythrocyte sedimentation rate (ESR) as assessed using an XN1000 hematology analyzer (Sysmex, Japan), high-sensitive C-reactive protein (CRP) (ng/mL), and TNF-α (pg/mL), both assessed by enzyme-linked immunosorbent assay (ELISA) (Vector Best, Novosibirsk, Russia). ESR Hyperlipidemias were classified according to the Fredrickson classification (1967) [18].

2.4. Research Ethics

All subjects gave their informed consent for inclusion before they participated in the study. The study was conducted in accordance with the Declaration of Helsinki, and the protocol was approved by the Ethics Committee of Siberian State Medical University (protocol No. 5596, 06.11.2017)

2.5. Statistical Analysis

A sample calculator was used in order to establish the required sample size. The minimum required size of a representative sample for a confidence interval equaling five was estimated to be 70 people. We also used a consistent strategy for calculating the sample size, taking into account the coefficient of variation (= standard deviation from the arithmetic mean in %). According to these calculations, the minimum required sample size for the main groups (patients with DM) was 61 people. Statistical analysis was performed using the SPSS Statistics ver. 23 software package (IBM Corp., Chicago, IL, USA). The Kolmogorov-Smirnov test was used to assess data distribution with the level of significance set at $p < 0.05$. Normally distributed parameters included glycated hemoglobin concentration, eGFR, transferrin, hematocrit and RBC. The remaining parameters, namely: age, duration of diabetes, body mass index (BMI), MA, serum creatinine, CRP, TNF-α, ESR, iron, ferritin, hemoglobin, reticulocyte count, leukocyte count, aspartate aminotransferase (AST), alanine aminotransferase (ALT), TC, HDL, LDL, VLDL and TG, did not obey the normal distribution law. For the sake of comprehensive and unified data presentation, all results were expressed as median and interquartile range (Me, Q0.25–Q0.75). A comparative analysis between two independent groups was performed using the Mann–Whitney criterion with the Bonferroni correction for multiple comparisons, the significance threshold being set at $p < 0.017$, alpha value = 0.05. Student's t-test was used for normally distributed data. Correlations were evaluated using the nonparametric Spearman rank correlation with the significance level was set at $p < 0.05$. Categorical variables were presented as numbers and percentages. Spearman's chi-square test was applied with a 5% significance level to test for differences between them.

3. Results

The study included 129 patients with either type 1 or type 2 DM, and 17 healthy volunteers with normal BMI and no evidence of carbohydrate metabolism disorders.

Among people with DM, 43 were men (33.3%) and 86 (66.7%) women. Within the main groups (groups 1 and 2), the ratio of men and women was comparable: in the group of patients with type 1 DM there were 19 (39.6%) men and 29 (60.4%) women, while the group of patients with type 2 DM comprised 24 (29.6%) men and 57 (70.4%) women ($\chi^2 = 1.276$; $p = 0.259$). The control group, just like the main groups, had fewer men than women (4 (23.5%) and 13 (76.5%), respectively). Table 1 shows the clinical characteristics of the study groups.

Table 1. Clinical characteristics of patients in the studied groups.

Variables	Type 1 DM n = 48	Type 2 DM n = 81	Control Group (Healthy Individuals) n = 17
Age, years	34.00 (26.00–52.00) **	60.00 (56.00–65.00) *	40.00 (32.00–58.00)
Duration of the disease, years	9.0 (3.00–17.00)	11.00 (8.00–15.00)	–
BMI, kg/m^2	23.67 (21.43–26.03) **	33.80 (29.55–38.82) *	25.10 (23.10–27.65)
HbA1c, %	8.80 (6.95–10.30) *	9.10 (7.97–11.03) *	5.20 (4.90–5.85)
eGFR, mL/min/1.73 m^2	95.00 (71.75–112.75) **	80.50 (63.00–93.00) *	96.50 (93.00–106.00)
MA, mg/L	20.50 (9.25–39.25)	13.55 (8.53–30.00)	–
AST (IU/L)	20.00 (16.60–27.00)	19.40 (15.00–28.00)	20.00 (16.50–22.50)
AST (IU/L)	16.00 (12.00–24.00) **	20.00 (14.00–29.75)	18.00 (11.50–21.00)

*—significant differences when compared to control group ($p < 0.017$); **—significant differences when compared to group 2.

As shown in Table 1, groups 1 and 2 were comparable in terms of DM duration, glycated hemoglobin concentration and MA. At the same time, patients with type 2 DM had significantly higher BMI compared to patients with type 1 DM ($p < 0.0001$) and control subjects ($p < 0.0001$). eGFR in patients with type 2 DM was lower than in patients with type 1 DM ($p = 0.006$) and healthy volunteers ($p < 0.0001$). Glycated hemoglobin concentration in the control group was significantly lower compared to patients with type 1 and type 2 DM ($p < 0.0001$ in both cases).

Among patients with DM, 94 people (72.8%) were suffering from hypertension at the time of inclusion in the study. Of these, 13 people (13.8%) did not receive antihypertensive treatment, while the remaining 81 patients (86.2%) were taking 1 to 4 hypotensive agents. People from the control group did not suffer from arterial hypertension.

At the time of inclusion, of all patients with DM, 106 (82.2%) people had no history of acute cardiovascular events (myocardial infarction/stroke), 17 (13.2%) patients had a history of myocardial infarction, five (3.8%) people had the anamnesis of stroke, and one patient (0.8%) suffered from both stroke and myocardial infarction. Cardiovascular events were more prevalent in patients with type 2 DM compared to individuals with type 1 DM ($\chi^2 = 8.049$; $p = 0.045$).

All patients with type 1 DM received basal-bolus insulin therapy. Among patients with type 2 DM, 22 people (26.2%) took oral hypoglycemic agents, 19 people (22.6%) received various modes of insulin therapy, while in 43 patients (51.2%) insulin was used in combination with oral antidiabetic agents.

As a result of a comparative analysis of inflammatory status, it has been shown that TNF-α level was significantly higher in patients with type 1 DM when compared to both patients with type 2 DM ($p < 0.0001$) and individuals from the control groups ($p = 0.004$). On the contrary, patients with type 2 DM demonstrated significantly higher CRP concentrations than patients with type 1 DM ($p < 0.0001$). Assessment of CRP in the control group was not performed due to technical reasons. It is worth noting that in type 2 DM patients, the ESR was also significantly higher than in their counterparts with type 1 diabetes mellitus ($p < 0.0001$) and in people from the control group ($p < 0.0001$).

Significant differences between groups were found in the concentration of ferritin, level being significantly higher in patients with type 2 DM compared to patients with type 1 DM ($p = 0.013$). There were no significant differences in other parameters of iron metabolism between the groups. The results of a comparative assessment of inflammatory status and ferrokinetics are shown in Table 2.

Table 2. Inflammatory markers and iron metabolism indices in patients with diabetes mellitus (DM) and in the control group.

Variables	Type 1 DM $n = 48$	Type 2 DM $n = 81$	Control Group (Healthy Individuals) $n = 17$
TNF-α, pg/mL	15.28 (12.41–24.41) *,**	8.54 (6.27–11.60)	9.68 (5.68–15.38)
CRP, ng/mL	2.00 (1.05–4.05) **	7.00 (3.00–11.85)	–
ESR, mm/h	14.00 (5.00–21.25) **	18.00 (9.00–27.00) *	7.00 (5.00–9.00)
Leucocyte count, ×10^9/L	6.55 (5.30–7.83)	7.38 (6.08–8.74)	6.08 (5.25–7.53)
Hemoglobin, g/L	138.50 (122.50–151.00)	141.00 (125.25–151.00)	146.00 (135.00–150.00)
Erythrocyte count, ×10^{12}/L	4.69 (4.38–5.09)	4.79 (4.39–5.19)	4.80 (4.49–5.02)
Reticulocytes, %	1.51 (1.12–1.75)	1.76 (1.54–1.91)	1.60 (1.40–1.66)
Hematocrit, %	40.95 (38.40–43.65)	42.05 (38.00–44.55)	42.70 (40.70–44.85)
Iron, µmol/L	12.00 (8.00–17.00)	13.00 (11.00–18.25)	16.00 (11.00–20.50)
Ferritin, ng/mL	44.48 (18.35–148.50) **	96.52 (42.93–189.0)	72.05 (43.23–148.60)
Transferrin, mg/dL	284.00 (250.00–334.00)	293.00 (267.00–321.50)	267.50 (208.75–306.50)

*—significant differences when compared to control group ($p < 0.017$); **—significant differences when compared to group 2.

Significant differences in certain indices of lipid profile were revealed depending on the presence and type of DM. In particular, patients with type 2 DM had significantly higher levels of VLDL-C ($p < 0.0001$), TG ($p < 0.0001$) and atherogenic coefficient values ($p < 0.0001$, as well as lower concentrations of HDL-C ($p < 0.0001$), when compared with type 1 DM patients (Table 3). At the same time, there were no significant differences in lipid profiles of patients with type 1 DM and healthy volunteers of the control group (Table 3). Comparative characteristics of lipid profile in three groups are presented in Table 3.

Taking into account the statistically significant differences in age of patients with type 1 and type 2 DM, as well as the correlations between age and lipid metabolism obtained during further research, it can be assumed that the differences in cholesterol and its components are caused not only by the type of diabetes, but the influence of age as well.

Table 3. Comparative characteristics of the lipid profile in patients with DM and in the control group.

Variables	Type 1 DM $n = 48$	Type 2 DM $n = 81$	Control Group (Healthy Individuals) $n = 17$
TC, mmol/L	4.98 (4.33–5.68)	5.41 (4.58–6.40)	4.90 (4.50–5.35)
HDL-C, mmol/L	1.50 (1.23–1.84) **	1.04 (0.90–1.30) *	1.60 (1.33–1.90)
LDL-C, mmol/L	2.95 (2.55–3.28)	3.25 (2.28–4.00) **	3.00 (2.25–3.24)
VLDL-C, mmol/L	0.50 (0.36–0.68) **	1.00 (0.73–1.31) *	0.41 (0.29–0.70)
TG, mmol/L	1.05 (0.73–1.58) **	2.20 (1.60–2.70) *	0.90 (0.65–1.45)
Atherogenic coefficient	2.38 (1.80–3.83) **	4.00 (2.95–5.11) *	2.30 (1.88–2.85)

*—significant differences when compared to control group ($p < 0.017$); **—significant differences when compared to group 2.

Among all persons included in the study ($n = 146$), hyperlipidemia was detected in 80.1% ($n = 117$). It is worth mentioning, however, that hyperlipidemia was not detected in any of the patients from the control group. Hyperlipidemia was present in 83.3% of patients with type 1 DM, and in 95.1% of type 2 DM cases (Table 4).

Table 4. Frequency of hyperlipidemia in patients with DM and in the control group.

Variables	Total ($n = 146$)	Type 1 DM $n = 48$	Type 2 DM $n = 81$	Control Group (Healthy Individuals) $n = 17$
Hyperlipidemia, %(n)	80.1 (117)	83.3 (40)	95.1 (77)	0.0 (0)
Absence of hyperlipidemia, %(n)	19.8 (29)	16.7 (8)	4.9 (4)	100.0 (17)

Among patients with hyperlipidemia ($n = 117$), only 27.4% ($n = 32$) received lipid-lowering therapy at the time of inclusion in the study. The only group of pharmacological agents received by the patients in our study were statins. Frequency of statin intake varied between groups, from 12.5% ($n = 5$) in patients with type 1 DM, to 35.1% ($n = 27$) in individuals with type 2 DM.

In patients with hyperlipidemia not receiving lipid-lowering drugs at the time of inclusion in the study ($n = 91$), Fredrickson's classification was employed to assess the type of lipid metabolism disorder. Analysis revealed the predominance of highly atherogenic type IIb hyperlipidemia in patients with type 2 DM. On the other hand, in patients with type 1 DM, less atherogenic phenotype of hyperlipidemia (type IIa) was more common ($\chi^2 = 34.051$; $p < 0.0001$).

Spearman's coefficient was calculated to assess correlations between lipid profile, parameters of metabolic control, markers of chronic inflammation, and iron metabolism indices in an overall sample of patients with DM ($n = 129$), as well as in individual groups of type 1 ($n = 48$) and type 2 ($n = 81$) DM, and in healthy controls ($n = 17$). The relevant data are presented in Tables 5–8.

Statistical analysis revealed a negative correlation between HDL-C concentration and microalbuminuria level in the overall sample of DM patients, which may reflect the mechanism of development and progression of endothelial dysfunction and, as a consequence, microvascular complications, as well as the role hyperlipidemia plays in this process (Table 5). In addition, regardless of DM type, there was a positive correlation between triglyceridemia and serum ferritin level. The mechanism of this relationship may be partly explained by the effects of functional activity of adipose tissue and an increase in the production of free fatty acids. Subsequently, this would lead to the development of nonalcoholic steatohepatitis, in which the inflammatory mesenchymal reaction would contribute to hyperferritinemia.

Table 5. Correlations between lipid profile, inflammatory markers and parameters of iron metabolism in patients with DM (independent of type).

			TC	HDL-C	LDL-C	VLDL-C	TG	Atherogenic Coefficient
Spearman r	Age	r	0.235 *	−0.287 *	0.256 *	ns	ns	0.308 *
	BMI	r	ns	−0.561 *	ns	0.529 *	0.524 *	0.502 *
	eGFR	r	−0.187 *	0.233 *	ns	−0.362 *	−0.385 *	−0.256 *
	ESR	r	0.200 *	ns	0.200 *	0.261 *	0.271 *	0.233 *
	TNF-α	r	ns	0.298 *	ns	−0.343 *	ns	−0.325 *
	CRP	r	ns	ns	ns	ns	0,276 *	ns
	Leucocytes	r	ns	−0.324 *	ns	0.322 *	0.238 *	0.253 *
	Ferritin	r	ns	−0.325 *	ns	0.365 *	0.415 *	0.402 *
	Transferrin	r	ns	0.362 *	ns	ns	ns	ns
	Reticulocytes	r	−0.346 *	−0.325 *	−0.504 *	ns	ns	ns
	ALT	r	ns	−0.200 *	ns	0.321 *	0.315 *	0.237 *

r—Spearman's rank correlation coefficient; ns—nonsignificant differences; *—$p < 0.05$.

Type 1 DM-specific correlations were also established (Table 6). For instance, TC levels and all of its fractions, with the exception of HDL-C, as well as the atherogenic coefficient, demonstrated positive correlations with serum creatinine and negative ones with eGFR. In addition, VLDL-C levels were positively correlated with microalbuminuria. These correlations reflect the role of hyperlipidemia in the progression of endothelial dysfunction and the development of microvascular complications, in particular, diabetic nephropathy. Positive relationships were also established between markers of chronic inflammation and the lipid profile parameters TC, VLDL-C and TG levels positively correlated with ESR, while CRP concentration positively correlated with TG level and atherogenic coefficient. The relationships between leucocyte count and VLDL-C and atherogenic coefficient were also revealed. In addition, positive correlations were observed between concentration of serum ferritin and TC, LDL-C and TG levels. As is well known, ferritin not only reflects total amount of iron stored in the body, but also acts as one of the acute phase proteins, with concentration increases in inflammation. Thus, it may be noted that in patients with type 1 DM, hyperlipidemia with an increase in atherogenic fractions of cholesterol is associated with chronic subclinical inflammation.

Table 6. Correlations between lipid profile, inflammatory markers and parameters of iron metabolism in patients with type 1 DM.

			TC	HDL-C	LDL-C	VLDL-C	TG	Atherogenic Coefficient
Spearman r	Age	r	0.436 *	ns	0.407 *	ns	ns	ns
	eGFR	r	−0.618 *	ns	−0.480 *	−0.490 *	−0.533 *	−0.459 *
	Creatinine	r	0.442 *	ns	0.417 *	0.387 *	0.436 *	0.550 *
	MA	r	ns	−0.293 *	ns	0.339 *	ns	ns
	ESR	r	0.371 *	ns	ns	0.642 *	0.546 *	ns
	CRP	r	ns	ns	ns	ns	0.567 *	0.592 *
	Leucocytes	r	ns	−0.331 *	ns	0.406 *	ns	0.391 *
	Ferritin	r	0.384 *	ns	0.361 *	ns	0.346 *	ns
	Transferrin	r	ns	0.490 *	ns	ns	ns	ns
	ALT	r	ns	ns	ns	ns	0.363 *	ns

r—Spearman's rank correlation coefficient; ns—nonsignificant differences; *—$p < 0.05$.

As for the group of type 2 DM patients, there was a positive relationship between BMI and VLDL-C and triglyceride levels. On top of that, negative correlation was revealed between BMI and HDL-C concentration, which reflects the role of adipose tissue in the development of hyperlipidemia. In addition, negative correlations between reticulocytes content and levels of TC and LDL-C were observed. At the same time, associations between inflammatory markers and indices of lipid profile were not characteristic for this group of patients (Table 7).

Table 7. Correlations between lipid profile, inflammatory markers and parameters of iron metabolism in patients with type 2 DM.

			TC	HDL-C	LDL-C	VLDL-C	TG	Atherogenic Coefficient
Spearman r	Age	r	ns	ns	ns	0.299 *	0.233 *	ns
	BMI	r	ns	−0.326 *	ns	0.255 *	0.230 *	ns
	MA	r	ns	−0.272 *	ns	ns	ns	ns
	TNF-α	r	ns	−0.440 *	ns	ns	ns	ns
	Ferritin	r	ns	−0.328 *	ns	ns	0.244 *	0.328 *
	Reticulocytes	r	−0.505 *	ns	−0.496 *	ns	ns	ns

r—Spearman's rank correlation coefficient; ns—nonsignificant differences; *—$p < 0.05$.

Correlations identified in the control group can be found in Table 8.

Table 8. Correlations between lipid profile, inflammatory markers and parameters of iron metabolism in healthy controls.

			TC	HDL-C	LDL-C	VLDL-C	TG	Atherogenic Coefficient
Spearman r	Age	r	0.519 *	ns	ns	ns	ns	ns
	BMI	r	ns	ns	ns	ns	ns	0.591 *
	Leucocytes	r	ns	−0.617 *	ns	ns	ns	ns
	Ferritin	r	ns	ns	ns	0.661 *	0.674 *	0.583 *
	Transferrin	r	ns	0.572 *	ns	ns	ns	ns

r—Spearman's rank correlation coefficient; ns—nonsignificant differences; *—$p < 0.05$.

Taking into account the statistically significant age differences in patients with type 1 and type 2 DM, correlations between age and the indicators of the lipid profile were studied. The result of studying these correlations was rather expected—in patients with DM there were positive correlations between age and the concentrations of atherogenic fractions of cholesterol, and a negative correlation between age and HDL-C concentration (only for type 1 DM). In the healthy control group, a positive correlation between age and TC remained. Moreover, in the overall sample of patients with DM, as well as in the group of people with type 2 DM, there was a weak correlation ($r = 0.175$ and $r = 0.278$, respectively $p < 0.05$) between age and ESR, which may confirm the potential effect of age on the severity of chronic subclinical inflammation. No other statistically significant correlations between age and iron metabolism and inflammation parameters were detected.

Thus, distinct correlations between the parameters of metabolic control, iron metabolism and chronic inflammation were obtained in both overall sample of people with DM and in patients suffering from specific types of DM (either type 1 or type 2).

4. Discussion

As a result of the study, it was possible to establish general (universal) relationships between the parameters of lipid profile and metabolic control in DM, regardless of its type, namely:

- a negative relationship between HDL concentration and the level of microalbuminuria, reflecting the primary role of HDL deficiency, rather than the increase in atherogenic lipid fractions, in the development and progression of endothelial dysfunction, ultimately leading to the development and exacerbation of diabetic nephropathy. The role of diabetic nephropathy in lowering plasma level of HDL-C was been established. Both hypotheses take into account the existing literature data;
- a positive correlation between triglyceridemia and serum ferritin concentration. This relationship can be explained by the effects of functional activity of adipose tissue and an increase in the production of free fatty acids leading to the development of nonalcoholic steatohepatitis with increase in the inflammatory mesenchymal reaction of the liver.

It is worth mentioning that a positive correlation between TG levels and serum ferritin content was evident not only in patients with type 1 and type 2 DM, but also in people from the healthy control group. The aforementioned control group subjects did not have hyperlipidemia or impaired carbohydrate metabolism. Therefore, the presence of this relationship in this subset of people characterizes it as strictly determined, resulting from the strong interdependence between the amount of adipose tissue, the level of free fatty acids and subsequent development of chronic liver inflammation and hyperferritinemia.

In patients with type 1 DM, atherogenic hyperlipidemia was associated with impaired renal function as assessed by decreased GFR, increased microalbuminuria and serum creatinine concentration, and chronic subclinical inflammation (evidenced by the increased ferritin, ESR and CRP). Revealed correlations are in agreement with the literature data and reflect the role of hyperlipidemia and chronic inflammation in progression of endothelial dysfunction and the development of microvascular complications such as diabetic nephropathy.

In the group of patients with type 2 DM, in addition to the universal relationships already noted previously, positive associations were established between an increase in atherogenic lipid fractions and BMI, which confirms the classical theory of the role of adipose tissue in the development of hyperlipidemia.

The results obtained in our study are in agreement with the existing literature data from both single-center comparative studies and multicenter cohort observational studies. Thus, a study conducted by Palvasha Waheed et al. showed the presence of a significant positive correlation between the inflammatory markers, hs-CRP and ferritin, and the parameters of dyslipidemia—TC, LDL-C and TG ($p < 0.001$, $r = 0.72$) except for HDL-C, which had an insignificant negative correlation with the inflammatory markers ($p > 0.05$ $r = -0.10$) [19]. According to the DCCT/EDIC study, lower LDL-C and TG levels were associated with reduced risk for progression from moderate albuminuria to severe albuminuria or end-stage renal disease [20]. A 2015 literature review provides a series of studies searching for new risk factors for developing diabetic nephropathy [21]. Among these factors, higher levels of proinflammatory cytokines and chemokines (interleukin 6, interleukin 18, and monocyte chemoattractant protein−1, hsCRP) are noted [22,23].

A large cross-sectional study (China Health and Nutrition Survey 2009) found that elevated serum ferritin levels were associated with the prevalence of hyperlipidemia among Chinese adults. There was a significant positive association between serum ferritin levels and lipid parameters independent of diabetes and insulin resistance in both genders. This study also showed that subjects with hyperlipidemia and diabetes had higher serum ferritin levels than subjects without hyperlipidemia and diabetes [24]. These results are in agreement with the results of correlation analysis conducted as part of our study.

It is well established that type 1 and type 2 DM are characterized by distinct lipid metabolism disorders manifested in the form of specific shifts in lipid profile. For instance, type 2 DM is characterized by a high TG level, low HDL-C concentration and denser LDL particles. Hypertriglyceridemia in type 2 DM develops as a result of insulin resistance and abdominal obesity. These changes serve as the background for the increase in the serum concentration of free fatty acids due to their augmented release from adipose tissue and reduced muscle consumption. As a response to these changes, liver increases production of VLDL and saturated TG, while the lipoprotein lipase-mediated hydrolysis of VLDL decreases. This ultimately leads to an increase in levels of TG-rich VLDL. The decrease in HDL-C concentration in type 2 DM is secondary, being attributed to the increased transfer of cholesterol esters from HDL to VLDL in exchange for TG. TG-saturated HDL are then rapidly destroyed by hepatic lipase. Moreover, in type 2 DM, the ability of HDL to inhibit LDL oxidation is disrupted, while the number of functionally defective HDL increases. Among the most important nonlipid proatherogenic factors in type 2 DM are oxidative stress due to overproduction of reactive oxygen species, accumulation of advanced glycation end products within the walls of blood vessels, increased endothelin production under the effect of hyperinsulinemia and apoptosis of smooth muscle cells of vascular walls. Combinations of these factors promote diffuse generalized endothelial dysfunction [25–27].

In patients with type 1 DM, lipid metabolism disorders are less common and often less pronounced. In the setting of adequate glycemic control, levels of TG and LDL-C are reduced in this category of patients. In addition, insulin therapy can increase the level of HDL-C, which is caused by stimulation of lipoprotein lipase activity in adipose tissue and skeletal muscles, resulting in the intense metabolism of VLDL. Furthermore, several studies have consistently shown that the severity of dyslipidemia increases after the development of diabetic nephropathy, manifesting in the form of elevated TG level and decrease in HDL-C concentration [28].

The significant differences obtained in the course of our study between the concentration of the lipid profile parameters in patients with type 1 and type 2 DM are consistent with the above literature data, though could also be influenced by age in our patient sample.

Glomerular mesangial cells, just like smooth muscle cells, express cell-surface LDL receptors. Under conditions of hyperlipidemia, these cells are capable of capturing and accumulating LDL and their oxidized forms. The presence of oxidized LDL promotes infiltration of mesangium by mononuclear cells and macrophages, which produce cytokines and growth factors. Oxidized LDL, growth factors and cytokines cause an increase in the synthesis of mesangial matrix and basement membrane components, thus advancing the development of glomerular sclerosis. In addition, lipoproteins can stimulate the activation of the transforming growth factor β (TRF-β) signaling pathway, which, in turn, promotes the production of reactive oxygen species that cause glomerular damage. In addition to the TRF-β signaling pathway, LDL have demonstrated the ability to activate monocytes and destroy cellular glycocalyx, causing increased glomerular permeability [29,30].

It should be noted that the development of diabetic nephropathy not only exacerbates atherogenic hyperlipidemia, but also accelerates the progression of endothelial dysfunction. As kidney function decreases, the synthesis of Apolipoprotein AI (ApoA-I) in the liver, which is the main HDL component, drops accordingly, leading to a decrease in the plasma level of HDL-C. Apo A-I is also an important activator of lecithin-cholesterol acyltransferase, an enzyme crucial for the conversion of HDL-3 to cholesterol-rich HDL-2. Inflammation of the vascular wall can subsequently cause structural and functional disorders of HDL. Thus, the most important antiatherogenic functions of HDL are disrupted, which in turn leads to a predisposition of vessels to oxidative stress [31]. According to published data, normalization of HDL levels can lead to the reduction in the risk of diabetes complications, in particular micro and macroangiopathies.

The suggested presence of shared molecular mechanisms of inflammation and insulin signaling pathways [32], supposedly resulting in insulin resistance, endothelial dysfunction and cardiovascular complications, provides a theoretical basis for the hypothesis of common causal factors for both diabetes and atherosclerosis (the theory of common soil) [33]. The concept that inflammation participates pivotally in the pathogenesis of atherosclerosis and its complications has gained considerable attention but has not yet entered clinical practice.

The literature review published in 2016 notes potential interventions aimed at preventing the progression of diabetic nephropathy, such as the use of pentoxifylline, silymarin, the endothelin-1A antagonist atrasentan, octreotide and statins [34]. In this case the use of statins has the most powerful evidence base.

It is worth mentioning that many studies have noted the effect lipid-lowering therapy exerts on the markers of chronic inflammation in DM patients. For example, in the CARE (Cholesterol And Recurrent Events) study, it was first shown that statin therapy causes a decrease in both LDL-C and CRP levels. Thus, after 5 years of pravastatin treatment, CRP concentration decreased by 35% compared with placebo [35]. According to the results of the PRINCE (pravastatin inflammation/CRP evaluation) study, pravastatin administration resulted in a decrease in CRP level by 15% within 12 weeks after the start of therapy [36]. In the JUPITER (Justification for the Use of Statins in Primary Prevention: An Intervention Trial Evaluating Rosuvastatin) trial rosuvastatin reduced both median LDL-cholesterol by 50% and hsCRP by 37% [37]. At the same time, the ability of fenofibrate to normalize HDL-C levels was demonstrated. Moreover, DAIS (Diabetes Atherosclerosis Intervention Study) [38] and FIELD

(Long-term fenofibrate therapy and cardiovascular events in people with type 2 diabetes mellitus) [39] studies showed decreases in the rate of occurrence and progression of microalbuminuria in patients receiving fenofibrate therapy.

Thus, the traditional use of renin–angiotensin–aldosterone system (RAAS) blockers alone is insufficient for preventing the progression of diabetic kidney disease in a large subset of patients. The results of our study are consistent with literature data, including those obtained in multicenter cohort studies, and suggest that it is necessary to develop an earlier and broader algorithm of action, as opposed to the existing clinical guidelines, for prescribing statins to patients with type 1 DM, with the aim of preventing the development and progression of diabetic nephropathy

5. Conclusions

Established relationships between the parameters of lipid profile, inflammatory status and microalbuminuria confirm the mutual influence of hyperlipidemia, chronic inflammation and nephropathy in DM. In addition, obtained results allow us to consider and justify a strategy for early hypolipidemic therapy initiation in patients with DM, including type 1 DM, from the point of view of preventing the development and progression of microvascular complications, diabetic nephropathy in particular.

The limitations of this study include the relatively small number of controls, which is planned to increase in the course of further research. Age differences between patients with type 1 and type 2 DM can also be considered as a limitation of this study. However, the formation of groups comparable in age can lead to the occurrence of statistical differences in the duration of DM or the severity of microvascular complications, including diabetic nephropathy between these groups.

Future perspectives of the study also include the study of the prospects for earlier intervention by means of lipid-correcting therapy for the course of diabetic nephropathy and the development and progression of anemic syndrome.

Author Contributions: Conceptualization, N.N.M. and T.V.S.; methodology, N.N.M. and T.V.S.; formal analysis, N.N.M.; investigation, N.N.M. and T.S.P.; resources, N.N.M., A.K. and T.S.P.; data curation, N.N.M.; writing—original draft preparation, N.N.M., A.K.; writing—review and editing, T.V.S., T.S.P. and A.P.Z.; supervision, T.V.S.; project administration, T.V.S.; funding acquisition, T.V.S. and N.N.M. All authors have read and agreed to the published version of the manuscript.

Funding: This research was funded by RFBR, grant number 19-315-90061 «Research of carbohydrate metabolism compensation parameters and glycaemia lability in ferrocinetics disorder among patients with diabetes mellitus».

Conflicts of Interest: The authors declare no conflict of interest. The funders had no role in the design of the study; in the collection, analyses, or interpretation of data; in the writing of the manuscript, or in the decision to publish the results.

References

1. Rabinovitch, A.; Suarez-Pinzon, W.L. Roles of cytokines in the pathogenesis and therapy of type 1 diabetes. *Cell Biophys.* **2007**, *48*, 159–163. [CrossRef] [PubMed]
2. Schneider-Brachert, W.; Tchikov, V.; Neumeyer, J.; Jakob, M.; Winoto-Morbach, S.; Held-Feindt, J.; Heinrich, M.; Merkel, O.; Ehrenschwender, M.; Adam, D.; et al. Compartmentalization of TNF Receptor 1 Signaling. *Immunity* **2004**, *21*, 415–428. [CrossRef] [PubMed]
3. Uno, S.; Imagawa, A.; Okita, K.; Sayama, K.; Moriwaki, M.; Iwahashi, H.; Yamagata, K.; Tamura, S.; Matsuzawa, Y.; Hanafusa, T.; et al. Macrophages and dendritic cells infiltrating islets with or without beta cells produce tumour necrosis factor-α in patients with recent-onset type 1 diabetes. *Diabetologia* **2007**, *50*, 596–601. [CrossRef] [PubMed]
4. Klimontov, V.V.; Tyan, N.V.; Fazullina, O.N.; Myakina, N.E.; о, А.П.; Konenkov, V.; Ва, .В.; Вооа, ..; оаа, Ф..; а, ..; et al. Clinical and metabolic factors associated with chronic low-grade inflammation in type 2 diabetic patients. *Diabetes Mellit.* **2016**, *19*, 295–302. [CrossRef]
5. Wang, Z.; Shen, X.-H.; Feng, W.-M.; Ye, G.-F.; Qiu, W.; Li, B. Analysis of Inflammatory Mediators in Prediabetes and Newly Diagnosed Type 2 Diabetes Patients. *J. Diabetes Res.* **2016**, *2016*, 1–10. [CrossRef]

6. Yamamoto, Y.; Yamamoto, H. RAGE-Mediated Inflammation, Type 2 Diabetes, and Diabetic Vascular Complication. *Front. Endocrinol.* **2013**, *4*, 4. [CrossRef]
7. Esser, N.; Legrand-Poels, S.; Piette, J.; Scheen, A.J.; Paquot, N. Inflammation as a link between obesity, metabolic syndrome and type 2 diabetes. *Diabetes Res. Clin. Pr.* **2014**, *105*, 141–150. [CrossRef]
8. Dandona, P.; Aljada, A.; Chaudhuri, A.; Bandyopadhyay, A. The Potential Influence of Inflammation and Insulin Resistance on the Pathogenesis and Treatment of Atherosclerosis-Related Complications in Type 2 Diabetes. *J. Clin. Endocrinol. Metab.* **2003**, *88*, 2422–2429. [CrossRef]
9. Donath, M.Y.; Gross, D.J.; Cerasi, E.; Kaiser, N. Hyperglycemia-induced beta-cell apoptosis in pancreatic islets of Psammomys obesus during development of diabetes. *Diabetes* **1999**, *48*, 738–744. [CrossRef]
10. Klüppelholz, B.; Thorand, B.; Koenig, W.; Gala, T.D.L.H.; Meisinger, C.; Huth, C.; Giani, G.; Franks, P.W.; Roden, M.; Rathmann, W.; et al. Association of subclinical inflammation with deterioration of glycaemia before the diagnosis of type 2 diabetes: The KORA S4/F4 study. *Diabetologia* **2015**, *58*, 2269–2277. [CrossRef]
11. Ammirati, E.; Moroni, F.; Norata, G.; Magnoni, M.; Camici, P.G. Markers of Inflammation Associated with Plaque Progression and Instability in Patients with Carotid Atherosclerosis. *Mediat. Inflamm.* **2015**, *2015*, 1–15. [CrossRef] [PubMed]
12. Soeki, T.; Sata, M. Inflammatory Biomarkers and Atherosclerosis. *Int. Hear. J.* **2016**, *57*, 134–139. [CrossRef] [PubMed]
13. Hameed, I.; Masoodi, S.R.; A Mir, S.; Nabi, M.; Ghazanfar, K.; Ganai, B.A. Type 2 diabetes mellitus: From a metabolic disorder to an inflammatory condition. *World J. Diabetes* **2015**, *6*, 598–612. [CrossRef] [PubMed]
14. Ganz, T. Anemia of Inflammation. *N. Engl. J. Med.* **2019**, *381*, 1148–1157. [CrossRef] [PubMed]
15. Kufelkina, T.Y.; Valeeva, F.; Kufelkina, T.Y. Anemia in patients with type 1 diabetes mellitus. *Diabetes Mellit.* **2010**, *13*, 49–53. [CrossRef]
16. Semakova, A.D.; Brykova, Y.I.; Silina, M.N.; Volynkina, A.P. Estimation of the anemia prevalence in patients with diabetes mellitus. *Cent. Sci. Her.* **2019**, *72*, 7–8.
17. Marynov, S.; Shestakova, M.V.; Shilov, E.M.; Shamkhalova, M.S.; Vikulova, O.; Sukhareva, O.Y.; Trubitsyna, N.P.; Egorova, D.; Bondarenko, O.N.; Dedov, I.I. Prevalence of anemia in patients with type 1 and type 2 diabetes mellitus with chronic renal disease. *Diabetes Mellit.* **2017**, *20*, 318–328. [CrossRef]
18. Frederickson, D.S.; Lee, R.S. A system for phenotyping hyperlipidemia. *Circulation* **1965**, *31*, 321–327. [CrossRef]
19. Waheed, P.; Naveed, A.K.; Farooq, F. Levels of inflammatory markers and their correlation with dyslipidemia in diabetics. *J. Coll. Physicians Surg. Pak.* **2009**, *19*, 207–210.
20. De Boer, I.H.; Rue, T.C.; Cleary, P.A.; Lachin, J.M.; Molitch, M.E.; Steffes, M.W.; Sun, W.; Zinman, B.; Brunzell, J.D.; White, N.H.; et al. Long-term Renal Outcomes of Patients With Type 1 Diabetes Mellitus and Microalbuminuria: An Analysis of the Diabetes Control and Complications Trial/Epidemiology of Diabetes Interventions and Complications Cohort. *Arch. Intern. Med.* **2011**, *171*, 412–420. [CrossRef]
21. Tziomalos, K.; Athyros, V.G. Diabetic Nephropathy: New Risk Factors and Improvements in Diagnosis. *Rev. Diabet. Stud.* **2015**, *12*, 110–118. [CrossRef] [PubMed]
22. Wołkow, P.P.; Niewczas, M.A.; Perkins, B.; Ficociello, L.H.; Lipinski, B.; Warram, J.H.; Krolewski, A.S. Association of urinary inflammatory markers and renal decline in microalbuminuric type 1 diabetics. *J. Am. Soc. Nephrol.* **2008**, *19*, 789–797. [CrossRef] [PubMed]
23. Stehouwer, C.D.A.; Gall, M.-A.; Twisk, J.W.; Knudsen, E.; Emeis, J.J.; Parving, H.-H. Increased urinary albumin excretion, endothelial dysfunction, and chronic low-grade inflammation in type 2 diabetes: Progressive, interrelated, and independently associated with risk of death. *Diabetes* **2002**, *51*, 1157–1165. [CrossRef] [PubMed]
24. Li, J.; Bao, W.; Zhang, T.; Zhou, Y.; Yang, H.; Jia, H.; Wang, R.; Cao, Y.; Xiao, C. Independent relationship between serum ferritin levels and dyslipidemia in Chinese adults: A population study. *PLoS ONE* **2017**, *12*, e0190310. [CrossRef]
25. Adiels, M.; Olofsson, S.-O.; Taskinen, M.-R.; Borén, J. Overproduction of Very Low-Density Lipoproteins Is the Hallmark of the Dyslipidemia in the Metabolic Syndrome. *Arter. Thromb. Vasc. Boil.* **2008**, *28*, 1225–1236. [CrossRef]
26. Krauss, R.M.; Siri, P.W. Dyslipidemia in type 2 diabetes. *Med. Clin. N. Am.* **2004**, *88*, 897–909. [CrossRef]
27. Krentz, A.J. Lipoprotein abnormalities and their consequences for patients with Type 2 diabetes. *Diabetes Obes. Metab.* **2003**, *5*, s19–s27. [CrossRef]

28. Reiner, Z.; Catapano, A.L.; De Backer, G.; Graham, I.; Taskinen, M.R.; Wiklund, O.; Agewall, S.; Alegria, E.; Chapman, M.J.; Durrington, P.; et al. ESC/EAS Guidelines for the management of dyslipidaemias: The Task Force for the management of dyslipidaemias of the European Society of Cardiology (ESC) and the European Atherosclerosis Society (EAS). *Eur. Hear. J.* **2011**, *32*, 1769–1818. [CrossRef]
29. Kawanami, D.; Matoba, K.; Utsunomiya, K. Dyslipidemia in diabetic nephropathy. *Ren. Replace. Ther.* **2016**, *2*, 225. [CrossRef]
30. Angel, P.M.; Spraggins, J.M.; Baldwin, H.S.; Caprioli, R.M. Enhanced Sensitivity for High Spatial Resolution Lipid Analysis by Negative Ion Mode Matrix Assisted Laser Desorption Ionization Imaging Mass Spectrometry. *Anal. Chem.* **2012**, *84*, 1557–1564. [CrossRef]
31. Kaysen, G.A.; Eiserich, J.P. The role of oxidative stress-altered lipoprotein structure and function and microinflammation on cardiovascular risk in patients with minor renal dysfunction. *J. Am. Soc. Nephrol.* **2004**, *15*, 538–548. [CrossRef] [PubMed]
32. Duncan, B.B.; Schmidt, M.I.; Pankow, J.S.; Ballantyne, C.M.; Couper, D.; Vigo, A.; Hoogeveen, R.; Folsom, A.R.; Heiss, G. Low-grade systemic inflammation and the development of type 2 diabetes: The atherosclerosis risk in communities study. *Diabetes* **2003**, *52*, 1799–1805. [CrossRef] [PubMed]
33. Stern, M.P. Diabetes and cardiovascular disease. The "common soil" hypothesis. *Diabetes* **1995**, *44*, 369–374. [CrossRef]
34. Montero, R.M.; Covic, A.; Gnudi, L.; Goldsmith, D. Diabetic nephropathy: What does the future hold? *Int. Urol. Nephrol.* **2015**, *48*, 99–113. [CrossRef] [PubMed]
35. Ridker, P.M.; Rifai, N.; Pfeffer, M.A.; Sacks, F.; Braunwald, E. Long-Term Effects of Pravastatin on Plasma Concentration of C-reactive Protein. *Circulation* **1999**, *100*, 230–235. [CrossRef] [PubMed]
36. Albert, M.; Danielson, E.; Rifai, N.; Ridker, P. Effect of statin therapy on C-reactive protein levels. The pravastatin inflammation/CRP evaluation (PRINCE): A randomized trial and cohort study. *ACC Curr. J. Rev.* **2001**, *10*, 30. [CrossRef]
37. Ridker, P.M.; Danielson, E.; Fonseca, F.A.; Genest, J.; Gotto, A.M.; Kastelein, J.J.; Koenig, W.; Libby, P.; Lorenzatti, A.J.; MacFadyen, J.G.; et al. Reduction in C-reactive protein and LDL cholesterol and cardiovascular event rates after initiation of rosuvastatin: A prospective study of the JUPITER trial. *Lancet* **2009**, *373*, 1175–1182. [CrossRef]
38. Vakkilainen, J.; Steiner, G.; Ansquer, J.C.; Aubin, F.; Rattier, S.; Foucher, C.; Hamsten, A.; Taskinen, M.R. Relationships between low-density lipoprotein particle size, plasma lipoproteins, and progression of coronary artery disease: The Diabetes Atherosclerosis Intervention Study (DAIS). *ACC Curr. J. Rev.* **2003**, *12*, 35. [CrossRef]
39. Keech, A.; Simes, R.J.; Barter, P.; Best, J.; Scott, R.; Taskinen, M.-R.; Forder, P.; Pillai, A.; Davis, T.; Glasziou, P.; et al. Effects of long-term fenofibrate therapy on cardiovascular events in 9795 people with type 2 diabetes mellitus (the FIELD study): Randomised controlled trial. *Lancet* **2005**, *366*, 1849–1861. [CrossRef]

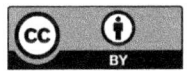

© 2020 by the authors. Licensee MDPI, Basel, Switzerland. This article is an open access article distributed under the terms and conditions of the Creative Commons Attribution (CC BY) license (http://creativecommons.org/licenses/by/4.0/).

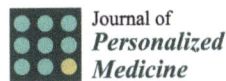

Article

Possible Differential Diagnosis of the Degrees of Rheological Disturbances in Patients with Type 2 Diabetes Mellitus by Dielectrophoresis of Erythrocytes

Margarita V. Kruchinina [1,*], **Andrey A. Gromov** [1], **Vladimir M. Generalov** [2] and **Vladimir N. Kruchinin** [3]

1. Research Institute of Internal and Preventive Medicine–Branch of the Institute of Cytology and Genetics, Siberian Branch of the Russian Academy of Sciences, B. Bogatkova Str., 175/1, 630089 Novosibirsk, Russia; gromov.center@rambler.ru
2. Federal Budgetary Research Institution "State Research Center of Virology and Biotechnology Vector", Rospotrebnadzor, 630559 Koltsovo Novosibirsk Region, Russia; general@vector.nsc.ru
3. Rzhanov Institute of Semiconductor Physics Siberian Branch of Russian Academy of Sciences, Lavrentiev Ave., 13, 630090 Novosibirsk, Russia; vladd.kruch@yandex.ru
* Correspondence: kruchmargo@yandex.ru; Tel.: +7-7913-728-1702

Received: 1 June 2020; Accepted: 2 July 2020; Published: 5 July 2020

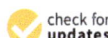

Abstract: Hemorheological disorders in structural and functional parameters of erythrocytes are involved in the pathological process in type 2 diabetes mellitus (DM). Aim: to investigate the feasibility of differential diagnosis of the degrees of rheological disturbances in patients with type 2 DM by dielectrophoresis of erythrocytes. Methods: 62 subjects (58.7 ± 1.6 years) with type 2 DM diagnosed according to the criteria of the ADA were subdivided into two groups: medium ($n = 47$) and high ($n = 15$) risk of microcirculatory disturbances (EASD, 2013). Electric and viscoelastic parameters of erythrocytes were determined by dielectrophoresis using an electric optical system of cell detection. Results: the progression of rheological disturbances in the patients with type 2 DM was accompanied by significant decreases in deformation amplitude; dipole moment; polarizability; and membrane capacity; and increases in conductivity, viscosity, rigidity, hemolysis, and formation of aggregates ($p < 0.05$). Combined use of the parameters increased sensitivity (97.8%) and specificity (86.7%) for diagnosis of rheological disturbances in type 2 DM. Conclusion: the proposed experimental approach possesses low invasiveness, high productivity, shorter duration, vividness of the results. The method allows to evaluate not only local (renal and ocular) but also systemic status of microcirculation using more than 20 parameters of erythrocytes.

Keywords: diagnostic method; severity of disturbances; rheology; diabetes mellitus; erythrocyte; dielectrophoresis

1. Introduction

Among patients with diabetes mellitus (DM), early disability and mortality, which are mostly caused by diabetic angiopathies, are the most important socioclinical problem of modern diabetology [1]. Timely detection of microcirculatory disturbances and reversal of hemorheological disorders are currently recognized as major components of modern diagnostic and therapeutic strategies in relation to patients with DM.

At present, in clinical practice, physicians use a variety of methods for the detection of microcirculatory disturbances in DM.

There are methods for the detection of diabetic microangiopathy that are designed strictly for local vascular analysis (e.g., in kidneys and eyes). To detect diabetic retinopathy, clinicians utilize several methods: slit-lamp examination of the conjunctiva, fundoscopy, retinal fluorescent angiography, quantitative perimetry, autocampigraphy, and examination of darkness adaptation. These methods allow visual evaluation of the state of retinal vessels and extrapolation of the obtained results to the vascular system as a whole. Nonetheless, these methods require specially trained personnel and ophthalmological equipment. The shortcomings of direct ophthalmoscopy are a small examined area, the absence of stereoscopy, close contact with a patient, and the inability to examine the extreme periphery of the fundus. In clinical practice, this approach is convenient as a screening method of medical examination. Contact binocular ophthalmoscopy by means of a slit lamp and contact lenses is the golden standard of diagnosis of fundus pathologies. Nevertheless, this method has limitations related to inflammatory processes on the eye surface, well-pronounced opacification or degenerative alterations of the cornea, and health state of the patient (e.g., convulsive disorder or epilepsy) [2]. A microalbuminuria test, urinary sediment analysis, measurement of glomerular filtration using endogenous creatinine, and other assays that only indirectly evaluate the presence of microvascular changes in kidneys during DM, are more informative at later stages, necessitate a set of expensive equipment, are costly, and require specially trained personnel [3].

Currently, the methods of capillaroscopy and capillarography and determination of vascular permeability allow us to answer the question about the systemic status of capillaries. Furthermore, capillaroscopy together with biochemical indicators is a cornerstone for diagnosing the preclinical stage of diabetic microangiopathy. In case of a combinatorial approach to the assessment of the microcirculatory bed, clinicians perform capillaroscopy in a resting state with subsequent evaluation of structural changes in capillary status. Additionally, they perform capillaroscopy and oxyhemometric analysis with four functional trials and the action of physical stimuli on the extremity being analyzed: cuff occlusion, assessment of cold exposure, assessment of heat exposure, and testing of raising the extremity. This technique ensures the most accurate diagnosis of microangiopathies in this group of patients because of comprehensive evaluation of the microcirculatory bed at early stages of a disorder on the basis of measuring the reserve properties of capillaries [4]. It should be noted, however, that these methods lengthen medical examination, and their results are affected by several factors (ingestion of liquids, food, or alcohol as well as cigarette smoking, vibration, or some medications) that alter the capillary state of extremities (fungal lesions of nail phalanx tissues, burns, traumatic or mechanical injury of hands (or finger cuticles) or feet or impaired light scattering by finger skin as a result of damage by aggressive chemicals) [5,6].

Abroad, in patients with DM, clinicians employ the method of microangiopathy diagnosis [7,8] that consists of examination of nail bed capillaries in ring fingers of patients at rest and assessment of their structural alterations by measuring the main capillaroscopic parameters using a computer-based capillaroscope equipped with a camera. This approach involves resting-state capillaroscopy with subsequent evaluation of structural alterations of the capillary state. A drawback of this technique is that the well-known method does not take full advantage of the diagnostic algorithm, thus limiting its application at initial stages of microangiopathy in patients with DM. At the same time, the physician is unable to detect pathological changes of capillaries in patients with first-time DM or with short duration of the disease; this situation precludes (i) assessing the status of the microcirculatory-system reserve and the degree of hypoxia of peripheral tissues, (ii) identifying a microangiopathy stage, and ultimately (iii) monitoring the capillary state in a patient with DM as a function of time.

Histochemical and electron-microscopic analyses of blood vessels in skin biopsies enable the detection of characteristic-for-DM alterations in vessel walls in the form of basal-membrane thickening, proliferation of the endothelium, and increased deposition of PAS-positive substances. A biopsy can be taken from any site of the skin by means of a special dermatome, from an ear lobe, or from the mucous membrane of the mouth or rectum. Nonetheless, because of the complexity and certain traumaticity of the method, it is used not so much for diagnosis but rather for studying the pathogenesis and prevalence of diabetic microangiopathies [9].

Various types of proteomics have been employed for pathoanatomical research on diabetic microangiopathy. Common proteomic techniques, including gel-based ones, possess limited sensitivity and reproducibility and are usually used to detect biomarkers of high or medium prevalence. Clinical samples from patients with diabetic microangiopathy, e.g., biopsy samples, are rather small. Therefore, the technologies of sample preparation, quantitative labeling, and mass spectrometry should be optimized for detecting a protein at a low concentration, for processing of multiple samples, and for accurate quantitation. Besides, signal transduction pathways are difficult to study because they contain many low-abundance proteins. At present, there are no biomarkers identifiable by proteomic methods that can be applied to the diagnosis of diabetic microangiopathy. It is noteworthy that the high cost of proteomic methods is another obstacle to their widespread use in clinical settings [10].

Shortcomings and limitations of the methods described above necessitate the development of new approaches to the detection of microcirculatory disturbances in DM.

The pathogenesis of microvascular complications in type 2 DM is linked with the pathological involvement of erythrocytes (red blood cells, RBCs), which not only perform the oxygen transport function in the blood–tissue system but also participate in the regulation of rheological properties of the blood and in interactions with endothelial cells [11].

At the capillary level, the state of RBCs is a determinant of microcirculation. Moreover, many changes in blood fluidity, for instance, deformability and aggregation of RBCs, are detectable much earlier than the obvious systemic symptoms [12].

Microrheological properties of RBCs, such as deformability, the aggregation ability, and production of vasoreactive factors, are determined by specific features of the molecular organization of the erythrocytic membrane and of the peri-membrane cytoplasmic matrix [13,14].

The dielectrophoresis method proposed by us for studying the electric and viscoelastic properties of RBCs is based on changes in cell parameters under the action of a nonuniform alternating electric field (NUAEF). The use of different frequencies of the electric field helps to assay the state of both RBC membranes (low frequencies: 10^5 and 5×10^4 Hz) and cytoplasm (high frequencies: 10^6 and 5×10^5 Hz). A brief dielectrophoretic assay (1–2 min.) helps to determine many parameters (>20) reflecting structural and functional status of RBCs (e.g., their surface charge, deformability, membrane stability, propensity for aggregation, and electric conductivity of membranes). The above characteristics of RBCs are tightly associated with a pathological process, as revealed by us previously in patients with a diffuse pathology of the liver [15] or a cerebrovascular pathology [16].

Such dielectrophoresis-measured parameters as cell deformation amplitude, summarized viscosity, and summarized rigidity reflect membrane alterations and an increase in internal rigidity as a consequence of a high concentration of glycated hemoglobin (HbA1c). On the other hand, the velocity of cell motion toward electrodes, dipole moment, and cellular capacity denote blood serum biochemical shifts associated with DM (e.g., disturbances of lipid and purine metabolism). Polarizability of cells and levels of hemolysis and aggregation are related to altered conditions of RBC maturation processes and indicate their lowered resistance to various factors; this drawback will later affect their interaction with the cells of a changed endothelium.

The RBC parameters in patients with type 2 DM were studied here for the first time by dielectrophoresis. This approach has several substantial advantages over the existing assays of microcirculation: low invasiveness (only 10 µL of blood is sufficient, collected by a method customary for the patients); the ability to evaluate the microcirculation state in the body as a whole rather than at a few sites; the use of high technologies; vivid results (the physician can visualize RBC behavior in a NUAEF); low cost without the need for expensive reagents and equipment; high reproducibility of the results; and possible the diagnostics as well as personalization of the therapeutic regimen for a patient.

Therefore, electric and viscoelastic parameters of RBCs, as measured by dielectrophoresis, help to obtain valuable information that is directly related to the development of rheological disturbances in DM.

The objective of this work was to test the feasibility of differential diagnosis of degrees of rheological disturbances in patients with type 2 DM by means of RBC dielectrophoresis.

2. Materials and Methods

2.1. Partisipants

In the clinical diagnostic department of the Institute of Internal and Preventive Medicine during 2016, we recruited patients with type 2 DM in accordance with the criteria of the American Diabetes Association (2016) [17]. Our inclusion criteria were as follows: patients aged 25–70 years with type 2 DM, who signed written informed consent to participate in the study. The following exclusion criteria were applied: age younger than 25 or older than 70 years; a decompensated pathology of the cardiovascular, pulmonary, and/or digestive system; or refusal to sign the written informed consent to take part in the study.

Sixty-two patients with type 2 DM at age 58.7 ± 1.6 years (mean ± SEM) were analyzed; 43 (69.4%) of them were females and 19 (30.6%) were males. The healthy control group consisted of 38 subjects at age 48.5 ± 2.2 years (24 (63.2%) females and 14 (36.8%) males) without DM, and without any other detectable pathology of internal organs, who visited our clinical diagnostic department for preventive purposes (Group 1). The subjects in the control group led a healthy lifestyle, did not smoke, and did not drink alcohol more often than once or twice a month, and the alcohol doses did not exceed 40 g for males and 20 g for females in terms of pure ethanol. In this group, the electric and viscoelastic parameters of RBCs were within the reference range appropriate for respective age.

Patients with type 2 DM were subdivided into two groups: medium risk (Group 2) and high risk of microcirculatory disturbances (Group 3) according to various indicators in keeping with recommendations of the European Association for the Study of Diabetes (EASD) (2013) [18] and recommendations cited in references [19,20]:

- Glycosylated hemoglobin (HbA1c): <7% for the medium risk and >7% for the high risk;
- blood pressure: <140/85 mm Hg for the medium risk and >140/85 mm Hg for the high risk;
- High-density lipoprotein (HDL) cholesterol: >40 mg/dL for the medium risk and <40 mg/dL for the high risk;
- Low-density lipoprotein (LDL) cholesterol: <100 mg/dL for the medium risk and >100 mg/dL for the high risk.

The Biomedical Ethics Committee of the federal publicly funded institution Institute of Internal and Preventive Medicine (session of 18 December 2015) approved the study protocol.

The patients underwent comprehensive clinical examination and instrumental analyses, including electrocardiography (Cardiovit AT-10/AT-2 (Schiller AG, Baar, Switzerland); ultrasonography of abdominal-cavity organs, kidneys, heart, and vessels (Vivid 7 Dimension (GE HealthCare, Norway); fundoscopy (ophthalmoscope PanOptic 11810-CE Welch Allyn, Skaneateles Falls, NY, USA); an assay of glycated hemoglobin (NycoCard READER II (Alere Technologies AS, Norway); and determination of the albumin/creatinine ratio in spot urine [21].

At admission of in-patients, fasting collection of venous blood from the cubital vein was conducted in the amount of 8 mL into two vacutainers (Becton Dickinson, Burlington, North Carolina USA): the first one (5 mL; SST II Advance) for biochemical assays, and the second vacutainer (5 mL; containing 0.109 M sodium citrate, 3.2%, in the 9:1 ratio) for determining the electric and viscoelastic parameters of RBCs by dielectrophoresis.

Biochemical indicators (total cholesterol, HDL cholesterol, LDL cholesterol, triglycerides, fasting blood glucose, uric acid, creatinine, urea, AST activity, total bilirubin, and albumin) were determined using KONELAB PRIME 30i (Scientific Oy, Thermo Fisher, Vantaa, Finland). RBC parameters (the number of RBCs, the hemoglobin level, color indicator, hematocrit, mean corpuscular volume (MCV), mean corpuscular hemoglobin (MCH), mean cell hemoglobin concentration (MCHC), red cell distribution width (RDW-CV) in %, and red cell distribution width (RDW-SD) in femtoliters) and leukocyte counts were determined on an automatic hematology analyzer, HT Micro CC-20 Plus (High Technology, Inc., USA). The RBC sedimentation rate was measured by Panchenkov's micromethod.

Blood fibrinogen was quantified by the Clauss method with reagents from Renam (Moscow, Russia). Immunoenzyme assays based on standard ELISA kits were carried out to quantitate serum C-reactive protein (Biomerica kit) on an immunoenzyme assay analyzer, Multiscan EX (Finland) [18].

2.2. Dielectrophoresis

Electric and viscoelastic parameters of RBCs were measured by dielectrophoresis by means of an electric optical system of cell detection [22]. The procedures for optical registration are explained in details in the Appendix A, which includes the functional scheme of the electric optical system of cell detection (Figure A1) and the makeup of the measurement chip containing an electrode quartet (Figure A2). For the assay, 10 µL of whole blood from the vacutainer with citrate buffer was added to a 0.3 M sucrose solution (pH 7.36) in the 1:30 ratio.

The measurements were conducted immediately after the resuspension of RBCs. In a measurement cell, the RBCs were exposed to an NUAEF at the following settings: electric intensity, 105 V/m; electric intensity gradient, 10^{11} V/m^2; and frequency range, 5×10^4 to 1×10^6 Hz. We analyzed cell polarizability, membrane capacity, electric conductivity, a position of crossover frequency, indices of aggregation and destruction of RBCs, velocity of cell motion toward electrodes, induced dipole moment, deformation amplitude of RBCs at a frequency of 10^6 Hz, the deformation degree of the cells at a frequency of 5×10^5 Hz, and summarized viscosity and summarized rigidity of RBCs. The data were processed using an original software suite, CELLFIND (developed by Federal Budgetary Research Institution "State Research Center of Virology and Biotechnology Vector", Rospotrebnadzor; www.vector.nsc.ru). Intertest repeatability of the method was 7–12%.

2.3. Statistical Analysis

Statistical analysis of the data was performed in the SPSS software, v. 22 (www.ibm.com/spss). The Kolmogorov–Smirnov test was employed to characterize the distribution of numerical variables. In case of a normal distribution, the average (mean) and standard error of the mean (SEM) were calculated (presented as mean ± SEM). In the case of the normal distribution, the significance of differences (or correlations) of parameters was assessed by Student's t test or Pearson's correlation analysis. If a distribution was not normal, then nonparametric tests were performed (Mann–Whitney U test, Kolmogorov–Smirnov test, and χ^2 test). In all the statistical analyses, the threshold of null hypothesis probability (p) was assumed to be 0.05. To evaluate the utility of RBC parameters for the stratification of severity of rheological disturbances in type 2 DM, receiver operating characteristic (ROC) analysis was carried out.

3. Results and Discussion

On the basis of the above-mentioned criteria, our patients with DM were distributed into two groups: a medium risk of damage to small vessels, i.e., medium severity of rheological and microcirculatory disturbances (Group 2; $n = 47$), and high risk of microcirculatory disturbances (Group 3; $n = 15$). The clinical parameters of the patients from these groups were found to be within the range corresponding to the risk of damage to large and small vessels.

The data on clinical examination and instrumental analyses of the groups are given in Table 1.

Table 1. Clinical and biochemical data in groups of patients with diabetes with varying degrees of risk of microcirculation disturbances (M ± m).

Clinical and Biochemical Indicators	Group 1, the Controls, $n = 38$	Group 2, with DM, Medium Risk of Microcirculatory Disturbances, $n = 47$	Group 3, with DM, High Risk of Microcirculatory Disturbances, $n = 15$
Age, years	48.4 ± 2.18	59.64 ± 1.18	57.8 ± 2.09
Gender (person)	F-24 M-14	F-35 M-12	F-8 M-7
Body mass index (kg/m²)	27.52 ± 0.61	31.74 ± 0.82 **	35.62 ± 0.97 ***^
Diabetes experience (years)	-	8.2 ± 3.2	14.2 ± 2.7^
Duration of hypertension (years)	-	9.8 ± 4.3	15.9 ± 3.9^
Family history of early cardiovascular disease, n(%)	2 (5.3%)	18 (38.3%) ***	9 (60%) ***^^^
The stages of diabetic retinopathy, n(%)			
0—no	38 (100)	14 (29.8)	0
1—non-proliferative	0	24 (51.1)	6 (40)
2—preproliferative	0	8 (17.0)	6 (40)
3—proliferative	0	1 (2.1) ****	3 (20) ****^^^
Stage diabetic angiopathy, n(%)			
0—no	38 (100)	0	0
1—I (asymptomatic)	0	24 (51.1)	0
2—II A	0	20 (42.6)	4 (26.7)
3—II B	0	3 (6.3)	
4—III	0	0 ****	
Glycosylated hemoglobin (HbA1c), %	4.78 ± 0.11	6.59 ± 0.025 ****	8.01 ± 0.07 ****^^^
Albumin/Creatinine ratio in a single portion of urine, mg/mmol	2.23 ± 0.06	3.34 ± 0.035 ****	4.1 ± 0.044 ****^^^
Total Cholesterol, mg/dL	183.7 ± 5.9	208.48 ± 6.35 ***	217.5 ± 11.7 ***
HDL Cholesterol, mg/dL	51.43 ± 1.92	49.33 ± 1.52	42.46 ± 2.74 **^
LDL cholesterol, mg/dL	77.38 ± 2.2	91.72 ± 2.8 **	112.46 ± 2.6 ***^^^
AST, U/L	12.52 ± 1.18	21.36 ± 1.26 *	28.53 ± 3.1 *^
Total bilirubin, μmol/L	11.88 ± 0.82	12.78 ± 1.4	19.24 ± 1.34 *^
Albumin, g/L	50.2 ± 1.2	49.1 ± 1.8	41.7 ± 0.94 *^
Triglycerides, mg/dL	126.08 ± 14.5	188.9 ± 27.7 *	222.3 ± 20.42 ***
Fasting blood glucose, mmol/L	5.76 ± 0.13	7.94 ± 0.33 ****	9.62 ± 0.69 ****^^
Uric acid (mg/dL)	360 ± 18	390 ± 15	420 ± 29
Creatinine, μmol/L	74.07 ± 1.58	74.94 ± 1.42	84.28 ± 5.43 **^
Urea, mmol/L	4.5 ± 0.28	5.51 ± 0.31 **	6.04 ± 0.34 ***
C-reactive protein, mg/L	3.0 ± 0.8	3.6 ± 0.9	5.5 ± 0.7 **^
Fibrinogen, g/L	2.4 ± 1.3	3.2 ± 1.8	5.1 ± 1.2 *^
The number of leukocytes, ×10⁹/L	4.56 ± 0.26	5.52 ± 0.42	6.75 ± 0.32
The number of red blood cells, ×10¹²/L	4.59 ± 0.096	4.63 ± 0.07	4.60 ± 0.17
Hemoglobin level, g/L	141.79 ± 2.25	140.93 ± 4.5	140.79 ± 2.25
Color indicator	0.92 ± 0.009	0.91 ± 0.008	0.87 ± 0.019 *
Hematocrit, %	42.41 ± 0.58	43.11 ± 0.64	44.79 ± 0.89 *
Mean corpuscular volume (MCV), fl	93.78 ± 0.52	92.89 ± 0.74	89.81 ± 1.46 ***^
Mean corpuscular hemoglobin (MCH), pg	31.21 ± 0.29	30.58 ± 0.31	29.4 ± 0.67 ***
Mean cell hemoglobin concentration (MCHC), g/L	333.11 ± 2.12	329.58 ± 2.2	326.4 ± 3.56
Red cell distribution width (RDW-CV), %	13.84 ± 0.08	14.11 ± 0.09 *	13.95 ± 0.18
Red cell distribution width (RDW-SD), fl	50.43 ± 0.36	50.17 ± 0.44	48.49 ± 0.65 ***^
RBC sedimentation rate, mm/h	10.20 ± 1.44	15.11 ± 1.58 *	19.8 ± 2.54 **^

Note: "M" is the mean, and "m" is the average error of the arithmetic average value; * significance (p) of differences from the control group (Group 1): * $p < 0.05$, ** $p < 0.02$, *** $p < 0.01$, **** $p < 0.0001$; ^ significance (p) of differences from the Group 2: ^ $p < 0.05$, ^^ $p < 0.02$, ^^^ $p < 0.01$, ^^^^ $p < 0.0001$.

There were no significant differences in age, sex, alcohol consumption style, and cigarette smoking between the groups of patients with DM. By contrast, in the group with the high severity of rheological disturbances (Group 3), DM duration and arterial-hypertension duration were significantly greater and there was greater prevalence of (1) a family history of early cardiovascular diseases and (2) a history of ischemic heart disease with myocardial infarctions. Systolic and diastolic blood pressure and the prevalence of cardiac rhythm and conduction aberrations ($p < 0.05$) were higher in Group 3 than in Group 2. All patients with DM received sugar-lowering therapy (targeted to healthy levels of glucose metabolism control) and hypertension medication.

The patients with high severity of rheological disturbances showed worse manifestations of DM and its complications: this group featured higher levels of fasting glycemia (9.62 ± 0.69 versus 7.94 ± 0.33 mmol/L in Group 2, $p = 0.018$), glycated hemoglobin, albumin/creatinine ratio in spot urine, stronger manifestations of hyperlipidemia (mostly type 2B hyperlipidemia), and disturbances of purine metabolism, liver function, and the excretory function of kidneys.

It is worth mentioning that the patients with well-pronounced rheological disturbances (Group (3) had a higher body mass index, severer diabetic neuropathy and retinopathy (in 60% of these patients, we detected pre-retinopathy and proliferative retinopathy), angiopathy (in 53.3% of the cases, it corresponded to the IIB stage, when pain in lower extremities presented after walking less than 200 m, $p < 0.0001$).

The analysis of RBC parameters did not reveal significant differences among the groups in the RBC count, a color parameter, and hemoglobin. Nonetheless, it was found that patients with DM had higher hematocrit and greater RBC distribution width, whereas the average corpuscular volume and average hemoglobin content of RBCs turned out to be lower than those in the healthy controls ($p = 0.047$, $p = 0.033$, $p = 0.002$, and $p = 0.009$, respectively).

3.1. Assessment of Viscoelastic and Electric Parameters of RBCs in Patients with DM

In the assay involving the NUAEF, RBCs of healthy controls (group 1) showed a high velocity of motion toward electrodes and high elasticity at frequencies of 5×10^5 and 1×10^6 Hz (Figure 1a). At low frequencies (5×10^4 and 1×10^5 Hz), we noted repulsion of the cells from the electrodes (negative dielectrophoresis) with hemolysis of some RBCs under the influence of the electric field.

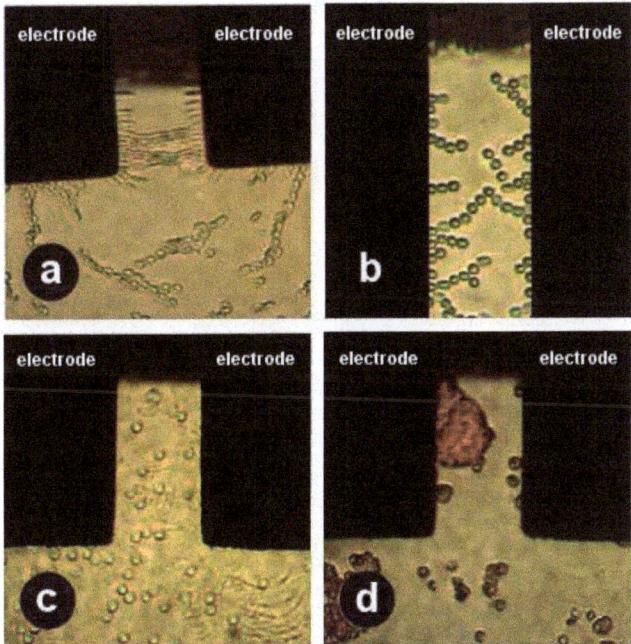

Figure 1. Behavior of red blood cells (RBCs) under the influence of the nonuniform alternating electric field (NUAEF) at a frequency of 10^6 Hz (**a**) in the healthy control group and (**b**–**d**) in patients with diabetes mellitus (DM) (see the main text).

In patients with DM, the behavior of RBCs in the NUAEF was substantially different: at high frequencies (5×10^5 and 1×10^6 Hz), deformability of the cells (m) and translational motion velocity of the cells (μm/s) toward the electrodes were found to be significantly lower ($p < 0.01$; Figure 1b). Pronounced destruction of RBCs was seen at all frequencies of the NUAEF (Figure 1c). Furthermore, the cells were prone to the formation of aggregates of various sizes ($p < 0.02$; Figure 1d).

There were differences in RBC characteristics associated with the severity of rheological disturbances in DM. In a solution of a dielectric, most RBCs from the patients with medium severity of rheological disturbances (Group 2) had a discocyte shape, and 24% ± 6% of the cells became spherocytes or assumed a shape of a "deflated ball." In patients with severe microcirculatory disturbances (Group 3), we detected an increase in the proportion of nondiscocyte shapes up to 48% ± 6% ($p < 0.001$), with ~25% of the discocytes becoming spikelike. It is known that the membrane integrity and biconcave shape of RBCs are mostly ensured by the energy of high-energy compounds [23], primarily by various forms of ATP arising during glycolysis, which is the main pathway of energy metabolism in RBCs [24].

A decrease in the APT level in RBCs is accompanied by blockage of ion pumps, thereby leading to shifts in the ion balance in a cell–environment system. This process contributes to a reduction in the surface area/volume ratio of RBCs, to spherocytic transformation of RBCs, and to the emergence of spikelike protrusions. Such alterations impede the oxygen transport from the RBC to tissues and aggravate hypoxia, which stimulates fibrogenic phenomena with internal remodeling of vessel walls, thus driving the progression of diabetic angiopathy [13,24].

With the increasing severity of rheological disturbances (from Group 2 to Group 3 of patients with DM), there were increases in electric conductivity, indices of aggregation and destruction, summarized viscosity, and summarized rigidity. At the same time, deformation amplitude of RBCs, polarizability at 10^6 Hz, dipole moment, electric membrane capacity of RBCs, and the velocity of cell motion toward the electrodes became significantly lower ($p < 0.001$–0.05; Table 2). The severity of microcirculatory disturbances in DM proved to be inversely related to deformation amplitude ($r = -0.652, p < 0.0001$) but directly correlated with summarized viscosity ($r = 0.680, p < 0.0001$) and summarized rigidity of RBCs ($r = 0.635, p < 0.0001$).

It is reported that the deformability of RBCs is determined by their viscoelastic characteristics [25]. According to our results, there was a decrease in RBC deformability with increasing summarized viscosity and summarized rigidity of these cells. These shifts may be associated with higher cholesterol content of the RBC membrane and a greater cholesterol/phospholipid index [26].

As a consequence of cholesterol exchange between RBCs and the lipoproteins adsorbed on their surface, cholesterol is incorporated into the RBC membrane. During this process, RBC size increases, and these cells change shape, with a substantial decrease in their filtration ability [27,28].

Such alterations cause microcirculatory disturbances and increase the risk of ischemic states including the diabetic foot. The decrease in cell elasticity under the influence of the NUAEF and progressive worsening of rheological disturbances in DM can be regarded as a "model" of RBC behavior at the level of capillaries, whose size is >2.5-fold less than the diameter of these cells [29]. On the one hand, "rigid and frail" RBCs, which are prone to aggregation, easily disintegrate under such conditions, whereas the aggregates damage the endothelial lining [27].

On the other hand, extensive regions of the capillary bed get "excluded" from the bloodstream and oxygen exchange because the aggregates and the rigid cells are unable to enter the zone of smallest vessels. The "rarefaction" of the capillary bed further aggravates hypoxia and ischemia at the periphery [30].

The propensity of RBCs for excessive disintegration and aggregation in patients with DM were found to correlate with low polarizability of the cells ($r = -0.60, p = 0.02; r = -0.53, p = 0.04$, respectively). Given that polarizability reflects biological activity of cells, its progressive decreases with increasing DM severity is possibly associated with activation of accelerated low-efficiency erythropoiesis in this disease. Activation of the renal juxtaglomerular apparatus, in conjunction with progressive narrowing of renal arteries, leads to increased production of erythropoietin, which is a stimulator of accelerated formation of RBCs [24]. Accelerated maturation of RBCs coincides with a peripheral release of the cells with altered membrane structure, including excessive presentation of carboxyl groups and a larger amount of structurally modified spectrin and phospholipid lysofractions. This state of affairs causes predominance (in the RBC population) of RBCs with lower resistance to various stressors. The changed structure of the RBC surface with signs of premature aging is a signal for immunocompetent cells to eliminate such RBCs from the bloodstream. During the destruction of RBCs, there is an intravascular release of intra-RBC ADP, ATP, and hemoglobin, which are potent inducers of the formation of aggregates, including mixed ones (leukocytic-thrombocytic-erythrocytic) [24,30]; this phenomenon can explain the high indices of destruction and aggregation at all frequencies of the NUAEF in our present study. Meanwhile, the increasing aggregation of RBCs is accompanied by the secretion (by the cell aggregates) of thromboplastic substances associated with the cell membrane, thereby creating a local hypercoagulative state. This process contributes to intravascular blood clotting and causes a secondary disorder of hemodynamics in microcirculation [11,31].

Table 2. Electrical and viscoelastic parameters of red blood cells in patients with diabetes with different degrees of microcirculatory disturbances (M ± m).

Electrical and Viscoelastic Parameters of Red Blood Cells	Group 1, the Controls, $n = 38$	Group 2, with DM, Medium Risk of Microcirculatory Disturbances, $n = 47$	Group 3, with DM, High Risk of Microcirculatory Disturbances, $n = 15$
The average diameter of RBCs, [μm]	7.55 ± 0.008	7.45 ± 0.011 ****	7.33 ± 0.013 ****^^^^
Deformation amplitude of RBCs at 10^6 Hz, [m]	(8.16 ± 0.11) × 10^{-6}	(6.18 ± 0.06) × 10^{-6} ****	(5.2 ± 0.04) × 10^{-6} ****^^^^
The Deformation degree of RBCs at 5×10^5 Hz, (%)	73.1 ± 1.97	41.55 ± 1.15 ****	25.86 ± 1.34 ****^^^^
Summarized rigidity of RBCs, [N/m]	(5.57 ± 0.16) × 10^{-6}	(8.62 ± 0.04) × 10^{-6} ****	(10.12 ± 0.03) × 10^{-6} ****^^^^
Summarized viscosity of RBCs, [Pa×s]	0.51 ± 0.009	0.70 ± 0.002 ****	0.78 ± 0.005 ****^^^^
Electric conductivity, [Cm/m]	(5.53 ± 0.11) × 10^{-5}	(6.83 ± 0.21) × 10^{-5} ****	(7.96 ± 0.38) × 10^{-5} ****^^^^
Electric membrane capacity, [F]	(7.3 ± 0.19) × 10^{-14}	(4.44 ± 0.42) × 10^{-14} ****	(4.10 ± 0.74) × 10^{-14} ****
The velocity of RBC motion toward the electrodes, [μm/s]	7.74 ± 0.19	4.57 ± 0.18 ****	4.2 ± 0.34 ****
The position of crossover frequency, [Hz]	(5.5 ± 0.58) × 10^5	(11.8 ± 2.2) × 10^5 ****	(16.0 ± 6.0) × 10^5 ***
Dipole moment, [Kl×m]	(12.4 ± 4.9) × 10^{-22}	(7.22 ± 0.15) × 10^{-22} ****	(4.5 ± 0.25) × 10^{-22} ****^^^^
Polarizability of RBCs at 10^6 Hz, [m^3], ×10^{-15}	0.574 ± 0.005	0.459 ± 0.017 ****	0.438 ± 0.005 ****
Index of RBCs destruction at 10^6 Hz, (%)	0	2.4 ± 0.1	3.4 ± 0.53
Index of RBCs destruction at 5×10^5 Hz, (%)	0	2.8 ± 0.4	3.11 ± 0.32
Index of RBCs destruction at 10^5 Hz, (%)	0	2.3 ± 0.5	5.0 ± 0.4 ^
Index of RBCs destruction at 5×10^4 Hz, (%)	0	2.0 ± 0.6	4.1 ± 0.32 ^
Index of RBCs aggregation, conventional units	0.62 ± 0.003	0.64 ± 0.005	0.65 ± 0.007 *

Notes: The magnitude of the dipole moment was determined at an electric field strength of 8.85×10^{-12} F/m.
* significance (p) of differences from the control group (Group 1): * $p < 0.05$, ** $p < 0.02$, *** $p < 0.01$, **** $p < 0.0001$;
^ significance (p) of differences from Group 2: ^ $p < 0.05$, ^^ $p < 0.02$, ^^^ $p < 0.01$, ^^^^ $p < 0.0001$.

We revealed correlations of RBC characteristics with several clinical and biochemical parameters and some parameters of RBCs. It should be noted that most parameters of RBCs were found to correlate with the fasting glycemia level ($r = -0.348$, $p = 0.005$, for deformation amplitude at 10^6 Hz; $r = -0.266$, $p = 0.034$, for the deformation degree at 5×10^5 Hz; $r = 0.439$, $p < 0.0001$, for summarized viscosity; $r = 0.338$, $p = 0.006$, for summarized rigidity; and $r = -0.32$, $p < 0.01$, for average RBC diameter), with glycated hemoglobin ($r = -0.551$, $p < 0.001$, for deformation amplitude at 10^6 Hz; $r = -0.677$, $p < 0.0001$, for the deformation degree at 5×10^5 Hz; $r = 0.601$, $p < 0.0001$, for summarized viscosity; $r = 0.63$, $p < 0.0001$, for summarized rigidity; $r = -0.49$, $p < 0.0001$, for the average diameter of RBCs; $r = -0.393$, $p < 0.001$, for dipole moment; and $r = 0.321$, $p < 0.01$, for electric conductivity), the urine ratio of albumin to creatinine ($r = -0.51$, $p < 0.0001$, for deformation amplitude at 10^6 Hz; $r = -0.567$, $p < 0.0001$, for the deformation degree at 5×10^5 Hz; $r = 0.517$, $p < 0.0001$, for summarized viscosity; $r = 0.451$, $p < 0.0001$, for summarized rigidity; $r = -0.482$, $p < 0.0001$, for the average diameter of RBCs; $r = -0.514$, $p < 0.0001$, for dipole moment; and $r = 0.247$, $p < 0.05$, for electric conductivity). It is known that higher excretion of albumin with urine develops as a consequence of damage to (and dysfunction of) the renal vascular endothelium, increased pressure in the capillary network of glomeruli (glomerular hypertension), disruption of structural integrity of the glomerular basal membrane, and dysfunction of the canalicular epithelium [32,33].

Because the last two parameters reflect the compensation degree of carbohydrate metabolism, their relation with electric and viscoelastic characteristics of RBCs is not surprising. Glycated hemoglobin noticeably raises internal viscosity of RBCs (by forming cross-links with the cell membranes) and summarized rigidity too [34,35]. These effects appreciably influence the deformability of RBCs. It should be noted that the deformation amplitude of RBCs significantly correlated with DM duration and arterial-hypertension duration ($r = -0.563$, $p < 0.01$, and $r = -0.42$, $p = 0.04$, respectively).

The observed correlations indicate the involvement of RBCs in the pathogenesis of diabetic complications. The observed associations with lipid profile parameters (for high-density lipoprotein cholesterol: with deformation amplitude ($r = 0.33$, $p = 0.013$) and with summarized viscosity ($r = -0.27$, $p = 0.043$); for triglycerides: with deformation amplitude ($r = 0.327$, $p = 0.008$), with summarized viscosity ($r = 0.325$, $p = 0.009$), with summarized rigidity ($r = 0.27$, $p = 0.03$), and with cell polarizability at 10^6 Hz ($r = -0.875$, $p < 0.0001$)) and with results of liver assays (for AST activity: with electric conductivity ($r = 0.33$, $p = 0.008$); for the total bilirubin level: with deformation amplitude ($r = -0.283$, $p = 0.025$), with summarized viscosity ($r = 0.27$, $p = 0.032$), and with summarized rigidity ($r = 0.248$, $p < 0.05$); for the albumin level: cell polarizability at 10^6 Hz ($r = 0.487$, $p = 0.028$)) confirms interactions of RBCs with serum components. The most revealing are the correlations of RBC characteristics with the severity of diabetic retino- and angiopathy (stages of retino- and angiopathy respectively correlated with deformation amplitude at 10^6 Hz ($r = -0.31$, $p = 0.013$, $r = -0.377$, $p = 0.002$), with the deformation degree at 5×10^5 Hz ($r = -0.228$, $p = 0.005$, $r = -0.414$, $p < 0.001$), with summarized viscosity ($r = 0.25$, $p = 0.046$, $r = 0.429$, $p < 0.0001$), with summarized rigidity ($r = 0.248$, $p = 0.048$, $r = 0.37$, $p = 0.003$), with the average diameter of RBCs ($r = -0.325$, $p = 0.009$), and with dipole moment ($r = -0.762$, $p < 0.0001$, $r = -0.454$, $p < 0.0001$). Probably, the shifts in the structural and functional properties of RBCs contribute to the progression of DM complications, in agreement with data from other investigators [36,37].

We uncovered associations of the urine albumin/creatinine ratio with electric parameters of RBCs, namely, with dipole moment, which correlated with the value and density of the surface negative charge of RBCs. A dipole reflects spatial asymmetry of the distribution of electric charges throughout the cell volume. Traditionally, measurements of microalbuminuria and of the albumin/creatinine ratio in spot urine are used in the clinic for diabetic-nephropathy screening. It should be noted that in recent years, the microalbuminuria level gained popularity as a marker of plasma membrane functions of highly differentiated cells, including determination of the severity of endothelial dysfunction. Normally, due to the presence of a high negative charge on the endothelial-cell surface, negatively charged albumin does not cross the renal glomerular filter. To some extent, this charge is predetermined by the phospholipid structure in the cell membranes that include polyunsaturated fatty acids.

A decreased number of double bonds in the acyl residues of phospholipids corresponds to a lower negative charge, thereby causing excessive filtration of albumin into primary urine. These aberrations have been detected during the development of atherosclerosis; accordingly, microalbuminuria develops in hereditary hyperlipidemias, arterial hypertension, ischemic heart disease, or DM in patients with aberrant glucose tolerance.

In DM, there are changes of phospholipid structure in the membranes of highly differentiated cells (e.g., RBCs, endotheliocytes, and renal cells); this phenomenon influences the surface charge of the membranes. The reason for the tight link between electric parameters of RBCs and the albumin/creatinine ratio is obvious; this ratio is being evaluated as an indicator of the initial stages of endothelial dysfunction, which is one of the major components of DM pathogenesis [1,11].

It was found here that in patients with DM, there is a shift of crossover frequency to a high-frequency range ($>5 \times 10^5$ Hz; $p < 0.01$; Table 2). Such alterations are probably caused by the increased electric conductivity of RBCs in DM. The latter parameter reflects the ability of membranes to conduct an electric current and is substantially related to the altered membrane structure, in particular to high cholesterol content. It is known that an increase in the cholesterol content of membranes raises summarized viscosity and summarized rigidity of the RBC [26], limits lateral diffusion of receptors, and changes permeability to dissolved substances and ion transport, thus resulting in higher electric conductivity of the cell [13,24].

The progression of rheological-disturbance severity in our patients with DM coincided with a decrease in electric membrane capacity ($p < 0.0001$), and this effect may indirectly indicate membrane thickening. This phenomenon is probably related to several factors, for instance, the enhancement of mutual exchange of lipids with blood serum, as confirmed by correlations of RBC membrane capacity with the levels of total cholesterol ($r = -0.51$, $p = 0.041$) and triglycerides ($r = -0.40$, $p = 0.03$). Another possible contributor is adsorption of high-molecular-weight proteins on the surface of membranes (e.g., globulins, fibrinogen, and fibrin) in conjunction with the well-pronounced inflammation in patients with DM. This notion is supported by the higher levels of some inflammation markers observed in the present study (C-reactive protein, fibrinogen, the leukocyte count, and RBC sedimentation rate, as shown in Table 1).

With increasing severity of rheological disturbances, dipole moment was found to decrease in the patients with DM and to reach the lowest values in patients with high severity of microcirculatory disturbances (Group 3). This effect is a sign of a decreased electric charge of RBCs. On the one hand, a possible reason is the alteration of average RBC corpuscular volume in patients with DM (Table 1); this change—due to redistribution of membrane glycoproteins and glycolipids on the cell surface—lowered the density of the surface negative charge [23,24]. On the other hand, another possible explanation is a decrease in the absolute membrane concentrations of sialic and neuraminic acids, which account for ~60% of surface charge density [30]. Finally, the greater amounts of high-molecular-weight proteins (as a consequence of systemic inflammation in patients with DM) can "shield" the negative charge of RBCs, via adsorption on the surface of their membranes regardless of the antigen type. A decrease in the surface negative charge of RBCs increases their propensity for the formation of persistent aggregates [27,31].

Thus, it was demonstrated here that DM progression is accompanied by a process of RBC depolarization. Meanwhile, amplitude and frequency parameters of RBCs in the NUAEF were found to be accurate indicators of physicochemical properties of the membrane and cytoplasm of these cells as well as markers of their biological activity.

3.2. Cutoffs of RBC Parameters in DM Patients for Different Degrees of Rheological Disturbances

To assess the usefulness of RBC parameters for the stratification of severity of microcirculatory disturbances in patients with DM, ROC analysis was performed (construction of ROC curves) for the various characteristics of RBCs.

The most accurate discrimination between the two severity levels of rheological disturbances in DM was shown by summarized viscosity and summarized rigidity of RBCs, deformation amplitude of the cells at the frequency of 10^6 Hz, the deformation degree of the cells at the frequency of 5×10^5 Hz, dipole moment, and electric conductivity of the cells. Less accurate discrimination was manifested by the polarizability of RBCs at the frequency of 10^6 Hz, morphology, structure of the RBC surface, and the velocity of RBC motion toward the electrodes (Table 3). Standard error for some parameters was in the range 0.018 to 0.093, and asymptomatic significance varied from 0.0001 to 0.168.

Table 3. Results of the analysis of ROC curves of erythrocyte indices in patients with diabetes by differentiating the degree of rheological disorders.

Electrical and Viscoelastic Parameters of Red Blood Cells	Area Under ROC Curve (AUC)	Asymptotic 95% Confidence Interval		Speci-Ficity, (%)	Sensi-Tivity, (%)
		Lower Bound	Upper Bound		
Summarized viscosity of RBCs	0.982	0.946	1.0	98.0	80
Deformation amplitude of RBCs at 10^6 Hz	0.979	0.939	1.000	98.0	93.3
Summarized rigidity of RBCs	0.967	0.92	1.0	08.0	93.3
Dipole moment	0.950	0.884	1.000	98.0	93.3
The Deformation degree of RBCs at 5×10^5 Hz	0.913	0.866	0.996	98.0	93.3
The average diameter of RBCs	0.890	0.98	0.982	77.6	86.7
Electric conductivity	0.713	0.565	0.861	83.7	86.7
Polarizability of RBCs at 10^6 Hz	0.696	0.566	0.826	71.4	66.7
Erythrocyte surface structure	0.696	0.549	0.843	80.0	40.8
Altered RBC morphology	0.626	0.463	0.788	60.0	32.7
The velocity of RBC motion toward the electrodes	0.618	0.436	0.801	71.4	66.7

The results of combined evaluation of a "panel" of electric and viscoelastic parameters of RBCs in patients with type 2 DM for determining the severity of rheological disturbances are presented in Table 4, in comparison with the risk assessment criteria for vascular complications in patients with DM as proposed by the EASD. Our panel has relatively high sensitivity (97.8%), specificity (86.7%), positive predictive value (95.8%), negative predictive value (92.8%), and accuracy index (95.2%). The higher accuracy of evaluation of rheological disturbances when the totality of RBC parameters is used (as compared with individual assays of stand-alone electric and viscoelastic parameters of RBCs) suggests that a panel of viscoelastic and electric parameters of RBCs should be employed for this purpose in type 2 DM.

Table 4. Diagnostic performance of the panel of electric and viscoelastic parameters of RBCs in patients with type 2 DM for assessing rheological-disturbance severity, as compared with the risk assessment criteria for vascular complications in patients with DM according to the EASD.

Results from the Panel of Electric and Viscoelastic Parameters of RBCs	Results of Analysis Using Risk Assessment Criteria for Vascular Complications in DM (EASD)	
	Group of Medium Severity of Rheological Disturbances in DM, $n = 47$ Cases	Group of High Severity of Rheological Disturbances in DM, $n = 15$ Cases
Group of medium severity of rheological disturbances in DM, $n = 48$ cases	True positive: group of medium severity of rheological disturbances, $n = 46$	False positive: group of high severity of rheological disturbances, $n = 2$
Group of high severity of rheological disturbances in DM, $n = 14$ cases	False negative: group of medium severity of rheological disturbances, $n = 1$	True negative: group of high severity of rheological disturbances, $n = 13$

Calculation of the main characteristics of the method according to T. Greenhalgh [38].; Sensitivity 46: $(46 + 1) \times 100\%$ = 97.8%; Specificity 13: $(2 + 13) \times 100\%$ = 86.7%; Positive predictive value 46: $(46 + 2) \times 100\%$ = 95.8%; Negative predictive value 13: $(1 + 13) \times 100\%$ = 92.8%; Accuracy index $(46 + 13)/(46 + 2 + 1 + 13) \times 100\%$ = 95.2%.

Our study has some limitations. Because of the experimental nature of this research, we recruited a relatively small number of subjects. Therefore, it is advisable to conduct an additional study on patients with type 2 DM featuring minimal rheological disturbances (recruitment of such patients is underway). Inclusion of such a group of patients with DM may increase the practical utility of this research because the rheological disturbances are reversible at the early stages.

A possible limitation of the proposed method of assaying RBC parameters is the necessity of taking into account various factors (alcohol, smoking, exposure to toxic compounds, an acute inflammatory process, and the acute stage of an infectious disease) that can affect these RBC characteristics.

The advantage of the proposed method over existing ones is that this diagnostic technique for rheological disturbances and diabetic microangiopathy allows to both identify this complication (regardless of the affected site) and determine its severity. The degree of changes in RBC parameters has the diagnostic value. Our method is barely invasive (involves only blood collection), thereby preventing serious complications in the patients and not requiring hospitalization. In relation to the physical and psychological state of a patient, there are no restrictions on our method. The evaluation of measured RBC parameters is objective and not affected by the qualifications and experience of the test operator. The dielectrophoresis assay requires only inexpensive widely available reagents thus increasing the accessibility of this method for a mass diagnostic program, including the one intended for screening. The proposed method is not labor-intensive and not costly. The high sensitivity, specificity, and clear-cut criteria for the evaluation of rheological-disturbance severity and diabetic microangiopathy are expected to facilitate diagnostics at an early stage of the disease.

4. Conclusions

Thus, our results on rheological disturbances in patients with type 2 DM lead to the following conclusions:

- worsening of rheological disturbances in patients with DM is accompanied by significant decreases in RBC deformation amplitude, dipole moment, polarizability at the frequency of 10^6 Hz, and membrane capacity and corresponds to increases in electric conductivity, summarized viscosity, summarized rigidity, and propensity for hemolysis and aggregation;
- we identified the most useful parameters of RBCs for the stratification of severity of rheological disturbances in type 2 DM: summarized viscosity and summarized rigidity of RBCs, deformation amplitude of the cells at the frequency of 10^6 Hz, the cell deformation degree at the frequency of 5×10^5 Hz, dipole moment, and electric conductivity of the cells (area under the ROC curve: 0.713–0.982);
- the proposed panel of electric and viscoelastic parameters of RBCs has the following analytical characteristics: diagnostic sensitivity 97.8%; diagnostic specificity 86.7%; positive predictive value 95.8%, negative predictive value 92.8%, and accuracy index 95.2% when used as a diagnostic test, in comparison with the EASD risk assessment criteria for vascular complications in patients with DM.

The application of dielectrophoresis to the diagnosis and severity assessment of rheological disturbances and diabetic microangiopathy will enable rapid detection (with minimal expenses) of the DM complications that determine the prognosis, risk of disability, and life expectancy of the patients. This feature denotes unquestionable economic efficiency of the proposed diagnostic method.

Author Contributions: Conceptualization, M.V.K.; methodology, M.V.K., V.M.G.; software, V.N.K.; validation, M.V.K., A.A.G. and V.M.G.; formal analysis, M.V.K., V.N.K.; investigation, M.V.K., V.N.K., V.M.G.; resources, A.A.G.; data curation, M.V.K.; writing—original draft preparation, M.V.K.; writing—review and editing, V.M.G., V.N.K.; visualization, V.N.K.; supervision, M.V.K., A.A.G.; project administration, M.V.K.; funding acquisition, A.A.G. All authors have read and agreed to the published version of the manuscript.

Funding: This research was done within the framework of the topic "Epidemiological monitoring of the population state of health and studies on molecular genetics and molecular biological mechanisms of the development of common internal diseases in Siberia for improvement of the relevant diagnostic, preventive, and therapeutic methods" in State Assignment No. 0324-2018-0001, registration No. AAAA-A17-117112850280-2.

Conflicts of Interest: The authors declare no conflict of interest.

Appendix A. The Procedure for Optical Registration

The procedure for optical registration

The electric optical system of cell detection allows to measure cell characteristics. It includes the following components: a computer, amplifier GZ-112/1, generator GSPF-052 coupled with the computer, a Micmed-6 microscope with a video camera, and a disposable measurement chip. A functional scheme of the electric optical system of cell detection is presented in Figure A1.

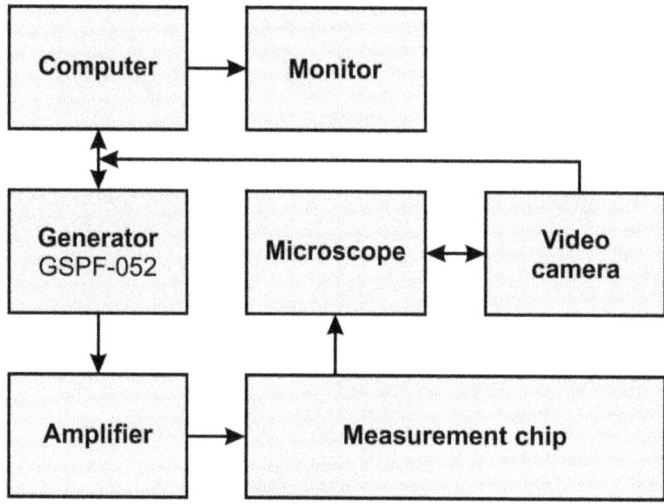

Figure A1. The functional scheme of the electric optical system of cell detection.

To monitor dielectrophoresis, a special measurement chip is used that is coupled with a light microscope. The measurement chip is illustrated in Figure A2. On one of its sides, chrome electrodes are created by photolithography. Between the electrodes, there is a small measurement chamber ($10^{-3} \times 54.10^{-6} \times 0.2 \times 10^{-6}$ m). Electrode thickness should be less than a cell radius (r_c). This condition ensures exposure of the cell to a nonuniform electric field. The measurement chip is installed on a movable stage of a microscope.

The procedure for optical measurements consisted of the following major steps. The measurement chip was installed on the movable stage of the microscope and was fixed in place with clamps. The microscope objective was focused (Micmed-6, magnification 40–1600×) on the measurement chip.

Next, a cell suspension was injected between the electrodes of the measurement chamber and was covered with a coverslip. The microscope was focused on the cells (particles) located between the electrodes. After the cells came to a standstill, electrode voltage was switched on. Video capture software recorded a video file of kinetic movement of the particles between the electrodes via a digital Sony video camera (with a 4.5 mm charge couple device) installed on the microscope as an add-on photo compoment; the digital frame rate was 25 fps. The observation and data registration were carried out with back-lighting. The sequence of frames in the video file enables a researcher to measure the average particle size, to trace the path traveled by each particle separately, and to calculate its velocity. Measurement of the particle radius is done by means of a size standard (scale bar).

Snapshots and the video allow to determine the size, velocity of kinetic or rotary movement, deformation amplitude of a cell being examined, frequency regions of positive and negative dielectrophoresis, and a boundary between them: crossover frequency. On the basis of the experimentally determined parameters, the computer calculates summarized rigidity and viscosity of the cells, their electric capacity, dipole moment, induced charge, and polarizability of the cell. The experimentally determined parameters had been validated by metrological testing.

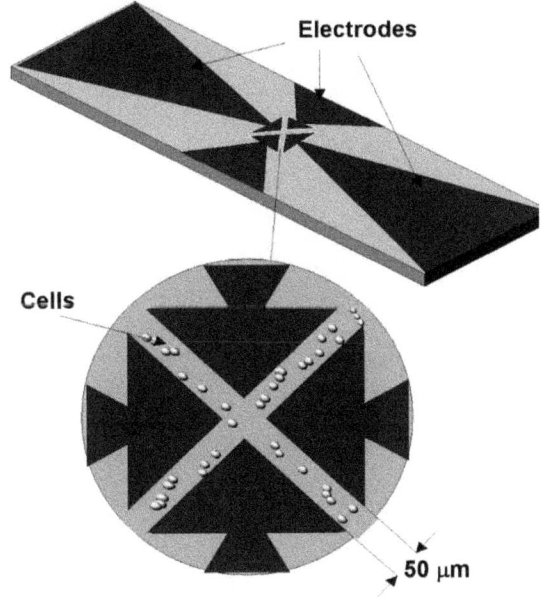

Figure A2. The makeup of the measurement chip containing an electrode quartet.

References

1. Fowler, M.J. Microvascular and macrovascular complications of diabetes. *Clin. Diabetes* **2008**, *26*, 77–78. [CrossRef]
2. Taylor, R.; Batey, D. *Handbook of Retinal Screening in Diabetes. Diagnosis and Management*, 2nd ed.; Wiley-Blackwell: Chichester, UK, 2012; pp. 89–103.
3. Bowker, J.H.; Pfeifer, M.A. *Levin and O'Neal's The Diabetic Foot*; Mosby: Philadelphia, PA, USA, 2008; pp. 256–264.
4. Krutikov, E.S.; Zhitova, V.A.; Tsvetkov, V.A.; Pol'skaja, L.V.; Polishchuk, T.F.; Krutikova, M.S.; Glushko, A.S. Diagnostic Technique for Microangiopathy in Diabetic Patients. Patent RUS. №2559640, 10 August 2015; Byul. №22.; application granted date 23.10.2014. (In Russian)
5. Bakirci, S.; Celik, E.; Acikgoz, S.B.; Erturk, Z.; Tocoglu, A.G.; Imga, N.N.; Kaya, M.; Tamer, A. The evaluation of nailfold videocapillaroscopy findings in patients with type 2 diabetes with and without diabetic retinopathy. *North. Clin. Istanb.* **2019**, *6*, 146–150. [PubMed]
6. Uyar, S.; Balkarli, A.; Kazim Erol, M.; Yesil, B.; Tokuç, A.; Durmaz, D.; Görar, S.; Hilmi Çekin, A. Assessment of the Relationship between Diabetic Retinopathyand Nailfold Capillaries in Type 2 Diabetics with a NoninvasiveMethod: Nailfold Videocapillaroscopy. *J. Diabetes Res.* **2016**, *2016*, 7592402. [CrossRef] [PubMed]
7. Kaminska-Winciorek, G.; Deja, G.; Polańska, J. Diabetic microangiopathy in capillaroscopic examination of juveniles with diabetes type 1. *Postepy Hig. Med. Dosw.* **2012**, *66*, 51–59.
8. Maldonado, G.; Ríos, C. Nailfold Capillaroscopy in Diabetes Mellitus: Potential Technique for the Microvasculature Evaluation. *Endocrinol. Metab. Syndr.* **2017**, *6*, e125. [CrossRef]
9. Chittenden, S.J.; Shami, S.K. Microvascular investigations in diabetes mellitus. *Postgrad. Med. J.* **1993**, *69*, 419–428. [CrossRef]
10. Ma, Y.; Yang, C.; Tao, Y.; Zhou, H.; Wang, Y. Recent technological developments in proteomics shed new light on translational research on diabetic microangiopathy. *FEBS J.* **2013**, *280*, 5668. [CrossRef]
11. Cho, Y.I.; Mooney, M.P.; Cho, D.J. Hemorheological disorders in diabetes mellitus. *J. Diab. Sci. Technol.* **2008**, *2*, 1130–1138. [CrossRef]

12. Schmid-Schonbein, H. Fluid dynamics and hemorheology in vivo: The interaction of hemodynamic parameters and hemorheological "properties" in determining the flow behavior of blood in microvascular networks. In *Clinical Blood Rheology*; Lowe, G.D.O., Ed.; CRC Press Inc.: Boca Raton, FL, USA, 1988; pp. 1–10.
13. Berk, D.A.; Hochmuth, R.M.; Waugh, R.E. Viscoelastic properties and rheology. In *Red Blood Cell Membranes: Structure, Function, Clinical Implications*; Agre, P., Parker, J.C., Eds.; CRC Press: Boca Raton, FL, USA, 1989; pp. 423–454.
14. Dupire, J.; Socol, M.; Viallat, A. Full dynamics of a red blood cell in shear flow. *Proc. Natl. Acad. Sci. USA* **2012**, *109*, 20808–20813. [CrossRef]
15. Kruchinina, M.; Voevoda, M.; Peltek, S.; Kurilovich, S.; Gromov, A.; Kruchinin, V.; Rykhlitsky, S.; Volodin, V.; Generalov, V. Application of optical methods in blood studies upon evaluation of severity rate of diffuse liver pathology. *J. Anal. Sci. Meth. Ins.* **2013**, *3*, 115–123. [CrossRef]
16. Kruchinina, M.V.; Gromov, A.A.; Generalov, V.M.; Kruchinin, V.N.; Shuvalov, G.V.; Minin, O.V.; Minin, I.V. Dielectrophoresis erythrocytes images for predicting stroke recurrence based on analysis of hemorheological parameters. In Proceedings of the International Symposium on Optics and Biophotonics VI; SPIE Saratov Fall Meeting 2018: Optical and Nano-Technologies for Biology and Medicine, Saratov, Russian, 3 June 2019; Volume 110650, pp. 1–6. [CrossRef]
17. Cefalu, W.T. American Diabetes Association Standards of Medical Care in Diabetes-2016. *J. Clin. Appl. Res. Ed.* **2016**, *39*, 119.
18. Rydén, L.; Grant, P.J.; Anker, S.D.; Berne, C.; Cosentino, F.; Danchin, N.; Deaton, C.; Escaned, J.; Hammes, H.P.; Huikuri, H.; et al. The task force on diabetes, pre-diabetes, and cardiovascular diseases of the European Society of Cardiology (ESC) and developed incollaboration with the European Association for the study of diabetes (EASD). *Eur. Heart J.* **2013**, *34*, 3035–3087. [PubMed]
19. Chew, E.Y.; Ambrosius, W.T.; Davis, M.D. Effects of medical therapies on retinopathy progression in type 2 diabetes. *N. Engl. J. Med.* **2010**, *363*, 233–244.
20. Baigent, C.; Landray, M.J.; Reith, C.; Emberson, J.; Wheeler, D.C.; Tomson, C.; Wanner, C.; Krane, V.; Cass, A.; Craig, J.; et al. The effects of lowering LDL cholesterol with simvastatin plus ezetimibe in patients with chronic kidney disease (Study of Heart and Renal Protection): A randomised placebo-controlled trial. *Lancet* **2011**, *377*, 2181–2192. [CrossRef]
21. Liewelyn, H.; Aun Ang, H.; Lewis, K.E.; Al-Abdullah, A. *Oxford Handbook of Clinical Diagnosis*; Oxford University Press: Oxford, UK, 2014; pp. 132–144.
22. Generalov, K.V.; Generalov, V.M.; Kruchinina, M.V.; Shuvalov, G.V.; Buryak, G.A.; Safatov, A.S. Medical and biological measurements method for measuring the polarizability of cells in an inhomogeneous alternating electric field. *Meas. Tech.* **2017**, *60*, 82–86. [CrossRef]
23. Park, Y.; Best, C.A.; Popescu, G. Optical Sensing of Red Blood Cell Dynamics. In *Mechanobiology of Cell-Cell and Cell-Matrix Interactions*; Johnson, A.W., Harley., B.A., Eds.; Springer: Boston, MA, USA, 2011; pp. 279–309.
24. Novitskiy, V.V.; Ryazantseva, N.V.; Stepovaya, E.A. *Fiziologiya i Patofiziologiya Eritrotsita [The Physiology and Pathophysiology of Red Blood Cells]*; Izdatelstvo TGU: Tomsk, Russia, 2004; pp. 123–136. (In Russian)
25. Ju, M.; Leo, H.L.; Kim, S. Numerical investigation on red blood cell dynamics in microflow: Effect of cell deformability. *Clin. Hemorheol. Microcirc.* **2017**, *65*, 105–117. [CrossRef]
26. Ercan, M.D.; Konukoglu, S.O. The effects of cholesterol levels on hemorheological parameters in diabetic patients. *Clin. Hem.-Orheol. Microcirc.* **2002**, *26*, 257–263.
27. Singh, M.; Shin, S. Changes in erythrocyte aggregation and deformability in diabetes mellitus: A brief review. *Indian J. Exp. Biol.* **2009**, *47*, 7–15.
28. Tomaiuolo, G. Biomechanical properties of red blood cells in health and disease towards microfluidics. *Biomicrofluidics* **2014**, *8*, 051501. [CrossRef]
29. Vahidkhah, K.; Balogh, P.; Bagchi, P. Flow of red blood cells in stenosed microvessels. *Sci. Rep.* **2016**, *6*, 28194. [CrossRef]
30. Schiffman, F.J. *Pathophysiology of Blood*; BINOM Publisher: Moscow, Russia; Nevsky Dialekt: Saint-Petersburg, Russia, 2000; pp. 69–87.
31. Li, Q.; Li, L.; Li, Y. Enhanced RBC Aggregation in Type 2 Diabetes Patients. *J. Clin. Lab. Anal.* **2015**, *29*, 387–389. [CrossRef] [PubMed]

32. Wu, H.Y.; Huang, J.W.; Peng, Y.S.; Hung, K.Y.; Wu, K.D.; Lai, M.S.; Chien, K.L. Microalbuminuria screening for detecting chronic kidney disease in the general population: A systematic review. *Ren. Fail.* **2013**, *35*, 607–614. [CrossRef] [PubMed]
33. Wu, H.Y.; Peng, Y.S.; Chiang, C.K.; Huang, J.W.; Hung, K.Y.; Wu, K.D.; Tu, Y.K.; Chien, K.L. Diagnostic performance of random urine samples using albumin concentration vs ratio of albumin to creatinine for microalbuminuria screening in patients with diabetes mellitus: A systematic review and meta-analysis. *JAMA Intern. Med.* **2014**, *174*, 1108–1115. [CrossRef] [PubMed]
34. Kung, C.-M.; Tseng, Z.-L.; Wang, H.-L. Erythrocyte fragility increases with level of glycosylated hemoglobin in type 2 diabetic patients. *Clin. Hemorheol. Microcirc.* **2009**, *43*, 345–351. [CrossRef] [PubMed]
35. Marini, M.A.; Fiorentino, T.V.; Andreozzi, F.; Mannino, G.C.; Succurro, E.; Sciacqua, A.; Perticone, F.; Sesti, G. Hemorheological changes in adults with prediabetes detected by hemoglobin. *A1c Nutr. Metab. Cardiovasc. Dis.* **2017**, *27*, 601–608. [CrossRef] [PubMed]
36. Shin, S.; Ku, Y. Hemorheology and clinical application: Association of impairment of red blood cell deformability with diabetic nephropathy. *Korea-Aust. Rheol. J.* **2005**, *17*, 117–123.
37. Brown, C.D.; Ghali, H.S.; Zhao, Z.; Thomas, L.L.; Friedman, E.A. Association of reduced red blood cell deformability and diabetic nephropathy. *Kidney Int.* **2005**, *67*, 295–300. [CrossRef]
38. Greenhalgh, T. *How to Read a Paper: The Basics of Evidence-Based Medicine*, 5th ed.; John Wiley & Sons Ltd.: Chichester, UK, 2014; pp. 203–219.

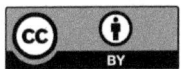

© 2020 by the authors. Licensee MDPI, Basel, Switzerland. This article is an open access article distributed under the terms and conditions of the Creative Commons Attribution (CC BY) license (http://creativecommons.org/licenses/by/4.0/).

MDPI
St. Alban-Anlage 66
4052 Basel
Switzerland
Tel. +41 61 683 77 34
Fax +41 61 302 89 18
www.mdpi.com

Journal of Personalized Medicine Editorial Office
E-mail: jpm@mdpi.com
www.mdpi.com/journal/jpm

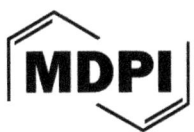

www.ingramcontent.com/pod-product-compliance
Lightning Source LLC
LaVergne TN
LVHW070631100526
838202LV00012B/776